Gerontology and Leadership Skills for Nurses

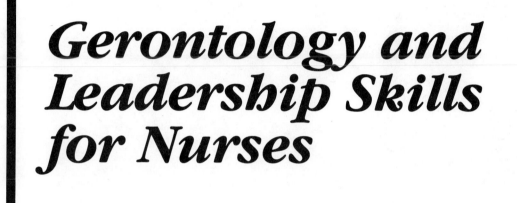

Gerontology and Leadership Skills for Nurses

Mary K. Ringsven, RNC, BA
Donna Bond, RN

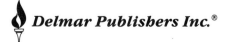

Delmar Publishers Inc.®

NOTICE TO THE READER

Computer Graphics: Ronald Ringsven
Cover Photo and Text Photos by: Donna Bond
Cover Design by: Backes Graphic Production Inc.

Delmar Staff
Executive Editor: Barbara E. Norwitz
Associate Editor: Marion Waldman
Project Editor: Carol Micheli
Production Supervisor: Larry Main
Art Supervisor: John Lent
Design Supervisor: Susan Mathews

Printed in the United States of America
published simultaneously in Canada
by Nelson Canada
a division of The Thomson Corporation

10 9 8 7 6 5

Library of Congress Cataloging-in-Publication Data

Ringsven, Mary K., 1940–
  Gerontology and leadership skills for nurses / Mary K. Ringsven,
Donna Bond.
      p.   cm.
  Includes bibliographical references.
  Includes index.
  ISBN 0-8273-3450-8 (textbook)
  1. Geriatric nursing.   I. Bond, Donna.   II. Title.
  [DNLM: 1. Geriatric Nursing. 2. Nursing, Supervisor.   WY 152
R582g]
RC954.R56   1991
610.73'65 — dc20
DNLM/DLC
for Library of Congress   90–13971
                                                              CIP

Contents

Preface

Gerontological nursing is just emerging from its infancy. The growth in this field of practice will mushroom as we enter the twenty-first century. The percentage of the population 65 years of age and older is climbing and will spiral upward in 2011 when the "Baby Boomers" begin to turn 65.

Many nurses practicing today did not have a gerontology course in their nursing education. Others were presented an overview of geriatrics with a focus on the frail elderly. Long term care facilities as sites for student clinical experience have developed only within the last two decades. When long term care facilities (nursing homes) began growing as a new industry it was believed that only nurses with "rusty" skills practiced in this setting. Today that idea could not work. Long term care facilities have more residents with acute as well as chronic conditions that require advanced technological medical treatment and skilled nursing care.

Nurses today need to be advocates for the aging population in their communities and nursing practice. They are using gerontological nursing skills in all practice settings. Examples include caring for a woman with a fractured hip in the hospital, a man having cataract surgery in the outpatient department, a man having his hypertension and congestive heart failure managed in the clinic, a woman with Alzheimer's in adult day care, or a woman experiencing late stage symptoms of emphysema in a long term care facility.

Gerontology and Leadership Skills for Nurses is designed to present nurses with information and learning tools to adapt nursing skills to the aging population receiving health care in a variety of settings. Leadership skills are introduced to assist nurse caregivers in long term care facilities. Job descriptions for these nurses include tasks relating to the role of a first-line manager nurse.

Section one introduces the nurse to the elderly as a population group. It identifies social changes and cultural influences that have affected the lives of the elderly and in turn their health. Projections for the elderly of the future are made by looking at the changing demographics and the influence of technology on health care and life expectancy.

Section two presents the active aging population. The details on signs of aging and physical conditions experienced by this group will assist the nurse practicing in clinics and other settings where the active elderly receive health care. A discussion of community services and approaches to patient teaching will guide the nurse in assisting the aging to remain active.

Section three identifies the dependent elderly population. The effects of chronic physical and psychosocial conditions that create a dependency are addressed. Dilemmas that face this aging group are introduced. Although the focus is on nursing practice in long-term care, these concepts for care of the dependent elderly may also be practiced in acute care or home care.

Section four introduces concepts of leadership and management for the first-line nurse manager/caregiver. Skills for organizing time are presented and responsibilities for managing a group of residents is discussed. Basic management levels and styles are introduced. Nurses are encouraged to expand nursing skills used in patient care to leadership roles.

Gerontology and Leadership Skills for Nurses is designed to build on the knowledge and skills of fundamentals acquired in nursing and medical–surgical nursing courses. Practicing nurses will find the text a helpful reference. Efforts have been made to present accurate information related to government regulations and nursing standards of practice at the time of publication.

Acknowledgments

We are grateful to the many people who helped us bring this dream to a reality. One of us has been a nurse educator for many years while the other has been a director of nursing in long-term care. We saw the need for students and practicing nurses to have a broader understanding of the elderly, the roots of their values and experiences, and more specifics related to their health care. We also saw the need to better prepare the LP/VN with the organizational skills required to manage resident units in long term care facilities.

Our families, especially our husbands Ronald Ringsven and Milton Bond, have been helpful and patient with this project. Ron turned our ideas and pencil scratches into wonderful computer graphics. Our children have been understanding when we could not join them: Sharon and Brian Ringsven, Steve and Shelly Bemel, and Doug Bond, Mike Bond, Laura Ingalls, Karen Seaquist, and their families.

We want to thank Leslie Boyer for her initial belief and support in this project. Our editor Marion Waldman has given us continued confidence through thick and thin. Additional thanks are in order to the Delmar reviewers: Cynthia Bence, Sarasota County Vocational Technical Center, Sarasota, Florida; Elaine Polan, VEEB School of Practical Nursing, Uniondale, New York; Joyce Bookout, Paris Junior College, Paris, Texas; Karen Ivers, Bullard Havens RVTS, Bridgeport, Connecticut; and Judith Conlin, Niagra Educational Center, Sanborn, New York.

Our colleagues at Dakota County Technical College, Rosemount, Minnesota, and Samaritan Bethany, Inc. and Maple Manor Nursing Home in Rochester, Minnesota, have been very supportive. We would also like to thank others who have contributed to this project: Leila Texer, Shelly Racek, Shirley Bailey, Sarah Oehlke, and the many people who have been willing to be photographed. Apple Valley Health Care Center, Apple Valley, Minnesota, Samaritan Bethany, Inc. and Maple Manor Nursing Home, Rochester Minnesota, Ostrander Nursing Home, Ostrander, Minnesota, and West Bend Health Care Center, West Bend, Iowa, also graciously permitted us to photograph in their facilities.

Our heartfelt thanks go to all the wonderful elderly we have met and assisted during their active and dependent years. They have taught us so much!

Mary K. Ringsven
Donna Bond
1990

Section 1
Introduction:
Aging at the Threshold of the Twenty-first Century

Unit 1: Reflecting on the Elderly in the Twentieth Century
Unit 2: Older Adults after 2000: Challenges for Everyone

What happened? Why is everyone getting so "worked up" over the elderly? Retail marketing offers discounts to people 65 years of age and older. The entertainment industry has discovered that women over 50 are box office hits. In the health care delivery system, it has been found that the costs of funding health care for the elderly are enormous and growing.

What is so extraordinary about this focus on the older population? First, the elderly age group is a relatively new social issue. Second, it is the growing number of this population who are living into their eighth, ninth, and tenth decades. In Biblical times Methuselah reportedly lived nearly one thousand years. But in modern times people have not lived long enough to experience physical, emotional, or social aging situations. The whole fabric of society has not needed goods and services tailored to the uniqueness of aging.

At the beginning of the twentieth century, a newborn could expect to live until age 47. By the 1980s, not only had infant mortality decreased, but newborns could expect to live until age 74. The *life span*, how long people can live under the most favorable conditions, is 115 years. Today, over 12 percent of the population, or 30 million people, are 65 years of age and older. Population projections estimate this number will double by 2030. Citizens of the United States over the age of 85 are the fastest growing segment of the population. Between 1980 and 1987, their numbers increased by 28 percent and they became the greatest users of health care services.

Why is it important for you, for all nurses, to learn this kind of information about the elderly? One reason is because health care has expanded beyond the hospital to a variety of other settings. In any area of nursing practice — the physician's office, clinic, home care, hospital, or long term care facility — you will use your knowledge of the aging process and its affects on the individual and society. You will be caring for larger numbers of elderly persons in all of these settings.

Another reason to have a basic understanding of the implications of population changes is that nurses need to be involved in the broader aspects of the health care delivery system. We are living in a global community; what affects another country affects us.

Why is the study of gerontology different from other courses in nursing education? It is unique because the one thing we all are experiencing is our own aging. In other course work some students will have experienced giving birth, having an operation, or perhaps receiving a transplanted organ. However, in this study of gerontology, regardless of your age today, you are experiencing aging!

Gerontology is the study of the possible causes of aging and the physical, emotional, and social results of the aging process. This study is very broad, encompassing all aspects of living and aging. It is different from geriatrics and geriatric nursing. *Geriatrics* is the branch of medicine that studies diseases of old age. This study of gerontology will include geriatric nursing; the care of older people with diseases that are experienced more often by the elderly. Studying gerontology will assist you in understanding your own aging, today and in the future. Also, as a resource person, you will be able to explain physical changes to a parent, grandparent, or neighbor.

To understand the events and practices that affect aging today, and project possible needs in the future, one must look at the influences of the past. A historical perspective can be fascinating; it can help us put the puzzle together by answering some of the "whys" in today's issues on aging.

Section one will set the stage for the remainder of the book. It will discuss briefly the events and changes in the United States and its people, that have influenced the lengthening of the life span. By reflecting on these events and their outcomes, hopefully, we can better plan for the next century.

Unit 1 will present influences of the twentieth century that affect today's elderly. Changing population groups have resulted from fluctuating birth rates and rapidly changing technology. This technological change has evolved from the importance of handwashing as a means of infection control to several generations of antibiotics. Social and family factors are introduced for you to see what events influences the elderly.

Unit 2 will look at events and issues of today and project what some of our needs might be in the first half of the next century. The increased numbers of older persons will affect every aspect of our lives. These older persons will be us! Those born in 1985 will be 65 in 2050! There will need to be changes in housing, packaging, advertising, and other experiences of daily living we consider commonplace; we have not yet thought about them in relation to aging needs.

The potential effects of increased numbers of older people on the health care delivery system will be considered. The care settings, costs, and funding are examples of health care issues of today and the future. The types of caregivers needed will be discussed, with emphasis on implications for nurses.

After reading this section you should have some basic understanding of lifetime influences on the aging of the people you will assist in your nursing practice. You should also have some ideas on factors that are influencing your own aging. Perhaps you will be better prepared for your own old age!

Unit 1
Reflecting on the Elderly in the Twentieth Century

Objectives

After reading this unit you should be able to:

- Discuss changing demographics in the twentieth century.
- List several influences of technology on the lengthening life span.
- Discuss the influences of social conflicts and social changes on the aging population.
- Identify effects of cultural and family traditions on the aging population.

Everyday the check-out clerk in a drug store in Florida or southern Arizona sees the growing numbers of people age 65 and older, figure 1-1. "Snow birds" migrate to the warmer climates of southern states every year between October and April. The *snow birds* are retired or semi-retired older adults. They have permanent homes in northern states that experience cold winters; they choose to live in warm southern states during these months.

This snow bird phenomenon is relatively new due to changing demographics in the United States. *Demography* is the statistical study of the population. Percentages and averages of age groups are studied to make projections for the future. Currently, studies show the 65 and older population comprises over 12 percent of our citizens with steady increases anticipated. Figure 1-2 demonstrates the growth in the population over age 65 since 1900.

When analyzing population groups, cohorts are studied. A *cohort* is a group of people born during specified years (the people are about the same age). The cohort currently analyzed and discussed the most is the "baby boom" generation. *Baby Boomers* were born between 1946 and 1964.

For purposes of analyzing data related to today's aging population, demographers divide

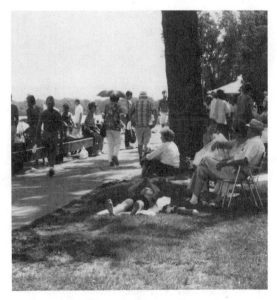

Figure 1–1 The elderly population in the United States is growing.

the older population into three groups. The *young old* are ages 65 to 74; the *middle old* are ages 75 to 84; the *old old* are ages 85 and older. This labeling may seem unfair, or inaccurate, since chronological age is often an unreliable gauge in observing aging. However, it does offer one method of evaluating characteristics and

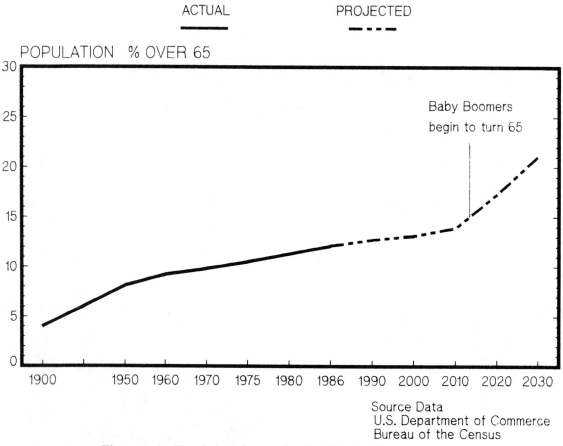

ACTUAL PROJECTED

POPULATION % OVER 65

Figure 1-2 Population changes for the 65 and older age group

needs of aging. The population changes within these three groups of older adults is demonstrated in figure 1-3.

The greatest influence on a cohort and its aging population is the birth rate. This influences the activities a society undertakes to meet the needs of the people. For example, in the late 1950s, many elementary schools were built to accomodate all the Baby Boomers entering school.

Technology has dramatically changed our lives. One area is our food supply. Seeds and soil conditions have been developed to provide a greater crop yield. Food processing now retains more nutrients. We have refrigerators to prevent spoilage. Other technology related to health has decreased infant mortality, increased the opportunities to recover from acute illnesses, and addressed services required to function with chronic conditions. This all brings us to old age and advanced old age.

Social change throughout the century has had a significant impact on today's elderly. Wars and military conflicts have influenced advancing medical technology. Surgical procedures were developed in response to complicated wounds. Wars have also initated changes in the family and the work place. More women working outside the home since World War II present issues for an aging population. Traditionally, women

AGE DISTRIBUTION OF PERSONS 65 AND OVER
1960 to 2050

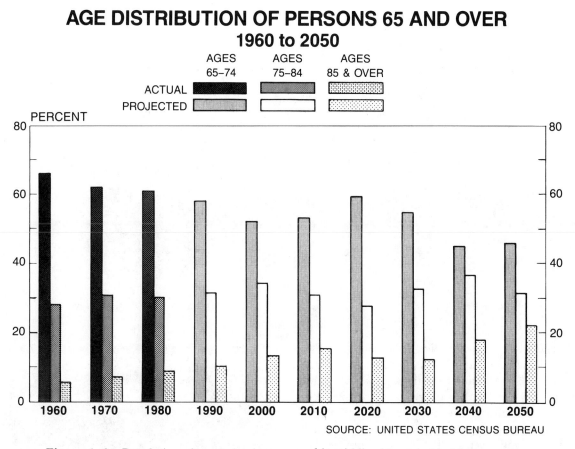

Figure 1–3   Population changes in the young-old, middle-old, and old-old age groups

were at home and were the caregivers for the young, old, and ailing.

Social and economic change has been influenced by the environment. For example, the winds and lack of moisture in the 1930s resulted in the drought and dust bowl era. In part, this led to government programs for all ages focusing on nutrition, maternal and infant care, and income for aging. These programs changed and expanded over the years. One example is today's Meals-on-Wheels nutrition program for the homebound. This unit will discuss some of the events that occured during the 1900s that bring to this country, for the first time, a large aging population.

Changing Demographics

Historical View

In 1900, when a newborn could expect to live until age 47, barely 4 percent of the population was 65 years of age or older. Approximately 75 percent of the population was under 40 years of age. This was a time of change in this country which involved hard physical labor by most people over ten years of age. Farming was not mechanized, figure 1–4, and the rapid growth of industry utilized even children for long, physically strenuous days.

With youth comprising a majority of the

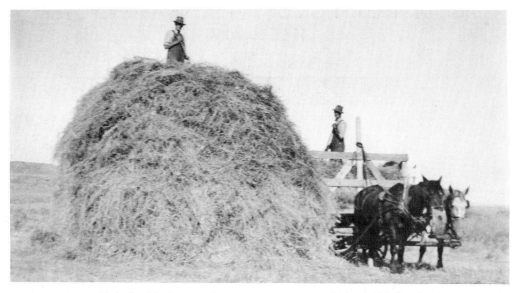

Figure 1–4 Today's elderly experienced many hours of physical labor in their youth.

population, medicine and the community did not have to address degenerative joint disease and other chronic conditions of aging. The cathedral pictured in figure 1-5 was built soon after the turn of the twentieth century. These steps, as well as those leading to libraries, courthouses, and other public places built during this period, did not need to consider mobility problems of aging. Today, new structures, figure 1-6, are more accessible to the greater numbers of elderly as well as other physically challenged citizens.

The newborns of 1900, who are in the 85 years and older group today, have experienced many personal and social changes in their lifetimes. One striking feature of this group is that they survived infections without antibiotics until their middle adult years!

Another way to look at the graying of America is the rise of the median age. *Median age* is the identified age at which half the population is younger and half the population is older. When George Washington was president, the median age was 16. Two hundred years later it has doubled and may be as high as 36 by the

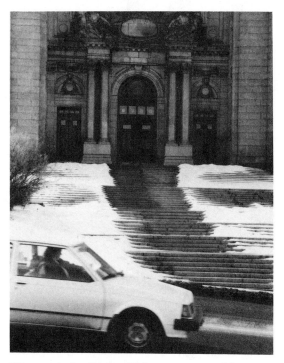

Figure 1–5 Early 20th century architecture had no need to consider mobility problems with aging.

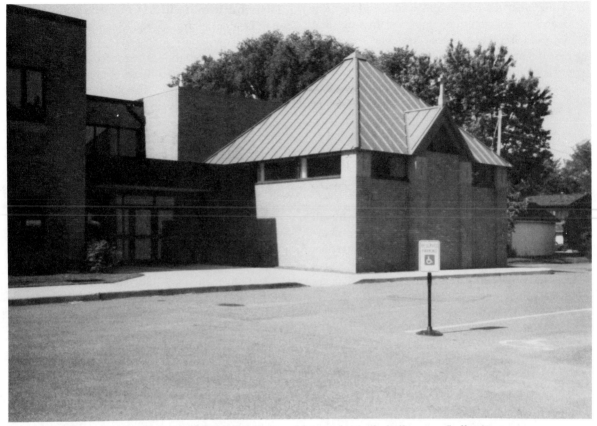

Figure 1–6   Today's public buildings address physical challenges of all age groups.

year 2000. The aging of the baby boomers will keep this median age continually inching upward.

The rise in median age affects us in many ways. For health care it means a shift away from a concentration of programs and health professionals serving infants and young people. We will need a greater number of physicians and nurses specializing in geriatrics and fewer specializing in obstetrics and pediatrics.

Influence of Technology

The birth rate is the major factor in determining a population group's needs and projecting the size of its elderly population. Demographer's also look at the death rate and the populations immigrating to this country. Nei-

ther has had a great impact on the size of a cohort.

In the 1930s, during the Great Depression in the United States, the birth rate was lower. As this group begins to join the older population in the 1990s it may provide some stabilizing, or a slower growth rate of the elderly. It is yet to be seen if this slower growth will, in any way, preserve resources for the rapid growth rate of the elderly population after the first decade of the next century.

If the birth rate increased at a gradual rate during the first four decades of this century, why are we already experiencing issues of aging? One reason is the rapid advancement of medicine. Another is scientific advancements that compliment the research in health and medical treatment. In addition, improved hygiene and nutrition have kept people healthier. When illness occurs, medical treatment provides recovery and, with it, a longer life.

Lister's support of Pasteur's "germ theory" was an 1865 landmark in the advancement of health and medicine. The practice had been that surgeons did not "wash up" until the end of the work day. The more blood and debris on the frock coat worn in the operating theatre, the more respected the surgeon! Surgeons began wearing rubber gloves in the 1890s.

In the early 1900s, causes of death for all age groups were infectious diseases such as tuberculosis and pneumonia for adults and diarrhea for children. Today, it is life style diseases, such as cancer related to cigarette smoking, that are the leading causes of death. Life style disease means that we do have some control over our probability of contracting the condition. Leading causes of death in the over 65 years population group are cardiovascular disease, malignancies, and cerebrovascular disease.

Once recovery from surgery and other illnesses was more probable because of infection control, the development of more sophisticated procedures began. The growth of pharmacology and drug therapy accompanied surgical advancements. These are perhaps the greatest influences related to health care that brought today's elderly through their infancy and youth into their early adult years. During the second half of this century, rapid advancement in technology through the use of computers in medicine, laser surgery, and specialized drugs has lengthened the lives of this population group. Coronary bypass surgery and antihypertensive drugs are two examples. Cataract extraction with intraocular implant has resulted in immeasureable improvement in the elderly's quality of life.

The threat of infection for the elderly, however, has not disappeared. With aging, the immune system weakens, leaving the elderly more vulnerable to infections. Pneumonia is a cause of death for many elderly.

Distribution of Elderly Population

Demographics of the distribution of the elderly population indicate that this 12 percent of the population is not evenly distributed throughout the United States, or between urban and rural areas. Where the elderly population is located has a great impact on the kind and amount of services needed.

In 1986, almost half of the older adult population lived in eight states. The states having the most elderly population were California, New York, Florida, Pennsylvania, Texas, Illinois, Ohio, and Michigan. In all of these states except California, Texas, and Michigan, this elderly population was the national average of 12 percent or higher. Florida has the highest with over 17 percent of the population over the age of 65. Figure 1-7 illustrates the distribution of the elderly state by state.

About 75 percent of the elderly living in their own homes, or otherwise independent, live in metropolitan or suburban areas. This weighs heavily on cities to provide a multitude of services. One advantage of metropolitan areas is that services available to all ages that are in place make the development of senior citizen programs somewhat more convenient. An example is the use of public transportation services to help the elderly get to physician appointments.

Rural areas have difficulties of a different nature. In recent years there has been a migration of young people from rural to metropolitan areas for education and employment leaving a very high percentage of old and growing old in these areas.

Health care for elderly in rural areas is becoming critical as the twenty-first century approaches. During the first half of this century, most rural communities had their own physicians. Recently, small community or regional hospitals have been closing. The increase in the costs of the health care delivery system and the shrinking economic resources of these communities have forced hospital doors to close and physicians to leave. Therefore, the elderly have further to go and more to pay for health care.

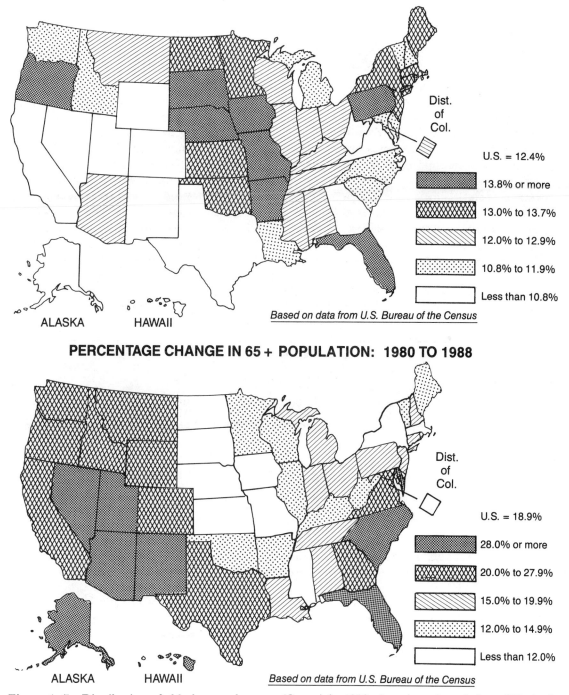

Figure 1-7   Distribution of elderly state by state (Copyright 1990, American Association of Retired Persons. Reprinted with Permission.)

These changing demographics indicate that nurses have been caring for increasing numbers of elderly people and that number will continue to grow. Nurses are seeing that the majority of their patients in the acute care setting are elderly. Exacerbations of congestive heart failure and chronic obstructive lung disease hospitalize the older adult. The acute symptoms of a stroke and surgery for hip fractures or malignant neoplasms will also bring the elderly to the hospital. In physicians' offices, nurses are assisting increasing numbers of elderly as they have chronic conditions monitored. The rapid growth of the long term care facility arm of the health care delivery system has required increasing numbers of nurses to care for the dependent elderly. Figure 1-8 summarizes demographic changes related to aging.

Influence of Social Change on the Aging Population

1900–World War II

The first social change to observe is the position of the elderly in society in the United States. During the first half of this century the elderly were not yet considered a separate population group. Society was oriented to keeping people working in the rapidly growing agricultural and manufacturing industries. The older adult was the landowner and therefore highly respected: his opinions were sought and valued.

World War II presents a dividing point when viewing the social influences on aging in America. It marks the close of the first half of the century as well as the beginning of countless chagnes affecting life styles in the United States.

CHANGING DEMOGRAPHICS

1900	Life Expectancy is 47 years for a newborn
	65 and older group is less than 4 percent of the population or about 3 million people
	40 years and under is 75 percent of the population
1990	Life Expectancy is almost 75 years for a newborn
	Life Span can be 115 years
	Birth Rate greatest influence on aging population
	65 and older group is more than 12 percent of the population or about 30 million people
	50 years and older is nearing 50 percent of the population

DISTRIBUTION OF ELDERLY

50 percent of the elderly live in eight states
Two million elderly live in the states of California, New York, and Florida
Some states have elderly populations greater than the national average of over 12 percent
75 percent of the elderly live in metropolitan or suburban areas
Population distribution has a great impact on health and social services

Figure 1-8   Summary of demographic changes related to aging

For example, in the 1940s at the time of World War II, farming was becoming mechanized. The tractor was replacing the horse as the power in front of the plow or wagon.

Beginning Government Assistance to Aging Population. The one event focusing on aging that occured before this time was passage of the Social Security Act in 1935. This public retirement fund was part of the recovery programs developed by the government in response to the economic disaster of the Great Depression. It was not until this time that the word retirement was even known or used in the work world. Social Security was based on the premise that a person who worked hard to build this country could share in the rewards without continuing to work.

A major problem with this idea is that the work ethic or pay-your-own-way philosophy of the immigrants building this country continued. This work ethic equated a persons value to society with his contributions or productivity. Here is a link with the label "useless old age": not working, not productive, and not valuable equals useless.

With this in mind, think about the 85-year-old you have assisted in the hospital or long term care facility. He was 30 years old during the Great Depression. Perhaps he was a farmer whose crops could not grow in the dry soil. Maybe he was a businessman who suffered from the stock market crash and the farmer's plight. He may be grateful, but not excited, that Medicare and Medicaid are paying for his health care. To his generation, the word is welfare, and to them that means NOT being able to pay your own way.

Next comes the magic age of 65! Some historians say the number was arbitrary; most people were working at age 60 and not very many were alive at age 70. Others indicate the concept, like many used by the framers of our Constitution, was developed from practices in Europe. In the late 1800s Germany developed Europe's first pension plan. It was decided that the pension plan would service the oldest 3 percent of the population. That population started at age 65. Today, if the same guidelines were used, Social Security and other retirement benefits would start at age 96!

World War II and Later

Veterans of World War II are now the in the young old and middle old cohorts. This war brought the United States from an isolated country into an international community, never to return to pre-war policies or life styles.

Advancing Medical Technology. Some of the events of this time that reflect on the elderly are the introduction of antibiotics and plastic surgery to repair the physical damage of more sophisticated weaponry. This brought more men and woman home with chronic and rehabilitative needs for medicine to address during their aging.

Pharmacology research and advances in drug therapy grew rapidly. The development of antibiotics, a polio vaccine, and sophisticated drug therapy for hypertension and other cardiovascular disorders are a few examples. With the invention of the electron microscope, viruses could be identified and genetic research with the study of the DNA began. The older adults who had survived on the strength of their own immune system now had a new lease on life with medical science ushering them into their old age.

Changes in the Home and Work Place. Woman were introduced into the work force in great numbers during World War II as men left the factories and other work places to join the military. After the war ended, not all women wanted to, or could afford to, return exclusively to "housework." Thus began the rise in the percentage of women in the work force. For the elderly, this meant fewer women remained at home to care for them during their dependent years. Most families had arranged for aging parents to live with the family of a son or daughter. The daughter or daughter-in-law was the primary caregiver.

As the United States became an international community, transportation moved from the horse, train, and car to the supersonic jet. Not only was the woman not in the home to assist aging parents, but families began living in other communities and other states. This is one of the events that contributed to the growth of long term care facilities.

Employers and society began to encourage retirement. Education and advancing technology were part of this wave. More and more education was required for entry level jobs. "Modernizing" was the forerunner of "high tech." There was no built-in mechanism on the job for the older worker to update job skills. The old age stigma entered, a belief that the older worker could not learn and performance would decline with age anyway. Employers retired older workers to make way for the increasing numbers of young and more educated workers. This all contributed to the lowering of the status of older people.

Despite society's marketing of retirement with "you've earned it" slogans, the work ethic prevailed. Self-esteem said it was more acceptable to retire due to health reasons than to accept mandatory retirement or choose to have more leisure time.

Federal Government Provides Elderly Health Care. The government began to address issues on aging. The White House Conference on Aging, held every 10 years, was first convened in 1951. Out of these conferences, the Older Americans Act was passed in 1965. Funds appropriated through this act provide many services to senior citizens. One example is Meals-on-Wheels, the hot noon meal transported by volunteers to homebound people.

During the social unrest of the 1960s President Johnson, in his "Great Society" programs, met the needs of the elderly primarily through Social Security amendments addressing costs of health care. We know these amendments as Medicare and Medicaid. *Medicare* is health insurance for citizens 65 years and older. *Medicaid* provides funds for health care for the financially oppressed of any age.

During the first White House Conference on Aging, it was identified that the health and health care of the growing elderly population was deteriorating. The elderly of that time, and many today, were employed when health and retirement programs were not yet employment benefits. They lived on Social Security income and personal savings. As their aging health needs increased, so did the costs of health care, and they could not afford to pay the bills. Many did not seek health care until a catastrophic event occured, such as a stroke from untreated hypertension. The health care delivery system saw the rising bills from a population group that did not have insurance and could not afford to pay.

Today, the elderly still need to purchase health insurance. The deductible, the amount a person pays before Medicare begins to cover charges, continues to rise. The elderly now need their own policy to cover costs that are not covered by Medicare. These supplemental plans are often called *Medigap* policies.

During the last quarter of this century the cost of health care for the elderly is the biggest issue facing every elderly person, the health care delivery system, and the United States economy. Most health care dollars are spent during the last weeks of life. This has stirred the waters of ethical issues as well as costs of health care.

Two events during the 1980s affected health care of the elderly. One was the prospective payment plan for patients receiving Medicare benefits. This law, passed in 1983, is commonly known as the Diagnostic Related Groups (DRG) system. *Diagnostic Related Groups* is a system of classifying general medical diagnoses for use in determining monies to be reimbursed to hospitals by a government payer. It was developed because, with the increasing numbers of elderly and the rising costs of health care, the twenty-year-old Medicare plan was running out of money. This DRG plan was designed for hospital costs. Instead of paying charges, Medicare would pay a fixed rate determined for the more than 400 identified admitting diagnoses.

To date, this system is still experiencing continual changes in regulations. For the elderly, this includes shorter hospital stays. Many must continue recovery at home or in an extended care or long term care facility. Many are caught in a gap between acute and recovery care. For a population group accustomed to a passive role when receiving health care, the discharge planning instructions are overwhelming. They need family members, friends, or others to be advocates as they struggle with the system. Home care agencies and community services are attempting to assist the elderly through this gap. Many elderly are still not aware of services available because the methods of communicating and linking services is not yet strong enough. Our health care delivery system is fragmented with gaps of service in one place and duplication of services in another.

For long term care facilities, the DRG system often means providing part of the acute care recovery. For example, a new admission may be a diabetic amputee or a hip nailing only a few hours or days postoperative.

The second event was the 1988 passage of the catastrophic health care bill followed by its repeal in 1989. This bill was intended to be another adjustment in the Medicare program. The concept was to assist elderly faced with enormous medical bills acquired in prolonged acute illnesses. The 1990s will no doubt demonstrate continued changes in government health benefit reimbursements and a "tug of war" for the health care dollar. Table 1-1 summarizes

Year	Government Intervention	Objective
1935	Social Security Act	Pension fund for citizens 65 years and older
1951	White House Conference on Aging begins	Address needs of elderly
1965	Older Americans Act	Social and health related programs for elderly
1965	Medicare and Medicaid Social Security Amendments	Health care insurance for 65 and older, and financially oppressed regardless of age
1983	Medicare Prospective Payment Plan (DRG)	Elderly health care cost containment measures
1988	Medicare catastrophic health care plan	Funding increases for prolonged acute care illnesses
1989	Medicare catastrophic health care plan repealed	Review long-term affects of government sponsored health care programs

TABLE 1-1
Government Intervention to Assist Elderly in Managing Health and Social Concerns

government programs to assist the elderly with health expenses.

Social Change Influences Housing for Elderly.

Housing for the elderly became another social issue during the second half of this century. When families were not so mobile and women did not work outside the home, aging parents moved in with adult children when they could no longer live independently. That situation still occurs in some families today. However, increasing numbers of elderly, often widows or widowers, live alone. Home maintenance and repairs decline as physical abilities decline unless families or community services can assist. Costs become prohibitive as taxes and utilities increase and the elderly remain on fixed incomes.

Leaving the family home is difficult, but often more so when there are high costs in apartments or other living arrangements. Remember, this is the pay-as-you-go generation. Many own their homes clear of any mortgage and are very apprehensive about "owing" anyone.

Housing in the last 25 years has also included long term care facilities. Until recently these facilities were called nursing homes. During the early part of this century, there were privately owned "boarding homes" where the more wealthy aged lived if they did not live with family members. Similar church sponsored homes began to emerge about this time. The beginning of proprietary (for profit) homes began following the passage of the first Social Security Act in 1935. Some financially destitute elderly lived in county "poor farms." According to the act, people living in public institutions could not receive the government assisted payments. Some elderly left to live in boarding houses, and others remained at the poor farms which were leased or purchased by individuals. These elderly were then qualified to receive Social Security payments.

The numbers of aged began to increase as did the numbers of long term care facilities, figure 1-9. In the early 1950s, there were about 7000 facilities, nearly 12,000 in 1965 when Medicare was instituted, and about 23,000 in 1980 prior to the first major adjustment in Medicare payments. Social changes that have influenced the aging population are summarized in figure 1-10.

Influence of Family and Cultural Traditions

Early Influences

The increasing number of elderly is the factor that has stimulated this country to look at the social and economic impact this is making, and will make, on all of us. There always have been, obviously, some elderly in a community. The family has been the basic unit of most cultures, and therefore the aged person was a family responsibility.

Anthropologists who study aging see a balance between costs and contributions. Those individuals not contributing to the growth or maintenance of society need to be subsidized in some manner. Years ago, all nonproductive people were grouped together: frail elderly, mentally incompetent, criminals, and others. They were considered burdens to society.

The elderly actually held a very high place in most cultures until modern times. A culture survived because of the stories told by the elders and their passing of tasks and traditions to younger members. The hunters and gatherers, early residents of this country, did balance cost and contributions. The grandparents tended and taught the young while parents were seeking fish and game or planting and harvesting food.

The invention of writing was a very early blow to the prestige of the elderly. No longer was story-telling the only method of passing on cultural customs and family traditions. This seems to have initiated a gradual process of devaluing the elderly. More recent modernization and advancements in technology delivered a two fisted blow to the elderly. The advance-

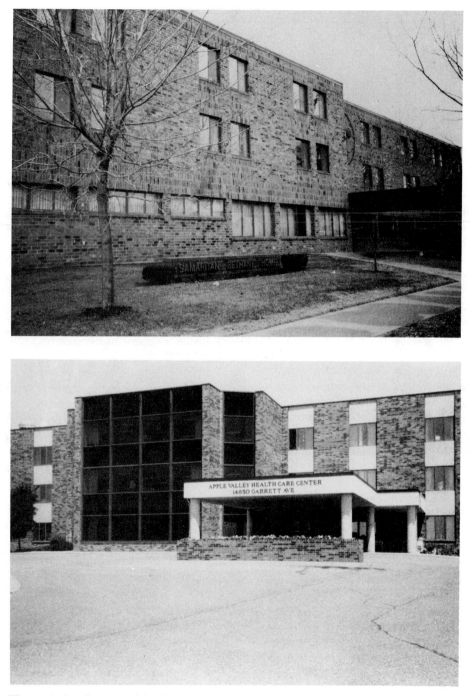

Figure 1–9 Communities began to have more long-term care facilities for elderly citizens.

PROFILE OF TODAY'S ELDERLY

- Highly respected landowner or industrial worker in early, largely agricultural and manufacturing society
- Opinions sought and valued by younger generations
- Work ethic philosophy and pay-your-own-way tradition of immigrants were foundation of rapid growth of U.S.
- Survived major health threats without antibiotics
- Experienced birth of automobile, jet airplane, computers

SOCIAL CHANGES INFLUENCING TODAY'S ELDERLY

- "Modernizing" and "High Technology" demanded more education; devalued experiences of older worker
- Introduction of "retirement" as commonplace tradition
- Social programs contradicted pay-your-own way philosophy
- Medical advances in diagnosis, surgery, and pharmacology prolonged life
- Increased number of women in the work force decreases caregivers in the home for dependent aging
- Home, in declining years, became long term care facilities

Figure 1–10   Social changes influence change in status of the elderly.

ments made them live longer and modernization retired them out of the main stream of productivity.

The United States has had three major work cultures: agriculture, followed by industry, and now information and service. Remember, the elderly owned the land. This work, as well as trades or crafts of the time, were learned on-the-job. As the country rapidly expanded, the pace of work, transportation, and life accelerated. Modernization required more education and technical skill. Historically, cultural beliefs would indicate that this eliminates the elderly from contributing to society and begins to be a cost to society.

Changing Family Structure

At the close of this century we are seeing a dramatic change in family structure. Guidelines for projecting needs for society had been based on a household defined as a family with a working husband, a wife who did not work outside the home, and two children. Today that definition fits less than 10 percent of all households.

In addition to more women working outside the home, there are more single parent families and blended and nontraditional family units. This adds many complexities to society's responsibility to aging members. Longevity has also produced the *sandwich generation*. This is the middle age population who are caregivers or support-persons for aging parents, young adult children, and often grandchildren.

Ethnic Perspectives

The United States has been called a "melting pot." With the exception of the Native Americans, all ethnic groups have been immigrants. There is usually an early period when most people new to this country strive to quickly blend into the "American Way," whatever that is at the time. But at some time, if it has not persisted from the beginning, people also struggle to maintain a cultural or ethnic identity. Even when people are not first-generation immigrants, there comes a time when they feel the need to reestablish cultural roots. Middle age often is that time: the time elapsed is adequate for reflection, and the need for a legacy for grandchildren is identified.

An elderly Native American woman was asked why there was not more teaching of traditional tribal dances to young Native Americans. Her reply was that the young people were more interested in rock music than traditional Indian music. She added that the interest in Native American customs today surfaces when members of the group are in their 30s and 40s.

Aging in Minority Groups.   People experience aging in different ways. There are differences in experiences between minority and majority group aging populations. There are differences between these elderly and the broader society. Two problems emerge when attempting to determine specific needs of aging minorities. One is that multiple ethnicities were catagorized under broad groups such as Asian, Black, and Hispanic. Each aging population can have different experiences and different needs. Also, various government agencies did not include the same nationalities or ethnic groups in their categories labeled Asian. Another problem is that until recently, detailed statistics regarding minority populations were not compiled.

There are, however, some similarities among all minority aging populations. First, their problems with declining health are more related to their general low socioeconomic status than the normal physical aging process. Second, the belief that the minority families take care of their aging is somewhat a myth. Their young people are becoming better educated and also relocate with their job opportunities.

Most problems can be traced to income and socioeconomic issues. Social Security benefits are based on income while working. Many minorities have had lower paying jobs, or part-time work with no benefits. This means fewer dollars for food, housing, transportation, and health care.

Culturally, people interact with families and society. The family provides a nurturing environment: belonging, self-esteem, and an identity. Society provides a sustaining environment: education, and goods and services for living. Society has generally failed the minority and aging minority.

Aging Asian Americans.   This population group represents many nationalities from countries in the Pacific Islands, the Far East, South East, and Near Middle East. There had been a quota system to immigration until 1965. The population of Asians increased by 50 percent between 1970 and 1980. Statistics are difficult to determine due to minimal research. Many immigrated to the United States because they had relatives here; they continue to live in extended families, figure 1–11.

Some of today's Asian elderly came at the turn of the century for industrial jobs. They were less educated and suffered from discrimination and isolation. In the 1970s, elderly from southeastern Asian countries fled with their children to the United States. Some, from rural areas, did not read or write their own language. It was emotionally and socially oppressive for these people to be away from their homeland and not be productive. They watched their children become "Americanized."

Over half of the Asian elderly live in western states: California, Hawaii, and Washington. Their major areas of need are in health care, income, social services, nutrition, and housing.

Some of these elderly tend to practice folk medicine; supplies may be available in larger metropolitan areas where the majority of them live. They underutilize social services partly because they are uninformed. Language is a barrier and they are not in the mainstream of activity to learn about the help that is available for their health care.

Aging Black Americans.   The elderly Black population continues to be disadvantaged by socioeconomic and racial discrimination. Unlike most immigrants, the first Blacks coming to this country did not come by choice. Elderly Blacks comprise about 8 percent of the Black population. They are the most poor of elderly minorities: there are three times as many below the

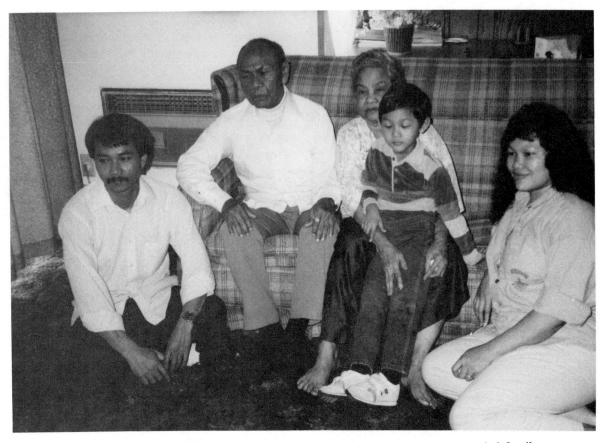

Figure 1-11   Elderly Asian Americans enjoy activities in an extended family.

poverty level as their white counterparts. Elderly Black females are the poorest of all elderly.

A majority of the elderly Black population live in the southeastern states, many of them in depressed rural areas. Although there have been increases in federal programs, these elderly have been hampered by inflation and fixed incomes. Transportation from remote areas to health centers is often a major problem. Their economic problems are compounded by loss of jobs due to new technology, increasing ill health, and young family members who grow up and move away.

They often see themselves in a powerless situation.

Many programs and services are needed to meet growing problems with aging, increasing chronic illness, and functional impairment. Without adequate funds, the elderly Black suffer from inadequate nutrition, housing, and medical care.

Aging Hispanic Americans.   This ethnic group also experiences the situation of multiple nationalities being labeled Hispanic. Those of Spanish origin include Cubans, Mexicans, Puerto Ricans, and others from Central and South America. Each group has had different experiences and has specific needs related to their aging.

The elderly of Cuban origin make up a greater percent of this minority population than do other Hispanic groups. This is, in part, due to the nature of Cuban emigration. Many middle and upper class people left Cuba following Castro's assumption of power in 1959. They represented skilled and professional sectors of the population. Later their parents followed these adult children. The Castro government welcomed this as they would soon be a dependent population group.

In 1980 there was another large migration of Cuban population to the United States. Unlike the earlier group, many of these people were educationally, occupationally, and economically deprived. The government also persuaded criminals and other institutionalized persons to leave. In these last two emigrations we can again see the cultural factors of cost versus contribution of a society's citizens.

A majority of the elderly Cuban population lives in the Miami area of Florida. Although these elderly have had more education than other groups, income is still a problem. Their age and number of work years in the United States influences their Social Security benefits.

The serious problems reported by these elderly include physical and mental health. Physical complaints include arthritis, circulatory, and eye problems. The mental health difficulties suggest a vulnerability and adaptation problems with social role losses.

Another elderly Hispanic group includes those of Mexican heritage. Gathering statistics on this group is difficult as this cohort includes a number of undocumented people. In 1986 amnesty regulations attempted to change this. However, since the objectives related to the workplace, the elderly statistics still may not be very accurate.

Socioeconomic concerns are the greatest for this elderly group. Next to the elderly Black Americans, they have the greatest numbers below the poverty level. Most were employed in low paying jobs, primarily in agriculture as migrant workers. Their poor health is related to inadequate nutrition, housing, and exposure to toxic substances used in growing fruits and vegetables.

Aging Native Americans. The elderly Native Americans represent several hundred tribes with many distinctly different languages and customs. Most of this population lives in western states with greater populations in New Mexico, South Dakota, Oklahoma, Arizona, and Montana. These elderly are not experiencing the longevity of other ethnic groups. They have the lowest percentage of elderly and the lowest median age.

Historically, elderly Native Americans have held a high position in their tribes. However, like other groups in the United States, they are experiencing changing culture and life-style patterns that are mostly influenced by younger members.

Economic issues also plague this elderly population. Lower paying jobs, unemployment, and other situations result in decreased Social Security benefits. Lower income results in inadequate nutrition, housing, and health care. In 1978 government grants were established for the development of social and nutrition services for older Indians.

Health problems that concern the older Native Americans include obesity, diabetes, hypertension, arthritis, liver and kidney disease, and dental problems. In providing health services, traditional care and folk medicine need to be considered.

Aging Minority in Traditional Health Settings. Aging minorities have generally underutilized traditional health settings. Some have not gone to the hospital even when it was recommended by a physician. The lower income elderly need care the most, and are most likely not to use it. Even with government insurance coverage, the deductibles are prohibitive and medigap insurance is unaffordable.

Another barrier in access to care is transportation. Appropriate health care may not be in the neighborhood and transportation may not be available or affordable. There are fears of doctors and hospitals. Health care in the United States is basically founded on the white culture's science and values. Folk medicine may be more comfortable to aging minority populations.

There are few minority aged represented in the population in long term care facilities. Reasons are related to cultural values. These elderly prefer receiving care in their home, by their family, if it is at all possible. There is also a lack of long term care facilities in minority neighborhoods.

Summary

Nurses practicing today and in the twenty-first century will need a broader understanding of gerontology. In all practice settings a majority of the patients nurses assist will be 65 and older. Birth rates have increased the population, and technology has kept people alive longer. For the first time, society has to consider meeting the needs of a large elderly population.

Advances in medicine that prolong life have included the development of antibiotics and other sophisticated drug treatments. Surgery was a "nightmare" a century ago. Today, procedures not even dreamed of are common-place. The ability to control infection and improve nutrition were two important factors in the first half of this century that influenced longevity.

The aging population is not evenly distributed, which influences the kinds of services and numbers of nurses and other professionals needed in specific areas. California, New York, and Florida have the greatest elderly population and higher populations of some elderly minority groups. The elderly are more socioeconomically

depressed. More elderly live in metropolitan areas. However, those living in rural areas have fewer services available.

Government intervention in addressing needs of the elderly began with the Social Security Act in 1935. This provided income for people over 65, and began the concept known as retirement. Health care insurance for this population sponsored by the government, came in 1965 in Social Security Amendments known as Medicare and Medicaid. Because of increasing numbers of elderly and a wide use of these benefits, the government began cost containment measures in the 1980s.

The lifetime experiences of today's elderly influence their response to their own aging and the physical, emotional, and social outcomes. They are a proud group that helped carve and develop this country. They are the "I'll-do-it-myself" and "pay-my-own-way" generation. Social programs developed in this half of the century are not always easy for this group to accept.

The changing family structure is making a difference in who takes care of the dependent elderly and where that care takes place. In the past, most elderly moved in with adult children when they could no longer be independent. Daughters and daughters-in-law were the primary caregivers. They still are, but are out of the home and in the workplace. These family changes, a more mobile society, and government payments for elderly health care were part of the growth of the long term care industry.

Aging for minority populations is more difficult than for their white counterparts. Their deteriorating health is a reflection of their depressed socioeconomic status. Social security benefits are linked to income during working years. Many of these elderly people had low paying jobs and were forced out of the job market with the growth of high technology. Ethnic neighborhoods are beginning to have more health services that focus on the needs of their elderly. These clinics receive funding from government sources and are less costly to the individual.

For Discussion

- Visit with a relative or neighbor who is 65 years or older. Learn about his/her lifetime experiences and values. How would this influence your nursing care if this person were your patient today?
- Determine characteristics and experiences of your cohort. How do these experiences influence the health care of this cohort today?
- Discuss cultural beliefs and traditions with someone whose background is different from your own. Identify two or three points that would assist you in providing nursing care for that population group.

Questions for Review

1. What is demography?
2. What is a cohort?
3. What advances in health care prolonged life in the first half of this century?
4. How did the Social Security Act help the elderly?
5. List two events of the World War II period that influenced today's aging population.
6. What is the major deterrent in health care for the aging minorities?

[Handwritten answers:]

12% — 65 & over

1. Statistical study of the population

2. Group of people born during specified years. "Baby Boomers" 1946–1964

3. ↓ infant mortality ↑ opportunities to recover from acute illnesses & chronic conditions. Pasteur's "germ theory" in 1865. Rubber gloves in 1890's.

4. Provided retirement fund

5. Long term care facilities — medication. Meals on Wheels. White House Conference on Aging 1965

Unit 2
Older Adults After 2000: Challenges for Everyone

Objectives

After reading this unit you should be able to:

* Discuss how projected changes in demographics may affect the elderly in the twenty-first century.
* Identify several potential effects of a population majority of elderly on industry in the United States.
* Discuss projected effects of a large elderly population on the health care delivery system.
* Discuss the implications of a large elderly population on nursing practice.

A few more steps (years) and we will be standing at the threshold of the twenty-first century. It is exciting and challenging, and a little bit frightening: it definitely indicates a lot of responsibility for everyone, including nurses. After looking back at some of the growth and change in the United States that has influenced issues of aging for today's elderly, it is time to project possible events of the future.

We can make some projections for the first half of the next century because those that will be aging during that time are now active in society. In the fall of 1987, television crews were busy filming the first day of kindergarten for many youngsters. They will be the high school graduating class of 2000. Those entering elementary school now will be the "young olds," those turning 65, in 2050.

During your study of anticipated events of the future and the determining of your own projections, it will be helpful to place yourself in a time line of current and future events. First, establish your cohort and determine the year you will be 65. Next, select some characteristics that identify your population group. You may consider memories from school that include favorite after-school activities, popular music, style of clothes, and entertainment personalities. Look at additional events in young adult and adult years. During these times what family, community, national, and world events influenced your activities and values? Reflecting on your cohort will guide you in determining what might be concerns and needs of your cohort as you age.

This unit will discuss the changing demographics in the next century. Population changes that are predicted today will probably be proven underestimated. We have already met earlier projections for 2000. Five thousand Americans reach age 65 everyday, and the elderly are expected to be 20 percent of the population in 2030.

The birth rate will continue to affect the aging population. The Baby Boom cohort will be reaching 65 years of age between 2011 and 2030. By that time, one out of five people will be 65 or older. Will most of those people be retired? How many will be dependent?

Technology will continue to affect our longevity. However, goals may be directed more toward the quality of life than on the length of life. Costs of technology will continue to be an issue. Will the technology focus on curative medicine, or the prevention and rehabilitation aspects of disease?

Industry will look at aging and technology. It will change our goods and services from a youth-oriented to an aging-oriented society. The "giant-economy-size" packaging will have to become the "small-economy-size," for the increasing numbers of singles and older couples. The smaller size packaging will move from the top shelf, figure 2–1, to the middle shelf where it can be reached by the majority of the consumers.

Cost of health care for the elderly is, and will be, a growing issue. Accompanying this issue is the access to health care for all. Will it be offered institutionally only in metropolitan areas? To what extent will health care be provided in clinics and the patient's home? Cost containment is part of the health care issue. Hospitals and long term care facilities have already experienced government intervention. States and the federal government are wrestling with approaches to provide all citizens with access to basic health care — a big challenge.

One of the problems that has persisted in this country is that all health care funding has focused on the medical model. The emphasis is on illness and the accompanying problems, treatments, and costs. A person may need to live in a long term care facility because of decreasing functional ability and limited support services, not because of a physical illness. Costs have been attached to prescribed treatments. For example, in long term care facilities, the costs of time and supplies for a nurse to change a dressing are easily justified for reimbursement purposes. However, the nursing time spent with an anxious, fearful new resident, or the time involved in reassuring a confused resident, is not easily quantified for reimbursement costs in the medical model system.

As citizens, how will people in the United States want health care to be managed? Most decisions are made by industry and lawmakers. There will be decisions made regarding limiting

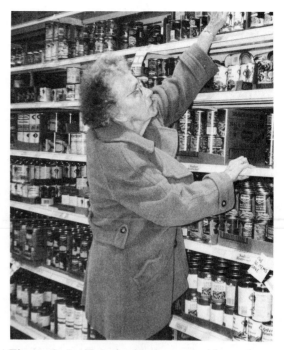

Figure 2–1   Today's elderly cope with marketing for a younger generation.

care to specific populations or conditions, limiting benefit packages with citizens paying more of their own health care, increasing taxes to pay for health care, and other possibilities.

How will the next century's elderly be described in the media and in nursing education? What impact will the increasing numbers have on the family, the workplace, and industry? Why does the health care delivery system need to consider health care and biomedical ethical issues today? Who will take care of the growing numbers of dependent elderly? What does the increased number of elderly persons mean regarding your nursing practice? These questions cannot be answered specifically today. But in this unit we will look at events that will give us some guidelines to start planning for aging in the twenty-first century.

Influence of Demographic Change on the Individual and Family

New Options for Aging Americans

A century ago people did not age, they died young. Aging today is becoming "stylish." Many of the older adults have options to explore after retiring at 65. President Carter's mother, Lillian, joined the Peace Corps and went to India at age 68. Entertainer George Burns, in his 90s, was in vaudeville at the turn of this century. He talks about the launching of his country music recording career in his 80s. Lesser known older adults also seek new careers or meaningful volunteer work. They develop new support systems and seek second careers as their children grow up and move away.

In the older life that provides new options, some are beginning school for the first time. Others are going to college or getting advanced degrees. The population today is becoming more educated. More people are completing high school and college or other post-secondary education. In the twenty-first century the elderly will have received more education and be more informed than the elderly of the twentieth century.

Many older adults seek second careers. Education and industry welcome the expertise of these experienced elders. Those with business experience are employed, or volunteer their time, to assist younger people starting their own businesses. Some are tutors for students. Others find a total change of pace enjoyable, figure 2–2.

The Changing Household

The structure of the family and household has changed in recent decades. This household includes a variety of family and friends and relationships. If this continues, a member of the household will also be an aging parent or friend. One projection related to families and households is the future need of eldercare as an employee benefit. Today, child care is a concern

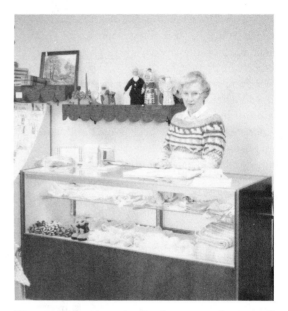

Figure 2–2   A retired educator enjoys retail sales employment.

of working mothers and employers. In the future this will change to the concern of eldercare for working daughters or other family members. Employers may offer flexible working hours, on-site services, or share the cost of adult day care, in-home meals, or other services for dependent elderly family members of their employees. This will occur because the admission criteria for long-term care placement will become very selective.

Changes in Personal Finances

Financially, the elderly will be more secure for a time. In the United States we are no longer paying our own way. Grandchildren of today's elderly may be the first generation that is not better off than their parents. The family income, after adjustments for inflation, had less spendable dollars in 1987 than it did in 1973. The standard of living in the 1960s that was based on a one income household needed two incomes in the 1970s. In the 1980s, this standard of living required two incomes plus credit cards.

Being thrifty has become outdated in the United States. The credit card, as we know it today, was born in the 1950s. Prior to that time some businesses offered credit in the neighborhood to well known customers. For example, the corner grocery store filed the receipts for groceries purchased by a neighborhood family. At the end of the month, or at a convenient time, someone went to the store to pay the bill. There was no formal billing process.

Today, only several decades after the initiation of credit cards, the average citizen has a credit debt of several thousand dollars. In the 1940s, about 35 percent of the elderly received financial support from their children. Social Security benefits have almost eliminated that need. It is more likely today that older parents provide some financial support to their children.

What does this mean to the elderly of the future? It probably means that there will be little or no savings to assist with health needs and other services during old age. Baby Boomers may enter into old age in debt. There will be an even greater financial responsibility for the young to pay for services for the elderly than there is today. The population of working Baby Boomers is largely supporting Social Security monies today. When the system started in 1936 there were 46 workers for every retired recipient of benefits. Today it is three workers paying into the system for each person receiving a Social Security check. Many elderly today receive benefit payments equal to 25 times more than they paid into Social Security during their working years. The average recipient of Social Security payments has has received his lifetime contributions in less than two years, yet many people live twenty years and more beyond retirement.

Some of this may seem to have political influence. It does. However, the general population has wanted, and bought, a standard of living greater than their resources. Baby Boomers are the cohort that demographers and futurists focus on the most. This group has many demands for goods and services for today and in the future. Many expect to live in retirement for 20 or 30 years. However, they are not saving or planning to meet these desires and demands. What will they expect and receive for health and social services in 2025?

Choices for the Generations

This initiates a projection of conflict between generations. Some are calling this "age wars" that will parallel or be greater than previous social conflicts between races, sexes, and socioeconomic classes. The thought is that, because of economic situations, decisions will have to be made where to spend the money, especially tax dollars. Will this be on health and social programs for the young or old? Will the money be spent on education for the young or housing for the elderly? Will the workplace focus benefits on workers or retirees?

These are examples of some projections for the future. They may seem discouraging, but the United States has always met the challenge. Looking at the last 50 years, we can anticipate new industry and new ways of meeting the needs of the people in the future. Figure 2–3 summarizes projected demographic influences on the individual and family.

Influence of Demographic Change on Industry and the Workplace

Some refer to the movement of the Baby Boomers through time as the "age quake." For this population, the United States has experienced the building of elementary schools, and then high schools. This was followed by bulging college and technical school classrooms. More recently the need for housing for this group was experienced, as well as their increased spending for goods and services. Soon after 2000, when the children of this cohort are grown, perhaps apartments or small homes will replace the larger homes demanded today. Travel and leisure activity industries will probably mushroom in response to the retiring Baby Boomers.

- Population over 65 will double by 2030
- 20 percent of United States citizens will be over 65
- Aging will become "stylish"
- More television programming, news articles, books, and films will focus on aging themes and concerns
- More second careers and educational opportunities will be experienced by older adults
- Credit card generation may not have finances to support desired life style and health care during elderly years
- Working households will have eldercare benefits from employers to assist with care of aging family members
- Potential conflict between generational values and the allocations of funds for social services

---

Figure 2–3 Projecting future demographic influences for individuals and families

Return to Older Workers

The general age in the workplace will be older. Currently, one third of the population is in the Baby Boom cohort and now in the work force. For the younger people, those born after 1964, the future job market is promising. Industry, however, sees a future shortage of workers. This means that more people will be in the work force into their 70s, filling employment gaps, figure 2–4. The numbers of older adults

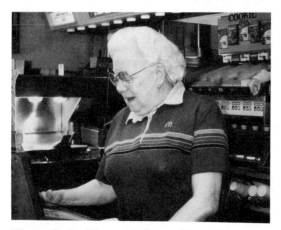

Figure 2–4 The workplace will employ many elderly workers.

over 65 in the workplace will nearly double by the year 2000. They will be about 20 percent of the work force compared to about 11 percent in the 1980s. Continually learning new skills will be common with all age groups, not just the elderly.

Employers will have to offer retraining and flexible or reduced schedules for older workers. More employers will offer educational preparation for second careers that will follow retirement. When mandatory retirement became illegal, offering early retirement with pension plans became a method of reducing the work force and saving corporate dollars. We will see if the trend reverses, moving retirement benefits to an older age to retain older employees.

Nearly one third of the over 65 population will be involved in unpaid or volunteer productive activity. This will include assisting family members having disabilities.

Public Places and Services Responding to Aging America

Public buildings and retail facilities will need to continue to meet the physical changes of aging, figure 2–5. Large warehouse-type grocery stores will be difficult to manage for those with arthritis and other mobility prob-

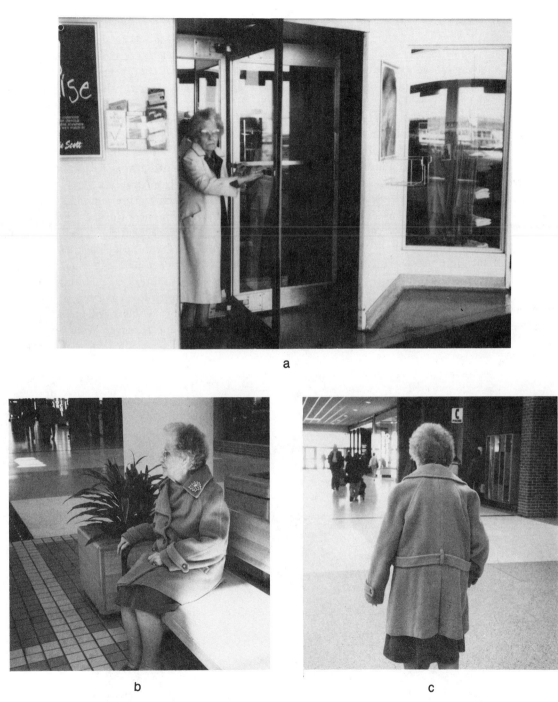

Figure 2–5 Public buildings will need to modify these aging challenges: (a) revolving doors are difficult for the elderly to manage; (b) shopping centers will need more seating areas for the elderly to rest; (c) shiny tile or marble floors are difficult for the aging eye and foot.

lems. Elevator doors will need to be timed to stay open longer. Revolving doors and escalators may no longer be the best choices for traffic flow. The revolving doors rotate too fast, and the older adults' pride prevents them from using the adjacent door that is marked for the handicapped. Escalators require a degree of good vision and timing. Shiny tile floors will be out of the question for the aging eye and foot. Nonglare lighting will be a must. Public buildings will need more handrails and seating areas. Older adults learning to pace themselves will need a place to rest for a a few minutes. The timing of traffic lights will have to be lengthened. Today, many elderly cannot walk across the street in the time allowed between "walk" and "don't walk."

Changes in Design of Homes

Homes will be designed more conveniently. People will choose homes with fewer levels to reduce the number of stairs. There will need to be improved lighting, particularly in hallways, stairways, and work areas. Thermostats, fuses, and directions on water heaters and furnaces will have to have larger print markings and directions. The dials and markings on stoves and other appliances will have to be larger and bolder for the aging eye to see.

Manufacturing and Marketing Response to Aging America

Some manufacturers are beginning to design products to meet the needs of the aging consumer. The Whirlpool Company has designed laundry appliances with large black lettering on a nonreflective background and enlarged dials and buttons. They also offer operating instructions in Braille or on audio cassettes, figure 2–6.

Marketing and retailers will need to shift gears as the country moves from a youth-oriented to an aging-oriented focus in market-

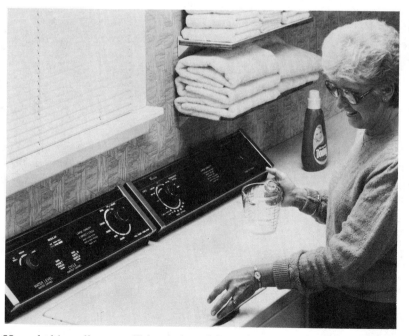

Figure 2–6   Household appliances will be designed for aging sensory deficits. (Photo courtesy of the Whirlpool Corporation)

ing. The advertising industry is studying the senior citizens market: some markets are on the leading edge of this new advertising. No longer are older people seen only in denture cleaning advertisements. Clara Peller was a hit in the early 1980s with her, "Where's the beef?"! Some of McDonald's television advertisements have shown older adults as customers and workers. This also demonstrates the individuality in the aging process regarding the decrease in finger dexterity and slowing of response and reaction time. A fast food restaurant is a busy place at meal time!

The 30-second advertisement on television will have to reduce the speed of the audio and video message to be caught by the aging ear and eye. Magazines will need to avoid shiny paper and use larger print. Catalogs will have to have larger letters and numbers for those wishing to telephone-shop from home. More newspapers will have to use larger print and a magazine style that is easier to hold.

Clothing manufacturers will become accustomed to an older market. For the first time there are grandmothers in blue jeans! However, the increased difficulty with small buttons, the small tab on zippers, and other clothing notions and designs will be considered. Labels and tags with size, fabric content, laundering instructions, and price will have to be in larger print. More designs will meet the preferences of the aging population. Sizing will be modified to fit narrowing shoulders and other changes in the aging figure.

Grocery store advertising will shift from offering specials and discounts on larger packages and multiple items marketed today to large young families. Manufacturers will package products in smaller containers, with caps, lids, and other opening devices that are easier to manage by fingers that have lost strength and dexterity. Directions will be in larger print on nonglossy surfaces.

Nearly every product will either change or add a product line for the aging population. Skin care products have promoted youth for

years. Greeting card manufacturers at one time stopped at age 21 on cards noting a specific birthday. With the Baby Boom approaching middle age, more cards with 40, 50 and other milestones were added to product lines. In 1988 Hallmark initiated a card line called "The Best Years," for the 55-and-older population. Greeting cards for great-grandchildren are also more in demand.

Other services in the community may expand, or shift their focus to address changing demographics. Currently many banking institutions provide checking accounts without service charges, or other free services, to senior citizens. Restaurants offer a discount on the bill to those with their "senior membership card." Some menus have selections for seniors that include smaller portions at reduced prices, figure 2-7. As the older population increases, more businesses and services may offer these kind of incentives. They save the elderly some money while encouraging customers from this age group. There is also the possibility that businesses will find that those programs are no longer profitable. There will be, regardless of the actual outcome, many types of marketing to this growing elderly population. Sample demographic influences of the aging population on industry and the work place are shown in figure 2-8.

Demographic Influences on the Health Care Delivery System

Historical Overview

Providing health care for an aging population will probably be one of the biggest challenges for the United States as we move into the next century. At one time health care was a responsibility of the community. Families, neighbors, and the church assisted people during times of birthing, illness, and dying. When people were poor, or without families, the community was still responsible. These less fortunate were cared for in "poor houses" or some desig-

Gerry Strandemo's

Sandy Point
Supper Club

THE OUT OF TOWN PLACE
**Open 7 Evenings and
at noon on Saturday and Sunday**

HORS D'OEUVRES

ONION RINGS .... ½ order $1.95   full $2.95
MEAT BALLS - BBQ - 15 .... 2.95
POTATO SKINS with cheese or BBQ 2.95
CHEESE CURDS batter fried .... ½ order 2.95   full 3.95
CHICKEN WINGS 3.95
HERRING cream sauce 1.95
EGG ROLL 2.50
BATTER FRIED CAULIFLOWER 3.95
BATTER FRIED MUSHROOMS 3.95
BATTER FRIED BROCCOLI 3.95
COMBINATION PLATE 3.95
Fresh cauliflower, mushrooms and broccoli
FRESH MUSHROOMS SAUTEED
  IN GARLIC BUTTER 4.25
  With Cheese 4.95
SHRIMP COCKTAIL 4.95

Party Platter	15 Meat Balls 12 Chicken Wings 1/2 order Onion Rings 1/2 order Cheese Curds	8.95

STEAKS

Petite Filet *Prime - 6 oz.* 10.45
Filet Mignon *With fresh mushrooms* 13.95
New York Strip Sirloin *16 oz.* 13.95
Ladies Strip Sirloin 11.95
Rib Eye Steak *With fresh mushrooms* 11.95
Chopped Sirloin Steak 7.95
  Broiled with mushrooms
Carol's Hungry Man Steak 16.95
  New York 24 oz.
Teriaki Steak 12.95

Prime Rib
Prime Rib *King's Cut* 12.95
Prime Rib *Queen's Cut* 10.95
Strandemo's 22 oz. Super Cut 17.95

*See back cover for our
Fine Selection of Dinner Wines*

GIFT CERTIFICATES
Available In Any Denomination For

Friends	Relatives
Neighbors	Favors Done
Secretaries	Business Acquaintances

SEAFOOD

Orange Roughy 10.95
  Broiled with drawn butter and lemon
Shrimp *Batter fried* 11.95
  Broiled 12.95
Avalon Stuffed Shrimp 10.95
  Stuffed with a tasty combination of bay shrimp, snow crab, and monterey jack cheese, on bed of blended wild rice or potato
Spanish Broiled Shrimp *Drawn Butter* 14.95
Walleyed Pike *Batter fried* 11.95
  Broiled with drawn butter 12.95
Cod *Deep fried or Broiled* 7.95
Combination Seafood Platter 15.95
  LOBSTER, Shrimp, walleyed pike and scallops. Drawn butter.
Deep Sea Scallops *Batter fried* 11.95
  Broiled with drawn butter 12.95
African Broiled Lobster Tail, drawn butter
  King 19.95   Queen 15.95
Broiled Halibut Steak 8.95
Pan Fried Cat Fish 8.95
  Garnished with broiled tomatoes.
Shrimp Scampi 12.95
  Sauteed shrimp in garlic butter, topped with Swiss and Mozzarella cheese.
Red Snapper Almondine 9.95
  Broiled with toasted almonds.

Ask About Our Fresh Fish

◦●◦ Senior Citizens Menu ◦●◦
Age 62 and older

Stuffed Shrimp $5.95
Broiled Orange Roughy 5.95
Beef Stroganoff 5.45
Bar-B-Qued Pork Ribs 5.95
Center-cut Pork Chop 5.95
Chopped Sirloin Steak 4.95
Smoked Ham Slice 5.45
Boneless Breast Chicken (Marinated) 5.45
Fried Chicken, ¼ chicken 4.95
Fried Shrimp, 4 shrimp 6.95
Walleyed Pike (Broiled or deep fried) 7.95
Baby Beef Liver (Onion or bacon) 4.95
Chicken Kiev (Bed of blended wild rice) 6.95
Cornish Game Hen 7.95
  (Bed of blended wild rice)
Cod (Deep fried or broiled) 5.45
Tenderloin Steak 6.95
Prime Rib 6.95
  —ALL DINNERS INCLUDE—
Appetizer, choice of tossed salad, potato, rice or vegetable, with bread sticks, garlic toast and rolls.

Figure 2–7 Some restaurants market to the elderly's appetite and wallet.

- Baby Boomer "age quake" begins to turn 65 in 2011
- Increased number of older workers in work force in response to a shrinking younger population
- Retirements and benefits may be pushed to later years
- Retraining in the work place becomes common for all ages
- Industry retools and adds new product lines to meet the demands of a large aging population
- Products have larger print directions on nonglossy surface to be managed by aging eyes
- Products have more manageable knobs, buttons, and tabs for fingers losing strength and dexterity
- Marketing reduces pitch and speed of audio advertising to be heard by the aging ear
- Public services and retail establishments arrange services, hours of business, and pace to meet the needs of the aging population

Figure 2–8   Sample projected changes in the workplace and industry

nated place in the community. Gradually the state and federal governments have taken over more of the funding and responsibility of health care for the elderly, the handicapped, and the financially oppressed. It has proven to be costly.

The United States is one of two industrialized nations that does not have a national health care policy. Every Congress since 1936 has vetoed this type of health care bill for the country. Our country was founded on individual and states' rights. Medicare is a type of national health care policy for a specific age group.

At the close of the 1980s nearly every newspaper and magazine reported the rising costs of health care in this country, and the impact on life, health, and the economy. We spend over one billion dollars per day on health care. Much of the focus is on the cost of health care for the elderly because of Medicare funding. This population group, especially those over 85, is the greatest user of health care services. Twenty-five percent of all government spending goes to the 12 percent of the population over 65 years of age. The government spends six times more on the elderly than on children. This is part of the health care dilemma and the potential conflict of values between generations.

Challenges to the Health Care Delivery System

Two parts of this challenge for the health care delivery system are costs and access to care. Costs have become unaffordable for employers in providing health care benefits. For the elderly and others, costs are not affordable because of the deductibles and other out-of-pocket expenses.

Increased costs are tied to the price of technology, the increased numbers of the population group that use the care, and the fact that we are not the healthiest nation in the world. Until recently, there was not a focus on wellness. Curative medicine is considerably more expensive than preventative medicine. Not very many years ago insurance companies did not cover the cost of a cervical pap smear, part of a cancer prevention examination for women. Benefits, however, did cover costs of a hysterectomy.

People are becoming more responsible for their own health. Part of this is by choice, and part by cost containment efforts. Home diagnostic kits or packets are a part of this movement. The ability to complete home testing for occult blood in stool specimens is an example of patient participation in diagnostics. There may be more development of this type of health care. The accuracy depends on patient teaching and the ability of people to correctly follow directions, figure 2–9.

In addition to the obvious increase in numbers of older adults, there is the frequency of use of health services by the elderly. This caught the payers of health care off guard. One example was the lack of Medicare funds in the Social Security system 20 years after the bill was passed. The increased cost of medical care was cited, but the number of elderly with benefits and the increased number of times they visited a physician for treatment were not anticipated.

Access to care is not only the elderly's geographical location in relation to health care services. It relates to costs as well. Minority elderly and poor elderly many times do not have access to care because of the inability to pay the deductible for Medicare. They can not afford medigap insurance to help pay for costs Medicare does not cover. An uncomfortable term that has surfaced is the "rationing" of health care. As our collective eyebrows raise at the thought of selective care, some are saying we already have rationing of health care in this country. Most of it is tied to the costs of care. Those who can afford the care have it; those who cannot, do not.

The increased spending on health care in this country is straining society's resources. Choices will have to be made. There are about 37 million non-welfare citizens who have no medical insurance. Many of those people are the working poor; about 20 percent are children. As the next century approaches, there are more people employed in low paying service jobs. These may be part-time workers with no health benefits. There will need to be some changes in the health care framework of the United States to open the door of basic health care to all people.

Medicare will probably continue to experience changes in coverage and policies. Some say there should be a means test rather than blanket coverage for people 65 and older. *Means test*

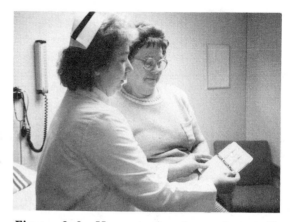

Figure 2–9 Home testing by patients will increase with nurses completing patient teaching.

identifies an income level before financial aid is granted. The idea is that the elderly who can afford to pay for their own health care, with their own insurance, should not receive Medicare reimbursements. Their Medicare funds would be used for the poor elderly who can not afford the Medicare deductible and other costs.

Settings for Care

Changing demographics in the next century will probably mean that more care of the elderly must be provided in their homes and similar settings. The elderly will receive health care and other services in their home in an effort to maintain a high level of functional ability. This home care will also eliminate the costs of meals, laundry, housekeeping, and other charges that are a part of the hospital or long-term care room rate. One of of the biggest costs in institutional care is the daily room rate.

In the future, more of the elderly will receive assistance with health care and other needs in a variety of settings. They may be able to stay in their own home with shared or cooperative housing. For example, a college student or other young adult may live with an elderly person who can no longer manage her house independently. The young person has room and board free, and the elderly person has help with home maintenance, meal preparation, or other tasks. Both individuals benefit from the companionship, figure 2–10.

Other options for care may include moving to the home of an adult son or daughter, sharing an apartment with other older adults, or moving into a retirement community for senior citizens. The elderly will continue to receive health care in traditional settings. Hospitals and long term care facilities will care for the acutely ill and those with chronic conditions that result in dependent situations. In both of these settings, the physical condition and functional ability of the individual will be more acute or severe than in the past.

Some projections indicate that the percentage of elderly requiring long-term care placement will be less at the beginning of the next century. It has been about 5 percent since the 1970s, but is projected to drop to 4 percent. However, the actual numbers of elderly in long term care facilities may be greater simply because of the increased number of elderly.

There will be ongoing changes in the regulation of long term care facilities. The growth in this industry has been rapid because of the increased medical technology and the lengthening life span. Today, many of these facilities could be labeled long-term-acute-care because of the more sophisticated procedures implemented. Some of these procedures include gastrostomy tube feedings, respirators and other oxygen therapies, and short-term intravenous therapies. Not many years ago, most of the elderly in long term care facilities were ambulatory and needed only minimal assistance with personal hygiene and health care. Those ambulatory elderly are managing in other settings today.

With the increased elderly population in the next century, there will be an increased need for services in all health care settings. The need for pre-admission screening will continue and the guidelines for services or long-term care placement will change. *Pre-admission screening* is an interview and assessment completed by nurses and social workers, figure 2–11, to determine health and social services needed by an individual. The findings are often the determining factor for government funding for the long-term care placement of this individual.

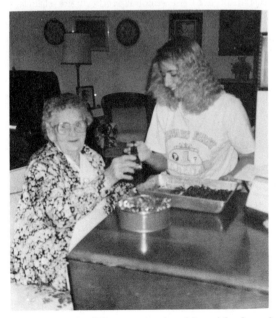

Figure 2–10   The companionship with shared housing benefits young and old.

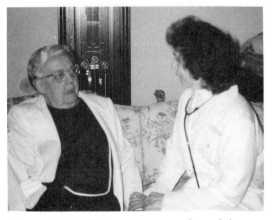

Figure 2–11   The nurse, a member of the pre-screening team, evaluates the elderly's abilities.

Gerontological Health Care Providers

The aging of the Baby Boomers in the twenty-first century will result in an expansion of health care services that is greater than today. It is projected that between 1980 and 2040, physician visits by the elderly population will increase by 160 percent. Other projections state that days of hospital care will increase by 200 percent, and the increase in elderly in long term care facilities will be 280 percent. The increase in hospitals reflects numbers of elderly being hospitalized rather than more days in the hospital per patient. In long term care facilities it is again the combination of advanced technology and increasing longevity with a large birth rate cohort.

These projections also indicate the increased need for all health care professionals — physicians, nurses, physical therapists, social workers, pharmacists, and many others. Every specialty area will have to have more education focused on gerontology and the needs of the elderly. Figure 2–12 summarizes the influence of a growing elderly population on the health care delivery system.

Demographic Influences on Nursing Practice

Nursing Education

As the population ages, the settings where nurses practice will include even larger percentages of elderly. Gerontological nursing will not be confined to long-term care settings. Greater numbers of patients in hospitals will be elderly as well as those seen in clinics, out-patient settings, and in home care.

Like other professions, nursing responds to the needs of society. In the past, nursing care has focused on needs of patients with tuberculosis and polio. As technology changed, nurses added new responsibilities, as well as changed the direction of care for patients with cancer, heart disease, and other conditions. Nursing education in the future will place a greater emphasis on the aging process and related situations. Care plan goals, methods of patient teaching, and other aspects of nursing care will be adapted to the special needs of the elderly.

- Costs of health care for elderly population continue to increase due to actual costs, and numbers of elderly
- Increased government intervention in payment for health care for elderly
- Continued changes in programs and policies for health and social services for the elderly
- Increased use of out-patient health care and social services in homes, day-care, senior centers, and other settings
- Increased use of traditional hospital and long term care facilities due to increased numbers of elderly; percent of elderly using these facilities will be reduced
- Costs and access to health care continue to result in unequal care for elderly citizens: a societal dilemma
- Rationing of health care: a troubling projection
- Advancing technology may focus on quality of life rather than length of life
- Increased numbers of physicians, nurses, and other health care professionals with gerontological education

---

Figure 2–12 Projected influences of an aging population on the health care delivery system

Employment Opportunities

More nurses will be needed in the twenty-first century. This includes nurses at the bedside, in the community, and in research. Although projections indicate increased use of hospitals, and more elderly in long term care facilities, there will be many other settings for gerontological nursing practice. More physicians will be in geriatric practice. Internists and other specialists will be monitoring chronic conditions of the elderly. This will provide more nurses with many opportunities to assist and teach older adults to monitor their own health and remain independent.

In the community, home care will expand as well as adult day care and other services for aging adults. Nurses may be employed by senior community centers or elderly apartment complexes. In these settings they will screen blood pressures and answer questions about therapeutic diets and side effects of medications, fig-

ure 2–13. As a resource person, the nurse will assure older adults they are doing fine or suggest perhaps they see their physicians.

Community nursing today, which is directed toward the future, includes nurses involved in their neighborhoods and churches. These nurses identify and respond to early cries for help. They may be employed or volunteer in "Block Nurse," or "Parish Nurse" services. These services may be funded by government grants, community monies, individual congregations, or ministerial associations.

Nurses practicing in these roles are not replacing but complementing home health nurses and other health and social services. In addition to their education and experience, they are acquainted with, and connect people with, community resources. The elderly feel comfortable with nurses from their church and community. The nurses explain physician instructions for medications or answer questions about other con-

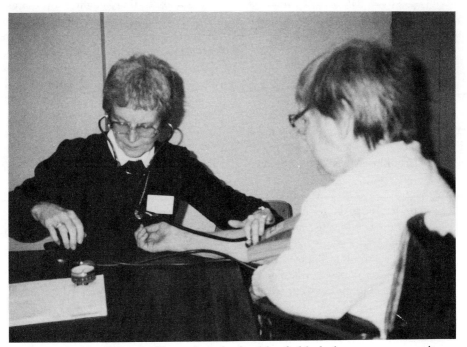

Figure 2–13   Nurses will monitor the health of elderly in more community settings.

cerns. For example, the elderly need continued reassurance that they are doing well in following hospital discharge instructions. When neighborhood or parish nurses are regular visiors, they are alert to potential problems and can make suggestions for the elderly to see their physicians.

Community and Advocacy Roles

Nurses have always been advocates for health issues and supported family and friends in times of health crisis. Often young mothers were the first to call a nurse friend or neighbor with concerns about a bump, scratch, or infant formula. As the demographics move the population to the older years, nurses will be a support for those facing issues with an aging dependent parent. An understanding of the aging process will assist the nurse in answering questions and supporting friends and family with their own aging. The nurse will be a resource person to direct them to other health care professionals and community services. Figure 2-14 includes examples of changes in nursing practice that will be influenced by the aging population.

Summary

The health care delivery system is on the edge of a new health care revolution. As a nurse you will be a part of the team, preparing to meet the challenges of health care in the twenty-first century. Perhaps the greatest part of that challenge will be meeting and assisting an aging population in meeting health needs and maintaining independence.

It is projected that by 2030 there will be twice as many people 65 and older as there are today. The most rapid increase will occur beginning in 2011 when the Baby Boom generation, those born between 1946 and 1964, begins to turn 65. By the time the last members of that cohort reach 65 in 2030, it is expected that the elderly will comprise over 21 percent of the population in the United States.

Today's focus on education for all people will be reflected in a more educated and better informed elderly population in the future. Many options will be open to these elderly, including opportunities for employment in their 70s and beyond, and education for post-retirement careers.

The structure of the household is changing to include a variety of members and relationships. In the past, the daughter or daughter-in-law was the primary caregiver to aging dependent parents. More of those caregivers are in the work place today, and will be in the future. One future projection is the addition of employee benefits for eldercare. This would provide assistance to those in the work force. There would be day care or other services for aging dependent family members.

Available funding for retirement living, leisure activities, and future health care will be

---

- Increased focus on gerontological theory and skills in nursing education
- More opportunities for nursing careers in an expanding variety of practice settings
- Unique community opportunities such as "Block Nurses" and "Parish Nurses" to utilize the nurse's gerontological nursing skills
- All practice settings will experience an increase in numbers of elderly patients receiving nursing care
- Increased opportunities to be advocates for the elderly in neighborhoods, the community, and in policy making

---

Figure 2-14 Sample projections of demographic influences on nursing practice

in question. The "cash and carry" generation of the early 1900s has been replaced by the "credit card" generation of today. People are not saving for a "rainy day" or their "old age." Part of this is due to a change in life style. Travel, communications, everything is moving faster. In this life in the fast lane, many want to "have it now." The "charge it" attitude of today will have a great financial impact on the elderly of the future.

Another factor is the passage of the Social Security Act of 1935. This government pension fund for the elderly has given some workers a sense of security for the future. Although many elderly today live only on Social Security income, it will not meet the needs of the elderly of the future. Social Security has experienced many changes. At the time of inception, over 40 workers payed into the system for each retiree receiving benefits. There are now only three workers contributing to Social Security benefits for each retiree. As those paying into the system decrease, the cost of paying for health care for an aging population increases. Medicare and Medicaid are Social Security programs to assist the elderly in paying for health care.

The United States, in approaching the twenty-first century, has two major health care challenges for the rapidly growing aging population. These are costs of health care and access to health care. In the 1980s there were major changes in the Medicare funding to help contain costs for elderly health care. No doubt there will be continued changes in programs and policies to curb costs in the future.

Access to care is tied to costs as well as geographic location of the elderly. Out-of-pocket costs (those not covered by Medicare) have also increased. Many cannot afford those costs, or the supplemental insurance that could cover them. This will probably not change in the future because of spending habits of the younger generation.

Manufacturing and marketing will meet the needs of the aging consumer. Many projections are made by watching the Baby Boom cohort. Society has addressed the needs of this generational wave as they moved through childhood, their teen and young adult years in the 1960s, and into middle life and careers. Futurists project the aging of this cohort will affect the design of homes and public buildings. Other examples of design changes will include the need for larger print directions on household appliances, and adaptations of knobs, buttons, and tabs on other products to be managed by less dexterous fingers.

For the health care delivery system, the projected change in demographics will mean the need for more health professionals. These professionals will need more gerontologically focused education to respond to the needs and treatment of the elderly. Nursing education will include an increased focus on the needs of an aging population.

Nurses will practice gerontological nursing in a variety of settings: hospitals, physician's offices, clinics, home care, and in long term care facilities. They will also be advocates for the aging in the community, working in neighborhoods and churches, and senior centers and elderly housing. It is an exciting time to stretch nursing skills to assist older adults and also learn from their rich experiences.

For Discussion

- Meet with several members of your cohort. Discuss experiences and values that describe your group. Project concerns and needs of your aging cohort.
- Interview one or two people from cohorts different from your own. Ask them to identify their concerns regarding life style and health needs during their older years.

- Interview a community mayor or other offical. What are the demographics of this community? What programs or services are planned or projected for the future that are directed specifically for the elderly population?
- In a local public building or retail store, identify several characteristics that make it easy and some that make it difficult for the elderly to manage the area.

Questions for Review

1. What is the projected population of the 65 and older age group by the year 2030? *21%   2+'s*
2. Why is the population of older adults expected to rise rapidly starting in the year 2011? *Baby Boomers*
3. What does "age wars" mean regarding the future of health care? *race-age- soc. ec.*
4. What are two projected changes in the workplace that are related to an aging population?
5. What were two efforts the government initiated in containing health care costs for the elderly in the 1980s?
6. What are examples of settings for gerontological nursing other than hospitals and long term care facilities?

Mean test — identify income level before financial aid is granted

Pre-admission screening — what government will pay for

Section 2
The Active Aging Population

Unit 3: Signs of Aging
Unit 4: Conditions Experienced by the Active Aging
Unit 5: Who are the Active Aging?
Unit 6: Community Services For the Aging
Unit 7: Patient Care Teaching for the Active Aging

The active aging population in the United States is the majority of the people 65 years of age and older. It is surprising for many people to hear that only 5 percent of this population group lives in long term care facilities. Due to the tremendous increase in numbers projected for the elderly population, the numbers living in these facilities will be even greater. There will also be many other older adults requiring some assistance to remain living in their homes, or the homes of their families. This still leaves a majority of the elderly population functioning independently, but needing health care services during their active aging years.

The major change for society in the twentieth century was the beginning of a large elderly cohort. When considering the thousands of years of history, the turnabout from a very young population to an elderly population occurred very rapidly. Life expectancy has the potential of almost doubling in this century. With the rapid advancement of technology, aging citizens have the opportunity for increased life expectancy and more active aging years.

No longer can people consider that old age and disability go hand in hand. The physical changes that have occurred do not seem to alter the functional ability for those young olds 65 to 74 years of age. Often, they are as active as they were during their 50s. Even half of the middle olds, those between 75 and 84, do not have health problems that limit their activity or require special care or monitoring. This is indeed becoming a nation of more active aging citizens.

This section will focus on biological aspects of aging as well as expanding on sociological issues. Psychosocial aspects of aging will be introduced. Physical changes in the normal aging process will be presented in Unit 3. Body structure and function changes that occur normally will be compared to those that result from a disease process. Some theories related to the causes of biological and psychosocial aging will be presented.

Unit 4 will discuss physical conditions generally experienced by the active aging population. These conditions occur because of the aging of the system, or because aging has accelerated a disease process. Since aging is a gradual process, people often do not seek assistance to manage a condition until it becomes a problem that affects functional ability. For example, an individual may attempt to manage diminishing vision until he can not pass the vision test for renewal of a driver's license. However, a symptom that develops in a short period of time is usually a result of an illness or disease rather than the aging process.

Who are the active aging? In Unit 5, this population group will be described. Some of the issues that concern the active aging will be presented. These include: retirement, health and financial concerns, family roles, and leisure activities and community participation.

Unit 6 will discuss community services provided for the elderly population. An overview of the history of the federal government's intervention in providing social programs for aging citizens will illustrate how communities can assist their elderly. Private organizations, professional groups, and state and local agencies develop programs and services to meet the needs of elderly in neighborhoods and communities.

Unit 7 addresses patient care teaching for the active aging. Nurses in all areas of practice today, and in the next century, will assist the active aging to maintain an independent functional level. To achievethis goal, nurses will be increasing the amount of time devoted to patient teaching. This includes addressing sensory deficits of aging in planning and implementing the teaching. The need to teach wellness concepts and saftey concerns is discussed.

Throughout this section, and others, the terms patient and resident are used when discussing nurses assisting people with health care needs. *Patient*, historically, has meant a person in a state of physical or emotional ill health who is receiving care or treatment from health care professionals. This indicates a passive participation by the individual. It is used primarily in acute health care settings such as hospitals, clinics, and other out-patient areas. *Resident* is more often used to identify people who live in long term care facilities. For most of these individuals it is their permanant home.

Client is a term traditionally used by social workers. It indicates a consumer, or purchaser of health services. Some clinics, home health agencies, and other health care providers refer to those seeking their services as clients. The use of the title client became more popular as people began to assume more responsiblity for their own health in the changing health care delivery system. The word client suggests a more active participation in health care.

Unit 3
Signs of Aging

Objectives

After reading this unit you should be able to:

- Identify your own views of aging.
- Describe theories related to biological aging.
- Discuss theories related to psychosocial aspects of aging.
- Identify changes in body systems' structure and function related to the aging process.
- Discuss symptoms related to the function changes.
- Discuss appropriate health teaching to assist people in maintaining their highest level of function during the aging process.

How old is old? Which birthday will you celebrate and then declare you are now old? How will you look and feel? Where will you be living? What will you be doing to occupy your time?

After you have considered those questions, what do you think influenced your answers? Was it the aging pattern of family members, messages received from advertising and media resources, or other influences?

In the United States it seems we spend more time and money to maintain or reclaim youth than to learn about and prepare for our own aging. Most of us have heard about Ponce de Leon's search for the Fountain of Youth. When Ferdinand sent him on his voyage in the sixteenth century, Ponce de Leon discovered Florida with its many pools and streams. Today, the older population has also discovered Florida and enjoys its water and sunshine!

Old. Webster's says it is having lived for a long time. Now, how long is long? People who have been in a crisis situation, such as being trapped in a car after an accident, state that minutes seem like hours and hours like days. So old, like time, can be a subjective measurement, figure 3–1.

Listen to someone's comments about daily activities and watch their body language. These comments will soon give you an idea of that person's definition of old. First, imagine a 75-year-old woman, with an apron over her arm, walking briskly to the senior citizen center to help cook a meal for the "old folks." Next, envision a 55-year-old man sitting hunched over in a lounge chair. He gazes at the television; he wonders if he should consider early retirement. It is the individual's perception of aging that influences the definition of old.

Many people stereotype when they are confronted with the word old. To *stereotype* is to have a fixed idea of behaviors or characteristics of a group of people. All people of this group will exhibit the behavior. Many stereotyped behaviors of the older population do reflect the aging process. It is true that aging changes in the ear result in diminished hearing ability for some, but not necessarily all, people. Have you noticed how many people automatically raise their voice when someone they think of as old enters a room?

Sometimes beliefs of ageism or behaviors demonstrating age discrimination grow out of stereotyping or being misinformed about older

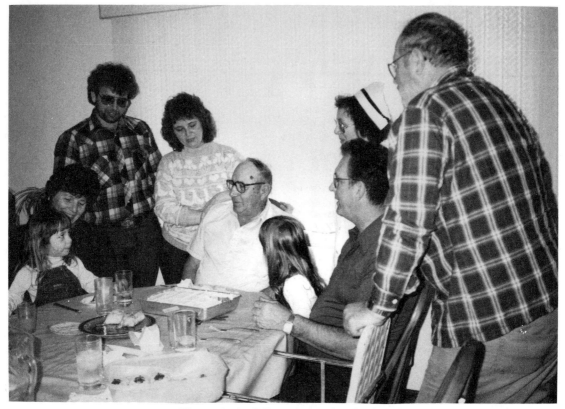

Figure 3–1 When does aging begin?

adults and their abilities. *Ageism* is a belief that older citizens should not be a part of the mainstream of society; they should step aside, or be forced out of jobs and other social roles to make room for younger people. *Age discrimination* is the unjust treatment of people only because of their age. Many organized groups of older adults include in their goals information and efforts to dispel these beliefs.

When does aging begin? Does it begin at birth? Or does it begin at that magic age of 65? Webster's says aging is to grow old. But mature, or full grown, is also included in the definition. This does provide some objective measurement. Our society tends to use physical appearance as a life span yardstick.

Growth and development changes are expressed in Aunt Ella's exclamation, "Johnny, you're getting so big!" Society views physical maturation as a beginning step of aging. Years later at the high school reunion, Sally whispers to a friend, "Look at John, he hasn't aged a bit." It is signs of physical deterioration that many people are looking for when they describe aging.

Nurses must examine their own definition and attitudes about aging, because these views will be reflected in the nursing care they provide for the older patient. How have you felt about people you define as old? What were your interactions? Have you been eager to visit a grandparent? Have you avoided starting a conversation with an older person you sat next to on a bus? What has been your approach to caring for an older patient in the hospital, nursing home, or other health care setting?

In this unit theories and signs of aging will

be discussed. *Theories* are ideas or plans about how something might work. Biological theories of aging present ideas on how and why body cells age. Psychosocial theories examine behaviors or responses to aging. In the study of gerontology, then, *aging* can be defined as the lifelong process of biological, psychological, and sociological change.

There are objective signs of aging related to changes in the structure and function of the body systems. They are not matched with a chronological age, but some tend to be observable in a general age group. For example, aging changes in the eye that require corrective lenses for reading occur at about age 45.

This unit will also include health teaching that has a focus on the aging process. The goal is to assist individuals in maintaining their highest functional level.

Biological Theories of Aging

What happens to the cells in tissues that result in a deterioration or aging of an organ or system? Those who research and study the aging process agree that there is no single theory or cause because there are many variables. All systems do not change at the same rate or to the same degree. For example, vision and hearing may undergo considerable changes that affect the independence of an individual. But for all the stress we place on our gastrointestinal system in a lifetime, it weathers aging remarkably well!

Genetic Cellular Theories

Genetic theories focus on the DNA. *DNA* (deoxyribonucleic acid) is the genetic part of the cell that controls the biological processes of life. One theory is that although cells are continually repaired, they are genetically programmed to divide or reproduce a fixed number of times. This could be called programmed aging. An example is to review the menstrual cycle. The onset of menarche is usually between the ages of 11 and 14 in young girls. Menopause — at the other end of the process — usually occurs around age 50. These events are "programmed" physical changes.

These genetic theories focus on the program that controls the biological development of the human being. Hereditary influences may be added to the human development factor. In the example above, women would most likely have a menstrual history and cycle pattern similar to their mothers'. This genetic clock may have a built-in timer that causes cells to cease functioning.

Other considerations in genetic theories of aging include mutations in the DNA. *Mutation* refers to change in form, quality, or characteristics. Recall your study and discussions of viruses. The reason last year's flu vaccine may not be effective with this year's flu virus is because of the ability of viruses to change their structure. The theory of aging is that if there are mutations in the DNA which increase over time with cell division, there will be changes in organs and systems that result in reduced function in body systems.

Another idea considers errors in DNA functioning. The errors would be like a computer that did not process the information correctly. The result would be a product that was not up to specifications and therefore would not function properly.

Nongenetic Cellular Theories

You have learned about some ideas of "built-in" aging influences on the cell. Other theories consider what happens to cells during a person's lifetime. One theory more commonly called the *wear-and-tear theory* suggests that the body, like machinery, can wear out. Cells functioning as a team in specialized tissues are confronted with numerous abuses. This results in impaired functioning. Degenerative joint disease is an example of the wear-and-tear theory. Weight-bearing joints suffer erosion over the years. The problem is compounded when the person is overweight, or when physical labor is injurious to the joints.

Some theories of cellular aging believe that environmental influences may be abusive to the cells. This can include radiation, such as extended exposure to the sun, and a variety of chemicals including prescription drugs. Products and waste products of industry are in the air, water, and soil. We are just beginning to see the results in acute and chronic disease. We know that the human fetus is vulnerable to a number of maternal environmental hazards. This is also true at the other end of the life span with the effects of air pollution on the aging respiratory system.

The effects of disease, inadequate nutrition, and stress are considered in the study of aging in the cell. During medical and surgical nursing courses, you have learned how these conditions affect the wellness or illness of an individual. Recall that two of the greatest contributions to longevity in this country are the control of infection and improved nutrition.

Collagen, a substance in connective tissue, is also being studied. It is thought that over time, molecules develop links between one another. The chemical change would affect cell function and result in loss of elasticity in connective tissue. This is visible in the skin of the face and arms as creases and wrinkles. Loss of elasticity also occurs in connective tissue in other body systems.

Immune System Theories

The immune system has come under more scrutiny and study in recent years. It is often difficult for people to understand the immune system because it can not be visualized like the heart or the kidneys.

In the aging process, it is believed that over time the body loses its ability to recognize deviations in the system. The cells that, in a younger person, would have been destroyed by the immune system survive. This could explain the increase in the incidence of cancer in the older population group. One theory on the prevalence of cancer is that many people have cancer cells circulating in their bodies and the immune system responds to them as antigens. In aging, the weakening immune system is not so sharp in its surveillance capability.

Another aspect of the immune system is the autoimmune reaction. In the aging, the system does not recognize the body as "self." Rheumatoid arthritis and Type II diabetes may be linked to this theory of aging.

When reviewing the biological theories of aging, remember they are only ideas. Everyone agrees that the aging process is complex and there is no single event or reason that initiates the process or governs its progression. The body has a remarkable recovery system from disease, stress, and other insults. It seems that one weakened system is supported by the strengthening of another. The body has its own support system for survival.

Accompanying the cellular aging theories is the emotional component. How does the individual and a culture respond to the aging process? It is difficult to isolate ideas or stages of aging into separate parts. Figure 3–2 summarizes biological theories of aging.

Psychosocial Theories of Aging

In learning about what happens to the body when it ages, results are described as "reduced function," "diminished abilities," or "impaired function." These results have a great impact on the social functioning of the individual.

There are as many variables in the psychosocial changes in aging as there are in the cellular theories. Family, ethnic, community, and other influences tend to direct an individual's emotional and social responses to the aging process. The individual's physical aging will influence social adaptations. For example, an elderly couple participated in a square dance club for many of their adult years. They became ballroom dance enthusiasts when degenerative joint disease made square dancing difficult.

GENETIC CELLULAR THEORY

- DNA programs cell to age
  - Examples are the onset of menarche and menopause
- Mutations in DNA alter quality and characteristics of cell
- Errors in DNA processing of information alters cell function

NONGENETIC CELLULAR THEORY

- Wear-and-tear theory: tissues and body wear out
  - Example is degenerative joint disease
- Environmental influences may be abusive to cells
- Waste products of metabolism may be toxic to cells

IMMUNE SYSTEM THEORY

- Body unable to recognize deviations in the system
  - Example is increased susceptibility of cancer in the elderly
- Autoimmune response does not recognize body as "self"
  - Example is linked to rheumatoid arthritis

Figure 3–2 Summary of the biological theories of aging

Disengagement Theory

This theory demonstrates a transfer of responsibility from older members of a community to younger members. It is a gradual, informal process that appears to be expected by all age groups and argued against by very few. An event that makes the process more formal and definite is mandatory retirement.

Society has not viewed all groups equally. In recent decades it has expected executives in business and industry to retire at age 65. Union contracts often had language addressing retirement and subsequent benefits. A physician specialist in a medical center may be expected to retire, but a small community hopes their "country doctor" never retires.

Supreme Court judges are nominated for life. Many legislators are in their 60s or older. Some studies have shown that a candidate's age has no bearing on the voter's decision. President Reagan was almost 70 when elected. In 1990, Senator Strom Thurmond, from South Carolina, ran for a seventh term in the United States Senate at age 87. Until his death at age 88, Florida Representative Claude Pepper was a well-known and outspoken advocate for the rights of older citizens. The oldest United States legislator was Rhode Island's Senator Theodore Green who left the Senate in 1961 at age 92.

A person demonstrating the disengagement theory would retire as society expected, lead a slower paced life style, include more leisure activities, and look for the younger generation to provide more services. This is the stereotyped image seen on television and in advertising of the elderly couple sitting on the front porch in rocking chairs.

Activity Theory

This theory is the opposite of disengagement. It is a denial of aging. The idea is to maintain the activity idealized in middle age. If the work place has encouraged retirement, other work must be found. Time previously spent on the job can also be replaced with similar community volunteer work. Changes in health, income, status, and other situations are to be resisted rather than accepted.

Aligning oneself with this role would not seem surprising in the United States where we place productivity and personal value very close together. This theory is not to be confused with activity and exercise which is promoted for a healthy life style.

An example of a person demonstrating the activity theory of aging would be an executive secretary who retires and then takes a position as the church secretary in her parish.

Continuity Theory

This theory focuses on the idea that an individual's behavior and beliefs are generally consistent throughout life. A person who has not enjoyed reading novels or playing golf when younger will probably not engage in these activities following retirement. Someone who has been actively involved in education may continue to be a volunteer tutor in an elementary school, and enroll in a community education course.

The continuity theory may seem the most comfortable. People continue to enjoy those activites that have always interested them. They adapt the pace to their changing physical abilities and social structure.

An example of the continuity theory is a man who ran in marathon races in his 30s. He continued jogging in his 40s and 50s, while assisting with marathon record keeping. Reducing the pace and distance, he continued a walking program into his 80s, and followed the successes of his favorite marathoners on television.

In reviewing these psychosocial theories of aging there are several ideas to remember. A person's lifestyle since childhood will probably determine his lifestyle in aging. We are creatures of habit. However, unexpected events can place someone in an unwanted role. A person may have a stroke, leaving many physical deficits which force the individual from a chosen activity role to disengagement. Figure 3–3 summarizes the psychosocial theories of aging.

Physical Changes in Aging

In an anatomy and physiology course you learned body structure and function. You memorized the parts and figured out how they worked. During a medical and surgical nursing course you adapted that knowledge by learning what

---

DISENGAGEMENT THEORY

- Gradual withdrawing from activity and community
- Time for reflection and leisure
- Accepted by individual and community

ACTIVITY THEORY

- Maintain activity of middle age
- Resist changes related to aging
- Denial of aging

CONTINUITY THEORY

- Maintain life-long behaviors and beliefs
- Continue desired activities at slower pace
- Adapt to aging changes in social structure

Figure 3–3   Summary of psychosocial theories of aging

happened to the structure and function of a system when disease or trauma occurred. For example, a 40-year-old may develop congestive heart failure as a result of cardiac damage following a heart attack. Now you will adapt the knowledge of normal anatomy and physiology to changes in structure and function related to aging. *Senescence* is the term sometimes used for this biological aging. An older person, for example, may develop congestive heart failure as a result of the aging process. The heart muscle becomes less elastic, valves become rigid, and contractions become weaker, resulting in reduced cardiac output. Aging changes in the heart set up progressive deterioration in function, which can lead to congestive heart failure. The heart wears out.

Musculoskeletal System

The major effects of time upon the musculoskeletal system are manifested by reduced bone and muscle mass. Various degrees of joint stiffness and immobility are also noted. The bone becomes more porous, like honeycomb, as the total amount of bone tissue is diminished. This makes the bones of the elderly person weaker and predisposes them to spontaneous fractures. However, the skeletal frame continues to be capable of supporting the body and protecting internal organs.

Joints undergo degenerative changes as cartilage erodes from wear and tear. The synovial membrane becomes fibrotic and joint stiffness occurs. Many active aging people have years of discomfort and varying degress of limitation in their physical activity.

Muscles begin to atrophy as the number of muscle cells are reduced in size and number. Protein building in the muscle also declines. A loss of muscle mass results in diminished strength. The center of gravity is altered as demonstrated in gait changes. Although those persons who remain physically active experience less atrophy, generally a man of 70 has about half the strength of a man of 30. These changes occur slowly and gradually and most people make adaptations that will compensate for the changes.

The symptoms that most people notice with aging changes in the musculoskeletal system are joint stiffness and reduced muscle strength. Older people say they are "growing shorter!" This can be true as intervertebral disks become dehydrated and compressed resulting in reduced height.

Health teaching appropriate to these changes and symptoms includes encouraging continued activity and exercise. Walking is the best exercise for older people, figure 3-4. Using the bones and muscles keeps them strong. Recall that muscle atrophy and disuse osteoporosis are complications of bedrest at any age. Wearing shoes that provide good support should be encouraged. Balancing activity and exercise will help joint stiffness. Weight loss, if indicated, will also reduce the stress on joints. Pacing activities to allow rest periods is a suggested adaptation for reduced muscle strength. Placing fewer

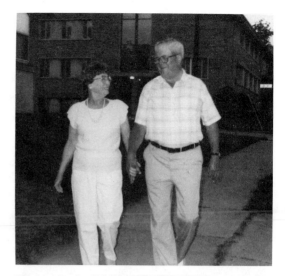

Figure 3-4 Walking is the best exercise for people.

items in smaller boxes or bags will help break up big jobs into more manageable tasks. Aging changes in the musculoskeletal system are illustrated in figure 3-5.

Respiratory System

There are definite changes that occur in the respiratory system as an individual ages. But, despite these changes, the individual's respiratory status is not compromised unless demands are placed on the system. For example, with increased physical activity, shortness of breath will occur much sooner.

The action of taking air into the lungs and then exhaling it is also compromised in aging by the changes in the musculoskeletal system. Kyphosis, calcification of costal cartilage, atrophy of respiratory muscles, and the flattening of the diaphragm are some of the changes. The rib cage remains in a more expanded position which results in the limited ability of the thoracic cavity to enlarge during inspiration. Vital capacity is also reduced.

The lungs begin to enlarge to fill the greater space of the thoracic cavity. The tissue becomes

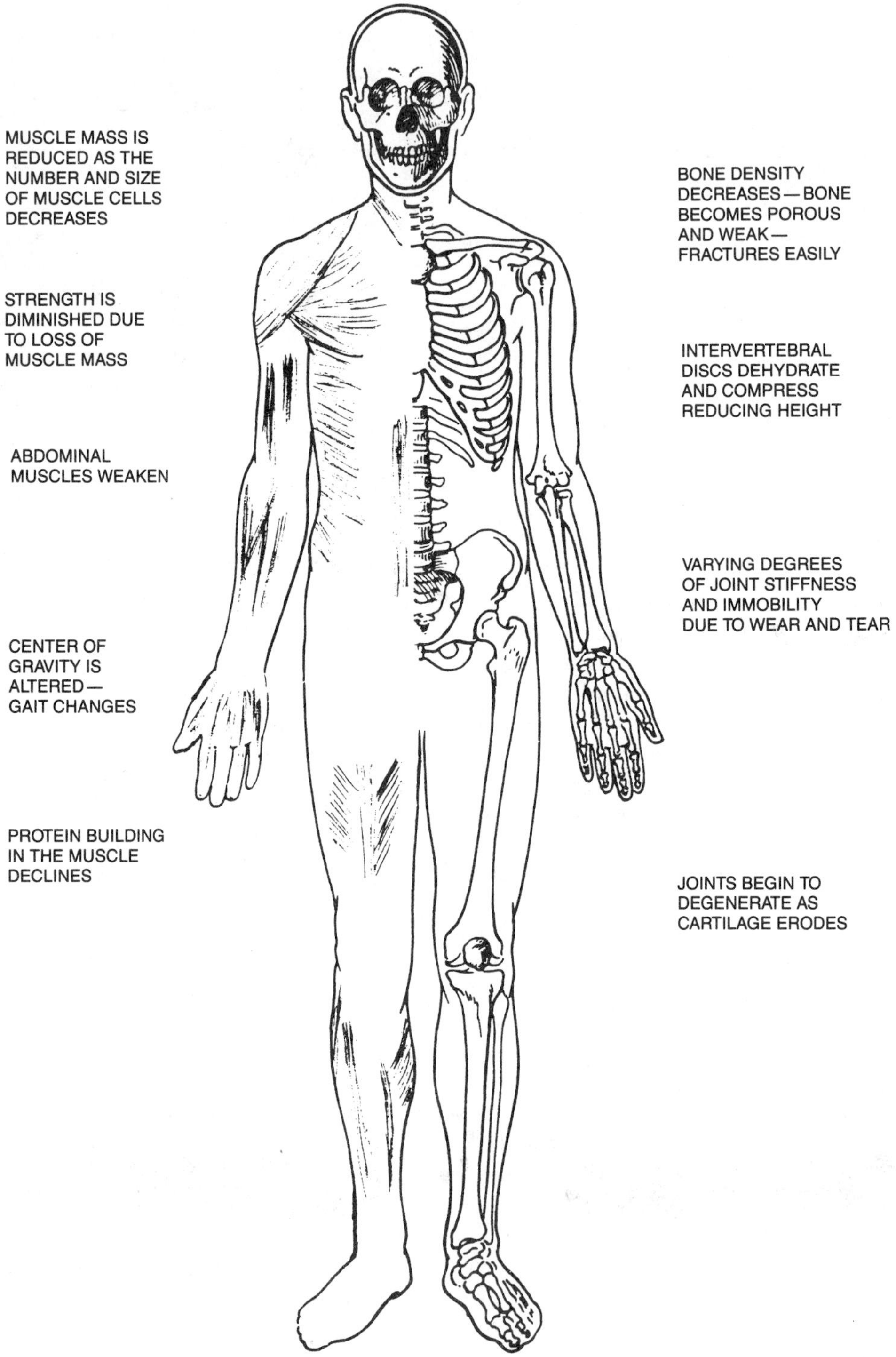

MUSCLE MASS IS
REDUCED AS THE
NUMBER AND SIZE
OF MUSCLE CELLS
DECREASES

STRENGTH IS
DIMINISHED DUE
TO LOSS OF
MUSCLE MASS

ABDOMINAL
MUSCLES WEAKEN

CENTER OF
GRAVITY IS
ALTERED —
GAIT CHANGES

PROTEIN BUILDING
IN THE MUSCLE
DECLINES

BONE DENSITY
DECREASES — BONE
BECOMES POROUS
AND WEAK —
FRACTURES EASILY

INTERVERTEBRAL
DISCS DEHYDRATE
AND COMPRESS
REDUCING HEIGHT

VARYING DEGREES
OF JOINT STIFFNESS
AND IMMOBILITY
DUE TO WEAR AND TEAR

JOINTS BEGIN TO
DEGENERATE AS
CARTILAGE ERODES

Figure 3–5 The aging musculoskeletal system

less elastic, more rigid, and results in more air remaining in the lungs leaving less available for ventilatory exchange. Many of the lung volumes are diminished with age, leaving the older person with a lower tolerence for oxygen debt.

In the alveoli, the membrane becomes thicker and there is a decline in the number of capillaries surrounding the alveoli. This results in less efficient O_2/CO_2 exchange. Also, more secretions remain in the lungs because of changes in lung and muscle tissue. Ciliary movement is reduced due to epithelial atrophy and an ineffective cough is the result. These lung changes make the elderly increasingly vulnerable to respiratory infections. Respiratory changes may not be entirely the result of the aging process. Environmental factors such as air pollution, occupational hazards, and cigarette smoking may influence or exacerbate other problems in the aging respiratory system.

Dyspnea and fatigue are the most prominent symptoms associated with aging changes in the respiratory system. A "barrel" chest and diminished chest movement may be noted as the respiratory muscles atrophy and the chest diameter increases.

Appropriate health teaching would include pacing activities to maximize respiratory effort. This reduces dyspnea by reducing the demand on the system. Other suggestions include deep breathing exercises and using the diaphram instead of chest muscles for breathing. Those who are at a greater risk for respiratory conditions should avoid irritants such as cigarette smoke and dust. They should use an air purifier, and stay indoors when respiratory alerts are announced. This is often during very cold weather or during peak hours of environmental pollution.

Older individuals should be advised to seek health care for respiratory infections that last more than a few days. Because the respiratory system is vulnerable to infections, annual flu vaccinations are often recommended. Figure 3–6 illustrates some aging changes in the respiratory system.

Cardiovascular System

The heart and arteries are affected the most by aging. Changes affect blood flow, therefore oxygen flow, to all parts of the body. Consequently, aging changes in the cardiovascular system have secondary effects in every other system.

In the heart, the endocardium becomes fibrotic and sclerotic. The left ventricular wall thickens and the mitral and aortic valves develop calcifications. There is myocardium muscle loss which results in muscle irritability. Functional changes in the heart include a reduced cardiac output, reduced strength in the heart beat, and development of dysrhythmias and murmurs. The heart rate at rest does not change much, but the maximum heart rate achieved during exercise is reduced by about 30 percent.

The inner coat of the arteries becomes thickened and fibrosed. They lose their elasticity and become more rigid, a process known as arteriosclerosis. This causes an elevated blood pressure in older individuals. Systolic pressures of 150 or slightly higher are expected and are often not treated with antihypertensives unless indicated by other pathological conditions.

Atherosclerosis, a result of a long-time diet of saturated fats, may be present. This condition compounds the problem of blood flow and provides a rough surface inside the artery. This increases the potential of clot formation. With the aging process, veins also lose their elasticity, resulting in varicosities and other lower extremity circulatory problems.

Symptoms associated with cardiovascular aging changes are fatigue and dyspnea that are chronic rather than short term. Complaints may be expressed in reduced stamina or inability to complete usual tasks. Light-headedness may be noted and reflected in postural hypotension.

Health teaching would again include suggestions of pacing activities and seeking health care for infections and sudden or more dramatic episodes of shortness of breath or any chest discomfort. Exercise, such as a walking program, is encouraged to help improve cardiac

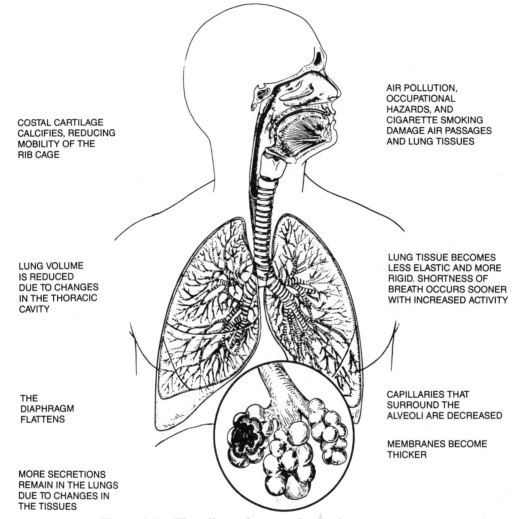

COSTAL CARTILAGE
CALCIFIES, REDUCING
MOBILITY OF THE
RIB CAGE

AIR POLLUTION,
OCCUPATIONAL
HAZARDS, AND
CIGARETTE SMOKING
DAMAGE AIR PASSAGES
AND LUNG TISSUES

LUNG VOLUME
IS REDUCED
DUE TO CHANGES
IN THE THORACIC
CAVITY

LUNG TISSUE BECOMES
LESS ELASTIC AND MORE
RIGID. SHORTNESS OF
BREATH OCCURS SOONER
WITH INCREASED ACTIVITY

THE
DIAPHRAGM
FLATTENS

CAPILLARIES THAT
SURROUND THE
ALVEOLI ARE DECREASED

MEMBRANES BECOME
THICKER

MORE SECRETIONS
REMAIN IN THE LUNGS
DUE TO CHANGES IN
THE TISSUES

Figure 3–6 The effects of age on the respiratory system

output. Suggestions for people to monitor and maintain their own cardiovascular system include regular blood pressure checks. There are many places to have blood pressure monitored, such as senior citizen centers and shopping mall health fairs. Health promotion should encourage reducing salt intake, losing weight, and cessation of smoking, if indicated.

Nurses should remember the effects of reduced oxygen supply to other parts of the body when assessing the older person and plan-

ning individualized health teaching. Examples of changes in the cardiovascular are illustrated in figure 3–7.

Gastrointestinal System

The nutritional status of an individual does not seem to be greatly affected by the aging process of the gastrointestinal system. Social factors probably play a larger role in influencing the nutrition of the body. These factors could include inadequate income or inability to

MURMERS AND IRREGULARITY
IN RHYTHM DEVELOP AS THE
MUSCLE WEAKENS

THE INNER COAT
OF THE ARTERIES
BECOMES THICKENED

THE MYOCARDIUM
LOSES MUSCLE
MASS, WHICH
RESULTS IN
REDUCED STRENGTH

ROUGH FATTY
DEPOSITS COLLECT
ON THE INSIDE
SURFACE OF THE
ARTERIES

MITRAL AND AORTIC
VALVES DEVELOP
CALCIFICATIONS

VEINS LOSE THEIR
ELASTICITY,
RESULTING IN
VARICOSITIES IN
THE LOWER
EXTREMITIES

THE LEFT
VENTRICULAR WALL
THICKENS

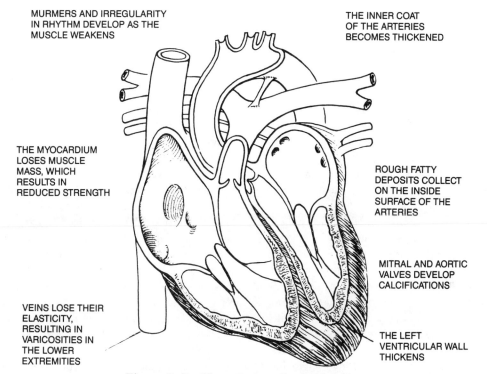

Figure 3-7   The aging cardiovascular system

get to a grocery store to purchase food. Mechanical difficulties such as improperly fitting dentures or pathological conditions that interfere with digestion may also alter the individual's nutritional status.

The gastrointestinal system, however, is the source of the most complaints! Distresses of indigestion, elimination, or weight gain or loss are frequent causes of complaints heard by physicians.

Elderly may not recognize the decrease in saliva and the diminished ability to taste. There may be delayed esophageal and gastric emptying related to the loss of smooth muscle tone. This can be a safety factor with the possibility of reflux action and aspiration. Gastric secretions and pancreatic enzymes decrease resulting in some indigestion and impaired absorption of iron and Vitamin B_{12}.

Abdominal wall muscles weaken as well as the muscles of the large intestine. With loss of

muscle tone and decreasing physical activity, persitalsis slows and complaints of constipation occur. Refined foods have often been the diet of choice. Water consumption is decreased with the idea it will eliminate urinary problems. These events compound the problem with stool consistency and resulting constipation. Loss of muscle tone in the perineal floor and anal sphincters result in diarrhea in some elderly persons.

Accessory organs in the gastrointestinal system demonstrate some changes in the aging process. The bile in the gallbladder is thicker, causing some problems with the emptying process. The incidence of cholelithiasis increases with age, probably due to this change. The stones found in the gallbladder are usually composed of cholesterol.

The liver does reduce in size during aging, but the greater concern is the decreased blood flow to the liver from reduced cardiac output.

The result can be drug toxicity from usual therapeutic dosages of medications.

Reduced pancreatic enzymes related to the exocrine function may also disturb the digestive process. Changes in the endocrine function are seen in Type II Diabetes, sometimes referred to as Adult Onset Diabetes Mellitus (AODM). There seems to be a decrease in carbohydrate tolerance with middle-age or older persons. The cells do not utilize the insulin that is produced. Type II diabetics are usually overweight and about 20 percent have a family history of this type of diabetes.

Common symptoms related to the aging of the gastrointestinal system include complaints of a dry mouth and diminished taste. The sweet and salty taste buds are reduced in number, resulting in a frustrating situation for those elderly people who have been instructed to limit their salt intake. Another complaint is difficulty in swallowing which is related to the decreased saliva production and drier mucous membranes.

Loss of appetite and resulting weight loss in the elderly is not clearly understood. It could be related to the gradual aging process and slowing of metabolism. Caloric requirements are reduced in older people and weight loss is seen after age 60. Social factors play a part in the loss of appetite. Most people of any age do not enjoy eating alone.

Functional bowel distress is the most common diagnosis related to the gastrointestinal system in people over 65. The complaints of constipation and other symptoms may be related to an organic problem as well as the aging process.

Health teaching that focuses on maintaining a functional gastrointestinal system includes following a basic four-meal plan. Individuals should be informed of suggested serving sizes. They may overeat if their perception of serving size is larger than recommended. Some elderly may feel that the servings suggested are beyond their appetite or income.

Additional health teaching includes maintaining or increasing fiber and fluids in the meal plan as well as a walking program which assists peristalsis. Individuals should be assured that daily bowel movements are not necessary, and they should avoid routinely taking laxatives.

Nurses providing health teaching to the elderly should be alert to symptoms that may suggest Type II Diabetes or signs of toxicity from medications. Figure 3–8 illustrates some normal aging changes in the gastrointestinal system.

Urinary System

Kidney function is reduced in a number of ways. During the aging process, nephrons are lost. This decline begins in middle age, and by age 75 half of the million nephron units in the kidney are lost; the filtering ability has also been reduced. Renal blood flow decreases due to reduced cardiac output and arteriosclerosis of renal vessels. The blood urea nitrogen (BUN) level will be increased. Drug toxicity occurs due to increased blood levels of medications usually excreted by the kidneys.

The muscular tissues of the ureters, bladder, and urethra lose their elasticity. This loss results in incomplete emptying of the bladder. There may be 100 cc of residual urine in the bladder after voiding. In addition, the bladder capacity declines from about 600cc to 250–300 cc and the signal to urinate does not occur until the bladder is nearly full.

In men the prostate enlarges, constricting the urethra and resulting in urinary retention. The muscles of the pelvic floor in women lose their elasticity due to childbearing and aging, resulting in a dropping of the pelvic organs.

Symptoms related to aging changes in the urinary system are primarily urinary frequency and urgency. Nocturia is one of the common symptoms of benign prostatic hyperplasia. Men, as well as women, having changes in pelvic floor muscles may express concerns regarding dribbling and stress incontinence.

Appropriate health teaching that focuses on the urinary system includes encouraging the older person to drink plenty of fluids during the day while lowering intake during evening hours.

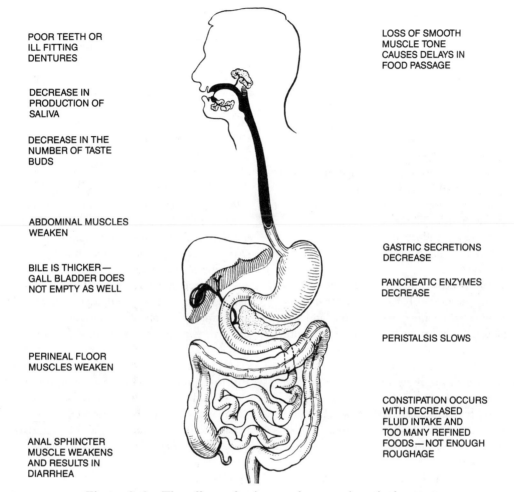

POOR TEETH OR
ILL FITTING
DENTURES

DECREASE IN
PRODUCTION OF
SALIVA

DECREASE IN THE
NUMBER OF TASTE
BUDS

ABDOMINAL MUSCLES
WEAKEN

BILE IS THICKER—
GALL BLADDER DOES
NOT EMPTY AS WELL

PERINEAL FLOOR
MUSCLES WEAKEN

ANAL SPHINCTER
MUSCLE WEAKENS
AND RESULTS IN
DIARRHEA

LOSS OF SMOOTH
MUSCLE TONE
CAUSES DELAYS IN
FOOD PASSAGE

GASTRIC SECRETIONS
DECREASE

PANCREATIC ENZYMES
DECREASE

PERISTALSIS SLOWS

CONSTIPATION OCCURS
WITH DECREASED
FLUID INTAKE AND
TOO MANY REFINED
FOODS—NOT ENOUGH
ROUGHAGE

Figure 3-8   The effects of aging on the gastrointestinal system

Explanations are focused on the fact that fluids prevent infection and increasing them will not produce incontinence. Health teaching should also include signs of urinary tract infection and toxic effects of medications excreted by the kidneys.

Reproductive System

In men, testosterone declines, the prostate becomes hypertrophied, and the testes become smaller. Sclerosing in the penile vascular network results in slower erections. In women, reduced estrogen production after menopause results in diminished fatty breast tissue and vaginal secretions. The results are sagging breasts and painful intercourse. Public hair thins in both men and women. Men develop more hair in their nostrils and on their ears while women develop facial hair primarily on their chin and upper lip.

As hormonal secretions diminish, the silhouette changes. Along with other aging systems, the extremities become thinner while body fat clings to the torso to protect vital organs. An older person may become discouraged with the changing body image. Symptoms of aging in the reproductive system are related to difficulties with intercourse. Women may also express concerns about physical and emotional changes with menopause. A flushed feeling or "hot flashes" is a frequent complaint. Changes in sleeping patterns and coping abilities may also be concerns.

Health teaching should focus on reassuring the older person that these changes and feelings are normal. The health professional may be the person to introduce the subject of difficulties with intercourse. Although the individual may have concerns, culturally it is not a subject that is easily discussed. Physicians may prescribe estrogen therapy for postmenopausal women. Age related changes in the urinary and reproductive systems are illustrated in figure 3–9.

Nervous System

The age-related changes in the nervous system are seen in altered behavior patterns. Neurons decrease in number as some die and are not replaced. Loss of neurons interferes with the integrating function of the brain. Due to vascular changes, the blood flow and oxygen supply to the brain is decreased. The myelin sheath degenerates, resulting in reduced conduction and transmission capabilities. The autonomic nervous system slows in its response time.

Results of these aging changes in the nervous system are seen as gradual forgetfulness. However, the person usually has recall within a few moments. Gait disturbances, head-nodding, or tremors may be observed. A slower reaction time and slower reflexes are noted. The individual may not realize that pain and other sensory signals are diminished. The deeper sleep cycle is reduced resulting in complaints of insomnia. Delta

Health teaching that is helpful with aging signs of the nervous system include allowing adequate time for tasks. The older person's ability to complete a task does not change. The time to complete the task to produce the same quality level does change. Timed assembly line projects would be frustrating to the older person. The body should be inspected for areas of injury due to the increased tolerance to pain. To improve sleeping patterns, individuals should be encouraged to

exercise during the day and avoid frequent napping. It may be helpful to avoid caffeine in the evening. Families should be informed that these changes are gradual and that any sudden change in behavior may be related to a disease process and should be investigated immediately.

Sensory Systems

Vision and hearing deficits that occur with aging are more evident as they greatly affect the person's ability to function in the environment.

The Eye. Aging changes in the eye occur primarily in the lens. The muscles weaken causing the lens to flatten and presbyopia results. *Presbyopia* is a far-sightedness due to aging and the changing shape of the lens.

Cataracts are due to changes in which the lens becomes yellow and opaque. These changes are common in older people and it is believed that everyone would eventually develop them if they lived long enough. Diminished color perception occurs and makes it increasingly difficult to distinguish between blue and green.

Blood supply to the retina is reduced and the macula begins to deteriorate. *Macular degeneration* is the gradual loss of the center of the visual field. The iris, a muscle, becomes more rigid, resulting in the decline in response to light accomodation. Glaucoma tends to occur in the earlier years of aging. *Glaucoma* is the increase in intraocular pressure resulting from an increase of aqueous humor. The exact cause of this is not known, but it is dangerous because the pressure on the optic nerve can result in blindness.

Symptoms reflected in the aging eye include the inability to do close-range vision tasks. Corrective lenses for reading, stitchery, or similar tasks are usually needed beginning during the mid 40s. Also, reduced secretions in the eye may result in complaints about eye irritations. Decline in depth perception, a slower recovery from glare, and night blindness make driving at night a more difficult and unsafe task. Not being able to drive is very threatening to the independence and self-esteem of the elderly.

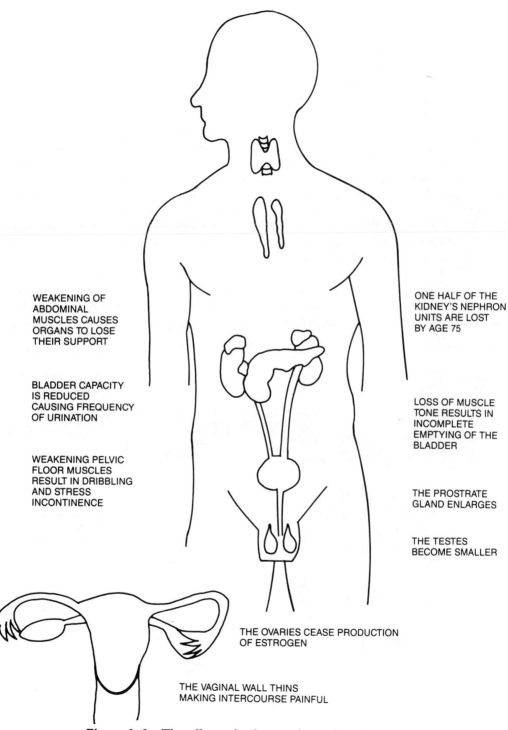

WEAKENING OF ABDOMINAL MUSCLES CAUSES ORGANS TO LOSE THEIR SUPPORT

BLADDER CAPACITY IS REDUCED CAUSING FREQUENCY OF URINATION

WEAKENING PELVIC FLOOR MUSCLES RESULT IN DRIBBLING AND STRESS INCONTINENCE

ONE HALF OF THE KIDNEY'S NEPHRON UNITS ARE LOST BY AGE 75

LOSS OF MUSCLE TONE RESULTS IN INCOMPLETE EMPTYING OF THE BLADDER

THE PROSTRATE GLAND ENLARGES

THE TESTES BECOME SMALLER

THE OVARIES CEASE PRODUCTION OF ESTROGEN

THE VAGINAL WALL THINS MAKING INTERCOURSE PAINFUL

Figure 3–9   The effects of aging on the genitourinary system

When promoting health for the aging, regular eye examinations should be encouraged. Corrective lenses may be expensive and the older person on a fixed income may "make do" with current lenses as long as desired tasks can be accomplished. Driving at night should be discouraged. Adaptations in the home that could help avoid accidents related to vision changes include increased lighting in hallways and other dark areas, placing a night light in the bathroom, and avoiding high gloss finishes on walls and floors. Figure 3-10 illustrates examples of aging changes in the eye.

The Ear.   A gradual decline in hearing acuity occurs with the aging process. Major changes occur in the inner ear where diminished blood supply results in deterioration of the cochlea and loss of hair cells in the organ of Corti. The tympanic membrane thickens, reducing sound transmission. Cerumen becomes harder and the transmission of sound may be impeded by the impacted ear wax. This is an example of conduction hearing loss or deafness.

A major symptom that occurs with these changes is *presbycusis*. This is a gradual hearing loss due to the aging process. Early changes result in the inability to hear high-frequency sounds, while there may also be difficulty later with the lower pitched sounds. The words heard may not be clear due to the difficulty in differentiating between S, T, Z, or other consonant sounds.

The exposure to loud noises at a younger age has been linked to sensineural hearing loss or deafness in older persons. Many elderly today were exposed to loud industrial noises before regulations demanded muffling devices on machinery, and protective ear pieces for the workers. Young people today, involved with high-

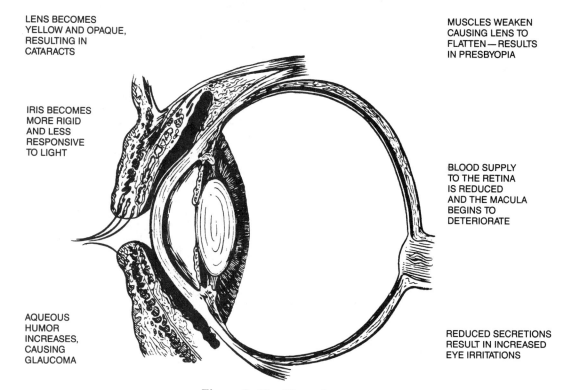

LENS BECOMES YELLOW AND OPAQUE, RESULTING IN CATARACTS

MUSCLES WEAKEN CAUSING LENS TO FLATTEN—RESULTS IN PRESBYOPIA

IRIS BECOMES MORE RIGID AND LESS RESPONSIVE TO LIGHT

BLOOD SUPPLY TO THE RETINA IS REDUCED AND THE MACULA BEGINS TO DETERIORATE

AQUEOUS HUMOR INCREASES, CAUSING GLAUCOMA

REDUCED SECRETIONS RESULT IN INCREASED EYE IRRITATIONS

Figure 3-10   The aging eye

frequency high-volume music, may have similar hearing loss problems when they are older.

Appropriate health teaching for presbycusis focuses on educating the family, friends, and others in social circles. Many people talk louder and at a higher pitch when they know or think someone has difficulty hearing. This makes it more difficult for the older person to hear and understand the conversation. The family and others should be instructed to speak in lower tones, and more slowly and distinctly, and face the individual to allow him to lip-read.

Persons beginning to notice hearing difficulties should be encouraged to have an ear examination and hearing assessment. This will rule out mechanical problems or disease processes and determine if a hearing aid would be helpful.

Difficulties with hearing lead to social isolation. An aging person feels threatened with everyday activities, such as shopping, telephoning, asking for directions, and other tasks. The individual may choose not to attend social events or, if attending, may seek a corner of the room to avoid interactions with others in a group. A person with a hearing deficit may ask to have a statement repeated once, but will probably not ask again if it is not understood. In figure 3–11, aging changes in the ear are identified.

Taste and Smell.   The number of taste buds and olfactory nerves are diminished. Remember the ability to taste sweet and salty flavors is reduced and the sense of smell is not as acute.

Health teaching should focus on safety factors as well as improving the psychosocial influences of taste and smell. The decreased ability to smell smoke to detect a potential fire is an example of a sensory related safety factor. Many older persons are on a low salt diet.

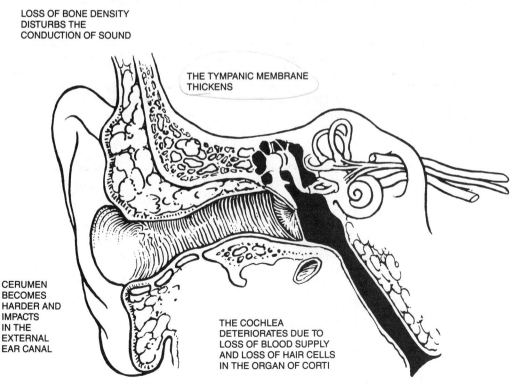

LOSS OF BONE DENSITY DISTURBS THE CONDUCTION OF SOUND

THE TYMPANIC MEMBRANE THICKENS

CERUMEN BECOMES HARDER AND IMPACTS IN THE EXTERNAL EAR CANAL

THE COCHLEA DETERIORATES DUE TO LOSS OF BLOOD SUPPLY AND LOSS OF HAIR CELLS IN THE ORGAN OF CORTI

Figure 3–11   Aging changes in the ear

These sensory aging changes intensify the complaints of "tasteless food." Individuals should be encouraged to try other spices to enhance the flavor of food. Enriching the environment with more strongly scented fresh flowers or the aroma of baked goods will provide stimuli to those with a diminished sense of smell.

The Skin, Nails, and Hair.   Aging skin is the most observable sign of aging. Photographers capture the effects of time in the facial crevices of the aging farmer or migrant field worker. As the tissues lose their strength and elasticity, the skin develops lines and wrinkles. First are the lines or "crow's feet" noted at the outer corners of the eyes. Areas of the body, especially the face and arms, that are exposed to the environment have more pronounced lines. It is known that exposure to the sun accelerates the aging of the skin as well as causing many skin lesions. Table 3-1 identifies and defines many of these conditions.

Sweat glands are reduced in number and functional ability, resulting in skin that appears dry and leathery. Subcutaneous fat deposits decrease in the face and extremities, revealing

Lesion	Description	Aging Factor
pigmentation increases		general aging of skin
seborrhea keratosis	irregular flat, light brown, crusted, rough, wart-like	connective tissue thickens
senile keratoses	cutaneous horn with reddened base	keratin accumulates
skin tags (neck, under arms)	colorless, color of skin, pedicle	connective tissue thickens
senile lentigo "liver spots"	brown, small or medium size	fragile capillaries
senile purpura (arms, legs)	reddish, purple, brown	hemorrhages due to fragile vessels
skin tears (arms, legs)	small area of epidermis displaced due to pressure, superficial bleeding	loss of subcutaneous fat, loss of skin turgor, fragile vessels
basal cell carcinoma	various shapes, sizes	years of exposure to sun
epidermoid cysts (scalp)	raised, marble-like, firm	composed of atypical epidermal cells

TABLE 3-1   Skin Lesions Related to Aging Changes

bony prominences. These deposits increase over the abdomen which gives the appearance of a "pot belly" to the changing figure.

Increased vascular fragility and decreased capillary circulation is manifested in delayed wound healing, risk of pressure sores, skin lesions, skin pallor, and graying and thinning of the hair. The nails become thicker, have ridges, and appear to have lines.

Changes in the skin may receive the brunt of comments of beginning aging, but generally present no symptoms or functional problems. The atrophy of sweat glands results in gradual intolerance of heat. Activities in hot weather have to be paced to be tolerated. Conversely, circulatory changes, decreased activity, and other changes result in the elderly feeling "chilly." Sweaters are commonly worn during warm weather.

Health teaching for the aging skin includes avoiding agents that are drying to the skin. Lotions may be applied to improve comfort and reduce the risk of opening the skin surface. A nutritious diet and adequate fluids will help keep the skin healthy.

Older persons should be encouraged to see a physician when they notice a change in a wart or mole or identify a new skin lesion so a benign or precancerous lesion can be monitored. Avoiding direct sunlight or using a sun screen lotion should be encouraged. Table 3–2 summarizes physical changes in aging and appropriate health teaching.

Summary

Signs of aging are manifested in psychological and sociological ways as well as biological changes. These changes are influenced by hereditary, cultural, and environmental factors. Acute and chronic disease are also factors. They are all interwoven, each influencing the other, making it difficult to separate biological changes from psychological or sociological changes.

Researchers in theories of aging generally agree that there is no single theory for the cause of aging. Beyond that agreement, many ideas are researched. The study of cells focuses on a genetic as well as a wear-and-tear theory. Genetically, the cells may have a built-in life span. Also, the continued abuse or environmental insult of specialized cells and tissues may eventually lead to changes in function.

An individual's perception of his or her own aging is influenced by expectations of the family and community as well as the status of physical health. Researchers studying the psychosocial aspects of aging see the older population: (1) gradually withdrawing from roles and activities, (2) attempting to maintain the roles and activities of middle age, or (3) adapting to changes in roles and activities as interests and physical abilities change. In most individuals, responses to aging are reflections of adaptation and coping abilities of youth and middle age.

Biological or physical changes may begin soon after the onset of physical maturity, following the phases of growth and development. Due to the many variables, it is difficult to place a chronological age on a specific sign of aging. However, the averages established by studies on aging provide the individual, as well as health care workers, guidelines to promote health and manage care.

Aging changes in different body systems have different effects on an individual's ability to function. Activities of daily living may be completed at a slower pace and leisure activities may have to be altered. As a nurse, your most important role may be in promoting appropriate health teaching to assist people in maintaining the highest level of functional ability during the aging process. You are a resource person for your family, neighborhood, and community. For many people, just understanding that a change is normal is reassuring.

STRUCTURE	FUNCTION	RISKS/SYMPTOMS	ADAPTATIONS/HEALTH TEACHING
A. Musculoskeletal			
bones become more porous		osteoporosis	exercise (walking program)
bone demineralizes		fractures of vertebrae, femur may be spontaneous	increase calcium in diet
intervertebral disks dehydrate	range of motion reduced	reduced height; back pain	back pain evaluated by M.D.
joint cartilage erodes		joint swelling, stiffness	balance activity and rest
synovial fluid thickens; joint fibroses			weight loss if indicated
collagen formation decreases	joint elasticity and resilience decreased	muscle decreased, flaccid	continue exercise program
muscle cells reduce in size and number; protein building in muscle diminishes	reduced muscle strength muscle mass decreased center of gravity altered	strength reduced	maintain protein in diet
B. Respiratory			
respiratory muscles atrophy	anterior/posterior diameter increases	fatigue	deep breathing exercises
diaphragm flattens		dyspnea	diaphragmatic breathing
costal cartilages calcify	chest wall mobility reduced	"barrel" chest	avoid irritants; use mask in cold weather
lung tissue elasticity reduced	vital capacity reduced		pace activities
pulmonary wall thickens	diffusion capacity declines		see physician promptly for upper respiratory infections
alveoli thicken	O_2/CO_2 exchange less efficient		
epithelial atrophy (aging changes in ribs and vertebrae)	ciliary movement reduced tracheal deviations chest movement diminished		

TABLE 3–2 Physical Changes With Aging

STRUCTURE	FUNCTION	RISKS/SYMPTOMS	ADAPTATIONS/ HEALTH TEACHING
C. Cardiovascular			
endocardium becomes fibrotic, sclerotic	cardiac output decreases	chronic fatigue, dyspnea postural hypotension	pace activities see physician for regular evaluations
left ventricle wall thickens	systolic murmurs develop		
mitral and aortic valves calcify: become fibrotic			
myocardium becomes irritable with muscle loss	atrial dysrhythmias slowed heart rate	palpitations	
inner coat of arteries/veins become thickened, fibrotic	vascular resistance increases	hypertension, varicose veins weak peripheral pulses	B/P monitored regularly prudent heart living: diet, exercise, no smoking.
arteries become rigid	arterial insufficiency		
changes in T-cells	immune function declines	susceptibility to infections	flu vaccine in fall
D. Gastrointestinal			
saliva production decreases	slows breakdown of starches	nutrition inadequate	reinforce Basic Four diet
smooth muscle tone lost	delayed esophageal, gastric emptying	difficulty swallowing heartburn, indigestion	
gastric secretions reduced	impaired absorption of vitamins and minerals	nutrition inadequate	reinforce Basic Four diet
abdominal muscle elasticity, intestinal mucosa secretions decreased	peristalsis slows	constipation	increase fiber, fluids in diet increase exercise
blood flow to liver decreases	detoxification reduced	drug toxicity	learn symptoms of toxicity

STRUCTURE	FUNCTION	RISKS/SYMPTOMS	ADAPTATIONS/HEALTH TEACHING
E. Genitourinary			
nephrons are lost	kidneys ability to filter blood is reduced	signs of drug toxicity	learn symptoms of toxicity
arteriosclerosis of renal vessels	renal blood flow decreased		
ureters, bladder, and urethra muscles lose elasticity	incomplete emptying of bladder	urine retention urinary frequency and urgency	teach signs of infections learn voiding patterns
	bladder capacity declines		
prostate enlarges	urethra constricted	nocturia	drink fluids during the day
F. Reproductive			
Men: testosterone declines prostate hypertrophied testes become smaller vascular network sclerosed	penile erections and ejaculation are slower	fears and frustrations related to intercourse	reassure not a sign of impotence encourage partners to share concerns, see physician
Women: estrogen declines vaginal secretions reduced fatty breast tissue diminishes	intercourse becomes painful	fears and frustrations related to intercourse "hot flashes" problems with coping	reassure changes are normal encourage physician visit to discuss estrogen therapy, vaginal lubricants
G. Nervous			
neurons decrease in number	brain's ability to integrate functions reduced	head-nodding, other tremor-type movements	see physician for sudden changes in memory loss
arteriosclerosis of cerebral vessels	blood flow to brain reduced	forgetfulness, gradual confusion, irritability	
myelin sheath degenerates	transmission capabilities reduced	slow reaction time, reflexes slower	plan more time for tasks

TABLE 3–2 Continued

STRUCTURE	FUNCTION	RISKS/SYMPTOMS	ADAPTATIONS/HEALTH TEACHING
E. Sensory			
1. Eye: lens flattens, becomes opaque, yellow	presbyopia cataracts, color perception diminishes	difficulty with close range tasks blurred, distorted vision difficulty with blue/green	obtain corrective lenses see ophthalmologist
reduced blood supply to macula	central vision diminishes	increasing difficulty with reading, seeing TV	physician to monitor vision changes
muscle to lens weakens, iris becomes more rigid	reaction to light declines	problems with night driving, glare on glossy surfaces	drive only during daytime; sunglasses, soft lights
2. Ear: reduced blood supply to inner ear	presbycusis	inability to hear high-frequency sounds, consonant sounds	see physician to assess for hearing aid
thickening of tympanic membrane	transmission of sound reduced	gradual hearing loss	family/friends to speak clarly, low tones, face person lip reading
decreased cerumen secretion	transmission of sound reduced; impacted ear wax	complaints of hearing loss	
3. Taste and Smell: number of taste buds and olfactory nerves diminished	sweet and salty tastes reduced acuity of smell diminished	complaints of "tasteless food"	suggested seasonings other than salt and sugar
4. Skin, Nails, Hair: loss of collagen in tissue, decrease in sweat glands, subcutaneous fat	skin loses elasticity inability to tolerate temperature changes	dry skin, lines, wrinkles feeling of chills, cannot tolerate warm temperatures	use humidifier, lotions pace activities, wear clothing for comfort
function of capillaries declines	wound healing delayed skin sensations decreased	cuts, scratches, will not heal nails thicken, hair grays	teach skin, nail care; see podiatrist if diabetic

For Discussion

- How have your views on aging changed since you began studying gerontology and the signs of aging?
- Ask friends or members of a social group their definition of old. When do they think aging begins?
- Reflect on the behaviors and responses of a parent, grandparent, or neighbor. Do they demonstrate the disengagement, activity, or continuity theory of aging? What factors influenced your decision?
- Consider your life style. Which psychosocial theory of aging do you think you will exhibit?
- What physical signs of aging do you observe in your parents or grandparents?

Questions for Review

1. What is the theory of programmed aging?
2. What is an example of programmed aging?
3. What is the wear-and-tear theory of aging?
4. What is an example of "wear-and-tear" aging in a body system?
5. What are the three psychosocial theories of aging?
6. Identify one sign of aging and the accompanying function change in each body system:
    a. musculoskeletal *↓ bone + muscle mass - Atrophy*
    b. respiratory *alveoli thicken, Dyspenea*
    c. cardiovascular *atherosclosis ;*
    d. gastrointestinal *indigestion - wt loss*
    e. urinary *loss of nephron, hypuphasia prostat*
    f. reproductive *— menopause — testes smaller*
    g. nervous *— ↓ brain cells*
    h. sensory *— smell, taste, hearing*
7. Why is health teaching important during the normal aging process?

Unit 4
Conditions Experienced by the Active Aging

Objectives

After reading this unit you should be able to:
- Discuss the gradual aging process related to changing functional abilities.
- Identify the most common physical conditions experience during the active aging years.
- Describe the physical symptoms that are most commonly related to the aging process.
- Discuss appropriate patient teaching to promote maximum functioning and independence.

Aging is usually a gradual process. It sneaks up on us! Our-day-to-day activities hum along until some event occurs that we perceive as aging. Perhaps it is the first gray hair you see in the mirror one morning. Maybe it is the first time a younger person calls you "sir" or "ma'am"! Whatever it is that gives you that inner feeling; and self exclamation "I'm getting old," it sets the wheels rolling for future self examination. For many, those first discoveries result in a sinking feeling. It takes the seasoning of aging, the later years, for most to feel good about the process they have experienced. They earned it!

This unit will discuss some of the more common physical conditions experienced by people as they age, figure 4-1. Your medical–surgical nursing texbook discusses these conditions for the general population. In this unit the emphasis will be on the relationship of the illness, or condition, to expected aging changes.

Depending on hereditary influences, most people have experienced some event they identify as aging by the time they reach their middle or late 40s. Most of these events do not interfere with daily activities. By the time an individual reaches age 65, the societal mark of young old,

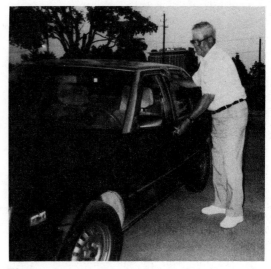

Figure 4-1 Aging begins during our active years

some complaint related to aging is being monitored by the family physician.

For the approximately 20 years between early signs of aging and the milestone of 65, the speed of change and degree of difficulty encountered is influenced by heredity and life style. Most of us can expect to demonstrate aging traits similar to our parents or grandparents. Our life style habits of eating, exercise, and managing stress will also influence or exacerbate aging symptoms.

Aging symptoms that result in changes in our lives are related to mobility, endurance, and sensory problems. Mobility problems related to joints may be signs of early degenerative joint disease. Joint stiffness and discomfort in hips, knees, or ankles are complaints expressed following usual work activities or hobbies such as gardening or the weekend game of touch football. Endurance complaints, combined with mobility changes, are usually related to the cardiovascular and respiratory systems. If a person has had a history of respiratory problems such as asthma, or vascular problems such as hypertension, normal aging changes will add limitations to the disease process. This will result in a weakening of physical endurance. Sensory changes affect interactions with the environment creating potential social isolation.

Between the ages of 65 and 75, the average number of chronic conditions experienced by individuals increases to 4. *Chronic* means ongoing, perhaps life-long, but not necessarily debilitating. These chronic conditions may seem insignificant to some people because problems develop gradually and most people adapt. The conditions have not been perceived as problems. For example, presbyopia, presbycusis, arthritic joint changes, and intermittent constipation may not be interpreted as chronic conditions related to aging. After age 75, the average number of chronic conditions increases to 5.

This unit will present conditions experienced by active aging people. Each system will be discussed, but not every person will experience every condition, nor to the same degree. As a person ages, particularly after age 85, the difficulties and number of systems involved will increase. Cancer in the elderly will be discussed as it is second only to cardiovascular disease in cause of death in old age. Emotional responses related to declining health and aging will be introduced. The focus of patient teaching will be identified in selected problems that will require patient self-care or family assistance.

Nurses in all areas of practice need to consider the aging process when providing patient care, and in the planning and implementing of expanded patient teaching. For example, a 60-year-old man is admitted to the hospital for a cholecystectomy. His history of osteoarthritis, indicated in the admission nursing interview, needs to be included in his care plan when considering postoperative ambulation. In the second example, a nurse in the pediatrician's office gives medication directions to the patient's grandmother or great-grandmother, figure 4–2. This nurse needs to incorporate knowledge of aging sensory changes to assure accuracy in patient and family teaching.

Patients, their families, and other support persons will be providing the continued care, and will be more responsible for their own health. By assisting people to understand their own aging and how to monitor their health, the nurse will promote continued active aging.

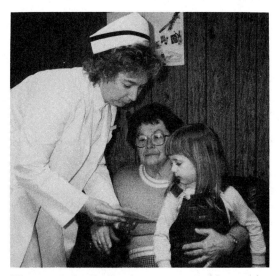

Figure 4–2 Pediatric nurse considers aging changes when giving directions.

Musculoskeletal Aging

Decreased muscle strength and joint aches and pains become common and more pronounced with increased age. There are many types of arthritis. Osteoarthritis, also called degenerative joint disease, is the type tied to the aging process. Gout, or gouty arthritis, is another chronic musculoskeletal condition experienced by the elderly. Bursitis can also occur from repeated stresses on joints.

Osteoarthritis

Osteoarthritis is a result of wear and tear on the joints, particularly the weight-bearing joints. Over time there is deterioration of the joint resulting in varying degrees of disability. This disability can range from stiffness after exercise to near incapacitation because of difficulty in walking. Usual symptoms are aching, stiffness, and limited movement of involved joints. The elderly sometimes call these aches and pains "rheumatism," and often state they can predict changes in the weather by changes in joint discomfort. Small nodules, called Heberden's nodes, may appear on joints in the fingers.

Physicians make the diagnosis of osteoarthritis by listening to the patient's complaints and examining the joints. Diagnostic tests and x-rays are not usually completed unless there is a need to rule out another problem. Often the elderly have self-treated and self-medicated these aches and pains for years. Gastrointestinal problems related to side effects of these medications, the appearance of joint nodules, or other complaints may be the reason for seeking medical attention.

Drug therapy for osteoarthritis is usually salicylates or ibuprofen analgesia. The elderly may be discouraged because they have previously purchased these medications at a drug store. They need explanations regarding dosage, time, and side effects. Additional medical therapy includes counseling related to pacing activities, a therapeutic exercise program, and weight reduction, if appropriate. Devices that help reduce stress on the weight bearing joints, such as a cane, crutches, or braces may be suggested, figure 4-3.

Surgical intervention — the replacement of diseased joints with artifical joints — has been very successful. Many people have experienced a new lease on life with pain free movement. Postoperative recovery includes prevention of infection and support in a physical therapy program. Nurses caring for these patients need to consider other osteoarthritic joints and additional aging symptoms in designing care plans.

Gout

Gouty arthritis can occur in the elderly and initiates many complaints. It often affects a joint in the great toe, which causes difficulty in fitting shoes and walking comfortably. Secondary gout may develop following another illness or as a side effect of medication. Drugs that would interefere with the excretion of uric acid would lead to its concentration in the blood. This results in urate deposits in joints or tissues.

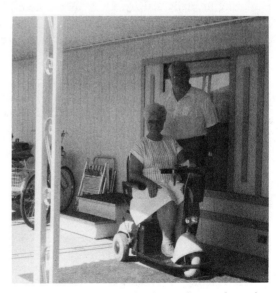

Figure 4-3 A motorized cart keeps the aging active in the community.

A gout attack may typically occur at night with an onset of excruciating pain. An inflammatory process is initiated and may result in intermittent mobility problems. Most people can provide vivid descriptions of an "attack" of gout pain.

Physicians diagnose gouty arthritis by patient history and examination of the involved joint. Aspiration of the synovial fluid will show intracellular crystals of sodium urate, and blood studies will demonstrate elevated serum uric acid.

Drug therapy includes prescribing allopurinol. One of the side effects of this medication is renal problems. This is a concern because of the decreased filtering capacity of the kidneys. Those who experience gouty arthritis may be placed on a diet that discourages alchohol and purine-rich foods such as organ meats and sardines.

Often compounding the musculoskeletal conditions are the circulatory problems created by the aging process. These may result from wearing round garters used with stockings, or crossing the legs while sitting. The elderly should be instructed to wear shoes that fit properly and to take other measures that promote adequate circulation. Mobility problems are the first to lead an older person to some degree of dependency.

In **Situation 1**, Mr. Bernard visits his family physician because his joint pain is interfering with his hobbies, figure 4-4. You are Dr. Winkel's office nurse. It is your responsibility to reinforce the doctor's recommendations which will improve Mr. Bernard's level of function.

Situation 1

Art Bernard is a 70-year-old retired railroad brakeman. During his five years of retirement he has enjoyed gardening and completing woodworking projects in his garage workshop. The last years of work he had pain in his knees, and his hips were painful when he kneeled to inspect the railroad cars. He recently visited his physician because of the pain experienced during his daily activity. Dr. Winkels prescribed Ibuprofen 400 mg p.o. qid.

SELF CARE TEACHING

PATIENT PROBLEM	GOAL	PATIENT TEACHING
Alteration in comfort: Chronic pain R/T* joint stiffness M/B complaints of pain, especially when standing at workbench, and kneeling in garden; increased during damp weather; joints enlarged.	Pain relief Reduced pain during activity	Pace daily activity. Plan rest periods. Purchase high stool to sit at bench. Take Ibuprofen as prescribed by doctor. Report any stomach problems. Use chair cushions. Wear supportive shoes.
Activity intolerance R/T joint stiffness M/B difficulty in completing usual daily activity	Restore function Maintain present activity	Pace activities. Continue moderate exercise, range-of-motion to joints. Avoid overexertion.

*R/T = Related to; M/B = Manifested by

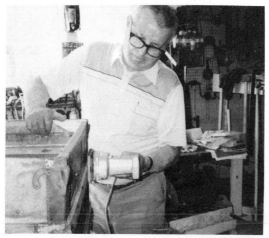

Figure 4–4 Joint pain often interferes with active aging lifestyle.

Respiratory Aging

The respiratory system and the cardiovascular system are keys to the well-being of the elderly as they are with other age groups. A difficulty with either system results in a domino effect. If there is a problem with the lungs in delivering oxygen to the blood stream, or a problem transporting the oxygen via blood vessels to cells, some or all of the body's systems are in trouble!

In addition to threats from the normal aging process, the lungs of older adults have experienced numerous environmental hazards. The lungs of elderly today have had a lifetime of toxic abuse. The first surgeon general's warning regarding the hazard of cigarette smoking was in 1962. During early wars and military conflicts, service organizations provided cigarettes free to service personnel. Most of those cigarettes were unfiltered. Mustard gas was used in World War I; each military conflict since then has used harmful chemicals. There were no early government regulations related to the inhalation of toxic substances in industry. People burned their trash in the backyard, and in the fall burned leaves in the street and coal in the living room stove.

The environmental insults, plus asthma or other respiratory conditions from childhood and the decreased surveillance in the aging immune system, lead to the increased vulnerability for infections in older adults. Pneumonia is the fourth leading cause of death in the elderly. Those with multiple respiratory risks may become victims of emphysema. The increased incidence of lung cancer may be a result of environmental irritants and the vulnerability of the aging immune system. Also more malignancies are identified today because of improved diagnostic tools. Early signs of lung cancer may be ignored because they are considered colds, influenza, or just aging complaints.

Emphysema in older adults usually will precipitate retirement from work becauseof a decreased level of endurance. These people manage at home with a decidedly decreased level of function. They receive medical treatment with bronchodilators and portable oxygen, and have frequent monitoring of their respiratory status by physicians and home health nurses.

Pneumonia and Influenza

Pneumonia or viral influenza may be a primary or secondary illness in the elderly. As a secondary problem it often occurs as a postoperative complication. It is also common in patients confined to bed due to a chronic condition or other debilitative problems. The need for nurses to encourage deep breathing, and a change in position to facilitate adequate lung expansion, can not be overemphasized.

Usual signs and symptoms of pneumonia are less prominent in the elderly than in younger people. Due to diminished neurological sensations, the complaints of chest pain may be a dull ache, rather than the sharp pain expressed by younger people. Elderly persons may not exhibit a fever due to normal lower body temperatures.

Diagnosis is made by history and physical, chest x-ray, and white blood count. A sputum specimen may be difficult to obtain in the elderly because of weakness and a decreased cough response with the inability to expectorate sputum.

Medical treatment for pneumonia in the elderly will follow the usual antibiotic and symptomatic therapy. The elderly will become dehydrated more rapidly and take a longer time to recover. There is less total body fluid because of age-related reduced intracellular fluid. Also, the elderly may reduce fluid intake because of fears of incontinence. Nurses need to be especially alert to prevent other complications such as paralytic ileus. Older adults are usually encouraged to obtain "flu" vaccines annually in the fall, figure 4-5. Those with chronic lung disease are also encouraged to obtain pneumococcal vaccine, a preventive measure against bacterial pneumonia.

In promoting wellness in the active aging, the nurse needs to be continually aware of potential problems with respiratory effort. Being aware of the patient's health history, previous employment, and environmental influences will assist the nurse in making appropriate observations.

In **Situation 2**, Mrs. Schultz has visited her physician with respiratory complaints for the third time in five months. You have been Mrs. Schultz's nurse during her hospitalization. She has responded well to antibiotics and has tolerated oral fluids following intravenous fluid therapy. It is your responsibility to reinforce the discharge plan while you are assisting Mrs. Schultz with her morning care. Your observations are to be reported to the primary nurse for further evaluation.

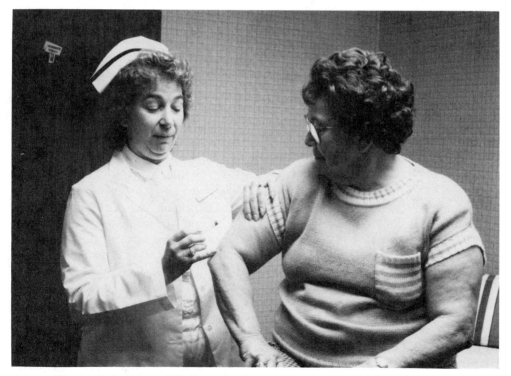

Figure 4-5   Annual "flu" vaccinations are recommended for all elderly.

Situation 2

Josephine Schultz is a 75-year-old widow who lives in senior citizen housing. She has a history of respiratory problems; they began with asthma when she was a youngster. On the third visit to her physician in five months, she complained of flu symptoms. He admitted her to the hospital with probable pneumonia. She was dehydrated and in a generalized weakened condition. Mrs. Schultz has had recurring complaints of cough and fatigue.

DISCHARGE TEACHING

PATIENT PROBLEM	GOAL	PATIENT TEACHING
Potential for infection R/T* compromised immune system, history of respiratory conditions M/B repeated flu symptoms, weakness, recent hospitalization	Reduce potential for future respiratory infections	Plan adequate rest. Avoid persons with upper respiratory infections. Obtain annual flu vaccination. Basic four diet.
Activity intolerance R/T disease process, loss of strength with aging M/B increased complaints of fatigue with usual activity	Resume/maintain usual activity	Pace self care activity; plan rest and activity time. Allow adequate time for recovery. Ask for help!
Potential fluid volume deficit R/T disease process, less total body fluid M/B diminished thirst, dehydration	Maintain adequate fluid volume: good skin turgor, stable weight	Drink 8 glasses of liquid every day; keep written record. Weigh weekly; call doctor with problems.

*R/T = Related to; M/B = Manifested by

Cardiovascular Aging

The problems with the aging heart and blood vessels are compounded by life style choices. Many of the middle and old elderly lived in a time when we did not know much about cholesterol and saturated fats. However, if this population consumed greater amounts of cream, butter, and fatty meats, they were a more active generation. Perhaps the young olds and pre-Baby Boomers are at greater risk because labor became more mechanized, but the eating patterns did not change. The wellness programs we know today have developed with the Baby Boomers and younger cohorts.

Essential hypertension has been labeled the "silent killer". Heart disease is the leading cause of death in people over 65. Many active aging live with, or ignore, cardiovascular problems until a crisis such as a heart attack or stroke occurs. Many others are alert to risks, and have their health routinely monitored.

Some elderly have developed cardiovascular problems in middle age which they carry into their later years. They may have hypertension, coronary artery disease, or peripheral vascular disease. With medical management, they have maintained an adquate level of function. Depending on heredity, extent of disease, aging process, and compliance with medical treatment, the older adult may avoid congestive heart failure until a more advanced age.

Cardiac Function

Angina/Myocardial Infarctions. Coronary artery disease is seen in greater numbers with advancing age. In angina, there is inadequate blood flow to the heart as a result of narrowed coronary vessels, and an increased demand by the heart for the oxygenated blood. This occurs more often with strenuous exercise. Myocardial Infarctions occur when a coronary vessel becomes occluded and there is no blood supply to a portion of the heart muscle. This can even occur at rest.

In the elderly the pain associated with these conditions may not be severe, or may even be absent. There may be a missed diagnosis if a "silent heart attack" occurred. Sometimes, when congestive heart failure symptoms are noted, diagnostic tests reveal small areas of myocardial necrosis. Diagnostic tests for cardiac conditions include numerous blood studies, ultrasound and scanning procedures, and physical endurance tests. These diagnostic tests have become very sophisticated in recent years.

During recovery from an acute phase of a myocardial infarction, the elderly may not be able to complete exercises and other protocols on the routine cardiac rehabilitation program. Nurses need to be alert to these limits and record and report specific observations.

Vasodilators, antianginals, and other therapy is implemented for the elderly on an individual basis. The elderly have a greater risk for congestive heart failure and other complications. Patient teaching that is clear and concise is vital to the elderly with cardiac problems. It is especially important with directions for medications. For example, many use outdated sublingual nitroglycerin because of their reluctance to throw away medication.

Arrhythmias. The aging heart may develop arrhythmias due to disease, sclerosing of valves and vessels, and side effects of medications such as digitalis. Older people may develop tachycardia, atrial fibrillation, or premature contractions. It is wise for the nurse to take apical pulses on persons with known cardiac problems, or when there is a question regarding cardiac function. Any change in the quality or character of the heart beat should be reported to the physician.

Blood Vessels

Hypertension. In older people, hypertension can occur simply from rigidity and other changes in aging vessels. Higher systolic and diastolic blood pressures (above 140 and 90, respectively) are often not treated in the elderly unless there are other symptoms. Central nervous system complaints such as headaches, dizziness, confusion, or epistaxis should be investigated.

When you are assessing the blood pressure of an elderly person, remember that the anxiety of a clinic appointment or out-patient diagnostic procedure will frequently elevate the blood pressure. Also, remember that careful assessment of the blood pressure includes several measurements — having the person in sitting, standing, and lying positions.

Drug therapy for hypertension has become more sophisticated, with a variety of antihypertensive medications. This therapy is not recommended as frequently for the elderly due to potentially toxic side effects. Renal problems in particular are a concern. It is also more difficult to stabilize and manage blood pressure in the elderly with antihypertensives due to circulation changes related to aging.

Peripheral Vascular Disease. Aging peripheral vessels often initiate discomfort in the lower extremities and difficulty in walking. Reduced efficiency in valves and arteriosclerosis can result in varicose veins, thrombi, and problems related to reduced blood supply. A complication that can occur is chronic stasis ulcers.

Amputation of a portion of a limb may be necessary when more conservative therapy is not successful.

Nurses are involved in a considerable amount of patient teaching in support of medical management with the elderly and their cardiovascular aging, figure 4–6. Diet, exercise, and drug therapy are important in each condition. Life-long habits are not easy to change. The nurse needs to understand the traditions of each person before supporting and reinforcing patient teaching. Often, small continuous steps for change are easier for the elderly to manage. The nurse must respect the elderlys' refusal to change dietary or other habits. It is their right to weigh the risks and make their own decisions.

In **Situation 3**, Mrs. Brown has decided to see a doctor. The salve in her medicine cabinet that has "cured everything for years," has not healed the sores on her ankle. Included in the physician's plan is saline wet to dry dressings to be applied three times a day. A telfa dressing with kerlix wrap is to cover the area at night. Ampicillin 1 gm p.o. qid is also ordered. As Dr. Gerber's office nurse you will teach Mrs. Brown aseptic technique, how to apply her dressing, and measures to improve circulation to her lower extremities.

Situation 3

Beulah Brown is a 68-year-old obese woman who recently retired from cooking at a neighborhood restaurant. Her legs have become increasingly painful in recent years; she can no longer tolerate the long hours of standing. She finally decides to visit a doctor because the open sores on her left ankle would not heal with her "tried and true" home remedies.

SELF CARE TEACHING

PATIENT PROBLEM	GOAL	PATIENT TEACHING
Alteration in comfort: Chronic pain R/T* fibrosed veins, insufficient circulation M/B painful legs when standing	Reduce pain in lower extremities	Elevate feet whenever sitting.
Potential for infection R/T impaired circulation M/B open areas on left ankle, purulent drainage on bandage and stocking	Prevent spread of infection; promote healing	Teach asepsis in caring for lesion, hygiene; continue through entire antibiotic therapy.
Alteration in tissue perfusion: peripheral R/T aging fragile capillaries, atherosclerosis, M/B dusky, scaly skin, reddened areas around ulcer lesions	Improved circulation to lower extremities	Elevate legs frequently, whenever sitting. Teach use and application of support stockings.

*R/T = Related to; M/B = Manifested by

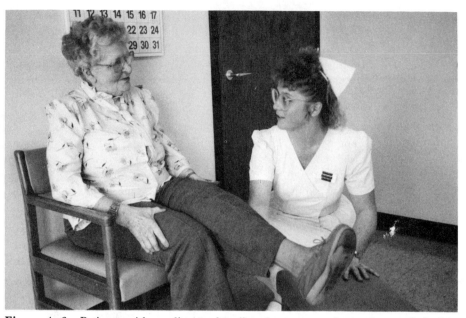

Figure 4–6 Patients with cardiovascular disorders are taught to elevate their feet.

Gastrointestinal Aging

Aging changes in the gastrointestinal system produce many complaints. Most of the active aging treat these complaints themselves with over-the-counter antacids and laxatives. Some elderly have joined the returning emphasis on high fiber diets. Others are reluctant to give up the more refined foods they enjoy. Many of the elderly today did not have dental care in their younger years and cannot afford that care or properly fitting dentures in their later years. This may contribute to inadequate nutrition.

Some of the conditions experienced by the active aging that result in complaints include indigestion, hiatal hernia, and diverticulosis. Cancer of the colon is increasingly common in the elderly. Tests for occult blood in stool samples are recommended and available for home testing.

Constipation

Constipation is a complaint even among the active aging. Reduced activity and exercise, less bulk and fluids in the diet, and growing dependence on laxatives lead to chronic constipation. Some elderly still have the idea that a daily bowel movement is necessary. This may lead to frequent use of over-the-counter laxatives.

During the nursing interview, in any setting, the nurse needs to ask appropriate questions to obtain an accurate assessment of nutrition and gastrointestinal functioning. A patient who has become accustomed to indigestion or routinely taking laxatives may not feel there is a problem. There may be a need for education regarding diet, fluids, and bowel elimination habits.

Genitourinary Aging

Loss of muscle tone is one of the problems in the genitourinary system that leads to complaints in the older adult. The decreased bladder capacity and stress incontinence often result in embarrassment. Situations that compound the problem include taking a diuretic for a cardiovascular problem, reluctance to drink fluids because of dribbling and nocturia, and retention of urine or inability to empty the bladder.

Incontinence

Women experience incontinence because of the relaxation of the pelvic floor muscles resulting from the weight of the uterus and other structures pressing on the bladder. Cystocele and rectocele can occur, and urinary infections become more common. Some women wear sanitary pads or panty liners to avoid the embarrassment of incontinence that occurs with a cough or laughter.

Women are taught perineal or Kegel exercises to improve bladder tone. This conscious effort to contract and relax muscles during urination helps to improve the tone of muscles involved in urination. Surgical procedures for repair of these relaxed muscles are common and effective. Preoperative teaching should include potential difficulties with early postoperative voiding. Some women may be dismissed from the hospital with a urethral or suprapubic catheter. They will need to be taught aseptic technique and how to measure residual urine.

Benign Prostatic Hyperplasia

Many men over 50 have some prostatic enlargement. The concern arises when the benign prostatic hyperplasia enlarges sufficiently enough to cause urinary obstruction. Early symptoms are difficulty in starting a stream, decreased force of urinary stream, nocturia, and retention of urine. Some men are reluctant or embarrassed to seek medical attention until they are alarmed by hematuria or symptoms of renal impairment. Treatment for an enlarged prostate is surgical intervention; a transurethral resection of the prostate (TURP) is performed. Two important aspects of postoperative nursing care are reassuring the patient that bladder spasms are causing the sensation to void when the catheter is in place, and that the surgery does not result in impotence.

Urinary Tract Inflections

Urinary tract infections are common in older adults. They are second to respiratory infections as a cause of fever in this age group. *Escherichia coli* (E. coli), a bacteria normally found in the intestinal tract, is frequently the causative organism. In women, a short urethra and the close proximity of the urinary meatus to the anus results in a higher incidence of cystitis. Older adults need to be taught or reminded of good hygiene practices to reduce the potential of urinary tract infections. In the hospital and other health care institutions, urinary tract infections may be the result of infrequent or poor perineal or catheter care given by caregivers assisting the patient.

The importance of adequate fluid intake must be emphasized. Fluids consumed early in the day, or at times that are convenient to the individual's schedule, should decrease the possibility of interrupted sleep or other problems. Hospitalized individuals may be in a weakened state and therefore not independent in consuming fluids. Nurses and other caregivers are then responsible for assisting with, and monitoring, fluid intake.

Nurses need to refine interview and observation skills related to the urinary system in aging adults. Often people are reluctant to discuss problems related to voiding due to the "private" nature of elimination. A societal response to elimination tends to reflect a repulsive activity rather than a normal body function.

In **Situation 4**, Mrs. Cooper's physician arranged for a home health nurse to evaluate the home environment and the ability of Mrs. Cooper's niece to manage her care. The case manager nurse developed a teaching and personal care plan. You are the home health nurse assigned to implement the plan during twice weekly visits.

Aging and Sexuality

Sexuality and sexual activity of the aging population may be more of a problem to

Situation 4

Ella Cooper is an 83-year-old frail woman who has lived with her 60-year-old niece for 3 years. Mrs. Cooper had lived alone until she broke her right hip. She has had recurrent urinary tract infections during the last six months. Her niece states that Mrs. Cooper has had some mild confusion in recent weeks and needs reminding to eat and drink and take care of herself.

HOME HEALTH TEACHING

PATIENT PROBLEM	GOAL	FAMILY TEACHING
Potential for infection R/T* delayed urge to void, bladder emptying, reduced oral fluids M/B recurrent bladder infections, inability to toilet self, or remember to drink water	Prevent further bladder infections	Encourage extra fluids during day; limit fluids at bedtime; call home health nurse when observing cloudy, foul smelling urine, elevated temperature.
Fluid volume deficit R/T inability to manage own intake M/B needing to be reminded to drink fluids; dark yellow urine	Increase oral fluid intake to 6–7 glasses per day; improve hydration status	Offer fluids between 7 a.m. and 7 p.m., keep record of intake on calendar.
Knowledge deficit R/T preventing urinary infections M/B inability to complete personal hygiene	Recalls purpose of personal hygiene, steps of handwashing, and perineal care	Teach patient, niece handwashing and personal hygiene practices.

*R/T = Related to; M/B = Manifested by

younger generations than to the aging themselves. Generally, our culture has maintained an attitude of intolerance for sexual behavior in the elderly, while accepting broad changes in sexual activity for younger people. Aging adults will adapt to changes in physical and emotional responses when they understand changes are normal. Adjustments are also easier when the elderly have had a healthy attitude regarding their own sexuality.

Sexual dysfunction in older adults may be related to side effects of medications or a chronic condition such as arthritis that prohibits previous sexual activity. Fears, such as having a heart attack during intercourse, can also cause sexual dysfunction.

Nurses need to recognize their own attitudes toward sexuality and aging when supporting the normal sexual needs of older patients. When a clinic nurse or home health nurse has established rapport with a patient, the patient may express concerns or ask questions about changing sexual function. Patients should be encouraged to make physician appointments for examinations and evaluation of symptoms and concerns.

Nervous System Aging

Hypoxia, related to aging changes in cerebral circulation, results in forgetfulness and other complaints in the active aging population. Many people in the United States have some cerebral atherosclerosis due to hereditary and life style influences. A 75-year-old has about 20 percent less blood flow to the brain than a 30-year-old. This decreased blood flow, plus the loss of neurons, may result in forgetfulness and slower reaction time. As a person ages, these difficulties become more pronounced. In addition, sensory losses compound problems and make the elderly more vulnerable to accidents.

The active aging manage well with gradual changes in the central nervous system and adapt accordingly. An 80-year-old woman, visiting with a niece, hesitates as she struggles for the name of the store where she shopped yesterday. "I just don't remember like I used to," she sighs. Many elderly realize it is normal to have moments when it takes longer to retrieve information. Sudden memory loss may be the result of an acute toxic illness. Progressive memory loss with no recall is related to dementias.

Because of the cerebral aging changes, older adults may have some postural hypotension, gait changes, fine tremors in their hands, or a growing irritability during interactions with others.

Transient Ischemic Attacks

Transient Ischemic Attacks (TIAs) can occur in the active aging population, and may be forerunners of more debilitating cerebral vascular accidents (CVA, stroke). A *Transient Ischemic Attack* is a temporary dysfunction of a brain activity due to reduced blood supply to a specific area. Symptoms may be slurred speech, visual problems, dysphagia, or difficulty in finger dexterity. These attacks may last only a few minutes and may not be detected; some elderly unknowingly call them "dizzy spells." When the elderly or a family member notices a change or difficulty in a usual activity, medical treatment should be sought.

Medical assessment of a suspected TIA can include a variety of diagnostic measures. Because of the fleeting nature of the attacks, the physician may not actually witness the symptoms. The examination may be initiated from events described by the patient and family. A lengthy, thorough neurological exam will test memory, calculating or problem-solving ability, motor response, and vision changes. Other diagnostic tests may include brain scans, examination of spinal fluid, and ultrasound or angiography to evaluate blood vessels.

Some people who have experienced TIAs are hospitalized for several days for evaluation while diagnostic tests are completed and the cause for interrupted blood flow to the brain is determined. Although a "cure" is not possible with this disease, it is often managed medically with anticoagulant therapy, or surgically with an endarterectomy. Other contributing conditions such as hypertension and atherosclerosis are reevaluated. Recent research indicates that salicylates (aspirin) are effective in preventing strokes. Many physicians prescribe five grains or less daily.

Nurses in all practice settings and in advocate roles in the community need to be aware of the subtle signs of impaired blood flow to the brain. It is often the nurse who senses and observes the change that leads to the diagnosis of TIA or stroke. It may be a shoulder that droops while the patient is sitting in a chair, the down-turned corner of the mouth, or a difficulty in buttoning a shirt or picking up a fork.

Nurses should encourage family members and neighbors to have their hypertension, diet, and other TIA risk factors monitored by the family physician. The nurse in the clinic may discover a TIA patient, who was noncompliant with hypertensive treatment in the past, asking more questions today after experiencing a frightening TIA event. In the elderly age group, many people know someone who has experienced a stroke. The thought to them is frightening because the word "stroke" translates to "burden" with the sudden loss of independence.

In **Situation 5**, Mrs. Shaw was admitted to the hospital for diagnostic studies. Her daughter had rushed her to the clinic emergency room when Mrs. Shaw's speech became slurred while they were visiting. Her condition has been stable with no identified episodes during the three days of testing and observation. Today you are assigned to Mrs. Shaw. She is to be discharged to her daughter's home for a week and then return home after seeing her physician.

Sensory System Aging

For the active aging population, changes in the sensory system are secondary to mobility problems in limiting usual activity. Vision and hearing loss, which are normal with aging, are often the conditions that initiate the change. Today's elderly did not have routine vision and

---

Situation 5

Mary Shaw, 80, was rushed to the clinic emergency section by her alarmed daughter. During a casual visit, Mrs. Shaw's speech became slurred. Dr. Fields examined her and found a blood pressure of 215/95, but no neurological deficits. He admitted her to the hospital for diagnostic tests. They were within normal range, but the hypertension persisted. Discharge orders included: ASA gr. 5 qd, and Captopril 25 mg. bid.

DISCHARGE TEACHING

PATIENT PROBLEM	GOAL	PATIENT TEACHING
Potential for impaired tissue perfusion: cerebral R/T* interrupted blood flow to brain M/B impaired speech or vision, dizziness, confusion	Prevent recurrence of cerebral symptoms	Teach importance of taking medications as prescribed; side effects affecting GI, CV, and CNS. See physician with visual, speech, or orientation symptoms.
Potential for injury R/T impaired sensory function, altered mental status, mobility or coordination, side effects of medications M/B changes in speech, thought processes, gait disturbances, GI bleeding, hypotension	Prevent injury associated with interrupted blood flow to brain or side effects of therapeutic medications	Teach family to be alert to sudden changes related to speech, vision, or mobility. Teach client/family to be alert to, and report side effects of medications.

*R/T = Related to; M/B = Manifested by

hearing screening in school, nor was periodic vision testing by the family doctor routine.

The diagnostic testing and surgical procedures today mean that the numbers of people experiencing vision and hearing loss should be considerably reduced. Because of untreated problems many people still become blind. Hearing aid mechanisms have become more sophisticated.

Other sensory changes relate to smell, taste, and touch. Changes in smell usually do not cause a great deal of stress in the active aging. A safety concern would arise, however, if a person did not detect food burning on the stove or food spoiling in the refrigerator or other storage areas. The decrease in sensory stimulation to smell may affect appetite and lead to anorexia. The ability to taste sweet and salty is diminished with aging. This, added to the less keen sense of smell, could also affect the elderly's appetite. Through the years we develop an opinion on how food should taste. Some elderly will, for example, increase the sugar on cereal or add more salt to vegetables in an attempt to have food taste the way it "should" taste. The nurse needs to be alert to these possibilities when making a nutritional assessment as these events challenge patient teaching that focuses on reducing sugars and salt.

Nurses reinforce the diet recommendations made by physicians and dietitians. When you are weighing a patient in the clinic, or observing ankle edema in the hospitalized active aging, you can begin to interview the patient about nutritional habits. Sometimes the independent active aging are aware that they are not being compliant with their diet. Others may not be aware of the sodium in processed foods or sources of refined sugars. This information may have been included in written meal plans, but the patient needs your continued teaching and support.

The decrease in the sensory perception of touch and the increase in tolerance for pain is a safety factor in the elderly. Unless water heaters in the home are well regulated, hot bath water could result in thermal injury to aging skin.

The Eye

Many of the active aging will have corrective lenses due, in part, to beginning presbyopia in middle age. Affording these lenses and periodic eye examinations are a concern of the elderly with fixed incomes.

As the eye ages, there is less secretion from the lacrimal glands. This may cause eye irritation as well as reducing the "sparkle" in the eyes; they appear more dull. Physicians may suggest artifical tears, which are eye drops that augment tear production. Nurses should be certain that the active aging know how to instill eye drops, how to prevent contamination of the solution, and the importance of using preparations that are specifically for the eyes.

Cataracts This is the most common condition of the aging eye that limits activity and that could result in blindness if not treated. By age 80, about 80 percent of the elderly have some clouding of the lens. Because the change is so gradual, many active aging do not seek treatment until they do not pass the vision test for driver's license renewal, or realize they can no longer read the newspaper or thread a needle.

The surgical removal of the cloudy lens and the insertion of an intraocular lens implant have been dramatically perfected in recent years. This procedure is completed in a few hours in outpatient surgery.

Nurses practicing in clinics, outpatient surgery, or other settings need to be alert to other aging needs of each patient. Lengthy preoperative and postoperative instructions are to be given in an office. The visual deficit, and a possible hearing deficit, may cause some problems in reading and following instructions. The nurse should suggest that a family member or other person be a part of the teaching process. Ideally, this person would be the individual driving the patient to the outpatient surgery site, or spending some postoperative time with the patient.

In **Situation 6**, Mr. Anderson is scheduled for a cataract extraction and intraocular implant in outpatient surgery. You are the office nurse

Situation 6

Gilbert Anderson, age 72, has just completed his eye exam with Dr. Radil. Mr. Anderson made the appointment because he did not pass the vision test for driver's license renewal. He drove himself to the clinic and stated, "I do just fine when I stay on the roads I know." Dr. Radil explained the cataract procedure to Mr. Anderson and stated he would schedule the surgery in the hospital outpatient department.

PRE-OPERATIVE TEACHING		
PATIENT PROBLEM	**GOAL**	**PATIENT TEACHING**
Sensory perceptual alterations: visual, auditory R/T* aging sensory changes M/B difficulty reading large print instructions, hearing aids, asks information to be repeated	Hears information clearly, repeats key information	Use examining room or other quiet area. Read instructions, with Mr. Anderson following along. Ask him to repeat key points. Allow time for his questions.
Knowledge deficit R/T preoperative activities M/B no experience with cataract or outpatient surgeries, states last surgery was "appendix operation when I was 25."	States he understands his responsibilities before surgery, repeats key activities: physical exam, NPO after midnight, someone must accompany him	Read and explain instructions. Verify family doctor to complete physical. Determine who will accompany him. State you will call him at home to answer questions.

*R/T = Related to; M/B = Manifested by

who is responsible for explaining the surgeon's preoperative directions. Consider Mr. Anderson's aging vision and hearing deficits when planning your patient teaching.

The Ear

Hearing loss in the active aging is usually gradual. It can be a conductive loss which is an obstruction in the sound waves. This is frequently a result of hardened cerumen. More often the hearing difficulty is perceptive deafness related to the change in hearing receptors in the inner ear. Thus presbycusis can begin during middle age and progress. There will be increasing difficulty in understanding high frequency sounds.

When assisting the active aging in any health care setting, the nurse should remember to face the patient to facilitate lip reading. Other aids include talking on the side of the least impaired ear, asking for clarification of information, and providing supplemental written information. When appropriate, nurses should instruct nursing assistants, family members of hearing impaired, and others in how to make their voice more easily understood.

Hearing Aids. Social isolation is a problem for some elderly with hearing impairment. They become embarrassed when they can not actively participate in a conversation. Hearing aids can assist, but the problem of isolation still occurs in large groups. This is because the hearing aid amplifies all sounds, making conversation difficult. The sounds are made louder, but not clearer. There are adaptors for hearing aids and telephones to improve telephone transmission. Headsets can be purchased for televisions so the volume can be lower for other listeners.

Once the initial adjustment of wearing a hearing aid is accomplished, the active aging can enjoy improved interaction with family, friends, and other social contacts. Today, most hearing aids are plastic. Their shape is taken from a mold of the person's ear. The amplifying mechanism and batteries are housed in this small package. The active aging manage well unless visual impairment or arthritic finger joints make it difficult to manage the device. Hearing aids, as well as the batteries that need to be replaced every few weeks, are expensive. They are not reimbursed by Medicare or by some insurance companies. However, they have qualified as deductions on income tax forms.

Endocrine System Aging

For the active aging, Type II diabetes is the endocrine system condition that will result in some life style adaptations. Type II diabetes becomes more prevelant in individuals over 40 years of age who are obese. At least 20 percent of the population over 65 have this type of diabetes. The increase can be attributed to longevity, more public awareness of the condition, and more sophisticated diagnostic tools.

In Type II diabetes there is adequate production of insulin, but the body is not utilizing it properly. There may be only mild complaints of thirst or hunger and vision problems may be attributed to aging. The onset may be so subtle, figure 4–7, that it is not detected until an individual has a problem with a chronic infection or perhaps early degenerative changes in the nervous or circulatory systems. Routine blood studies will demonstrate an elevated glucose. Once an acute condition such as an infection is resolved, the glucose may return to normal levels. A diet and exercise program could manage diabetes in this person.

In aging, the fasting glucose rises because the body's ability to utilize glucose decreases. Active elderly may not be treated aggressively for slightly elevated glucose levels.

The goal for the active aging Type II diabetic is the same as the younger Type I diabetic — the goal is to control the blood glucose levels. If the aging individual is compliant with treatment, the condition can often be managed with appropriate diet and exercise programs, and perhaps an oral hypoglycemic.

DIABETES IN THE ELDERLY

- Symptoms may be vague or absent
- Complaints of sleep disturbances
- May be related to high or low blood sugar and nocturia
- Blood glucose levels are commonly over 400
  Testing not dependable in this age group
- Complaints of vision changes; blurred or decreased abilities
- Complaints of fatigue; signs of anemia
- Unsteady gait
- Slurred speech
- Complaints of cramps, burning feet or toes, especially at night
- Complaints of vulvular itching in females
- Signs of confusion, disorientation, convulsions

Figure 4–7 The onset of diabetes in the elderly

When the individual remains hyperglycemic with this management, insulin therapy may be initiated. Hospital and clinic nurses may be involved in diabetic teaching or the patient may be referred to a diabetic clinic. Costs of devices and supplies for blood glucose monitoring as well as syringes and insulin are covered by Medicare and most insurance payers.

Nurses involved in teaching the new elderly diabetic, or supporting the teaching of others, experience a challenge in patient teaching. The elderly of today have called this condition "sugar diabetes." Some may still use this term and have a misconception of their body's use of carbohydrates. When following the protocol of patient diabetic teaching, remember to adapt teaching objectives to the aging learner.

Diabetes in the elderly compounds and exacerbates nearly all normal aging processes. There is increased renal impairment, infections are more difficult to overcome, and cardiac and cerebral problems occur secondary to circulatory problems. Complications can advance and deteriorate the physical status of the diabetic elderly very rapidly. Complications of diabetes are usually the factors that move the active aging adult to dependent aging.

Cancer in Aging

Cancer is the second leading cause of death in persons over 65 years of age. One theory related to the increase in cancer in the older population focuses on the immune system. If the immune system is not the protective fortress it once was, then cancer cells have the opportunity to multiply rather than be destroyed. It may be difficult to determine an early sign of cancer in the elderly. For example, a change in bowel habits, one of the danger signals, may be attributed to the slowing of peristalsis, the usual decrease in activity, or reduced fluid intake.

The aging population has been exposed to carcinogens for many years. Two body systems that demonstrate higher incidences of cancer in the elderly are the gastrointestinal and respiratory systems. Colon cancer and rectal cancer are more prevalent and may be ignored. The person may attribute problems to old age or hemorrhoids.

Cancer of the lip related to pipe smoking, cancer of the esophagus related to alcohol intake, and cancer of the stomach may also affect the elderly. Lung cancer is seen in more men than women in today's elderly. The situation may be different for the elderly in the twenty-first century. This is projected because of the smoking habits of women today.

Breast cancer is more common in elderly women, and bladder cancer is seen in older men. Although most prostate enlargement is benign, men should have periodic rectal examinations after age 60. Skin cancer is also a concern with the elderly population. There are many aging changes with the skin, and each should be evaluated. Some elderly, such as lifelong farmers, are subject to malignancies on their faces and arms after years of exposure to the sun.

The American Cancer Society and the media have presented a variety of extensive educational opportunities for the American public. President and Mrs. Reagan, during their years in the White House, each had two cancer surgeries. They shared their experiences to encourage everyone to be alert to sings of cancer. Some people, however, continue with the "it won't happen to me" syndrome of ignoring the danger signs of cancer.

Society generally expects the elderly to accept the diagnosis of cancer as if it were to be anticipated. This is unfortunate, as the word cancer is just as devastating to the elderly as it is to the young. Diagnostic tests are completed to evaluate the type of cancer and the extent of growth. Surgery, radiotherapy, chemotherapy, or a combination of the treatments may be recommended depending on other conditions and the general health of the elderly person. Someone in a weakened condition from a chronic respiratory disease may not be able to tolerate a general anesthetic or the side effects of chemotherapy. The way healthy active aging repond to cancer treatments demonstrates a remarkable resilience.

It is challenging and rewarding for nurses to assist patients of any age who have cancer. Nurses assisting the active aging need to continue patient teaching in preventive measures as well as the warning signs of cancer. For those who have experienced cancer, the nurse assists each individual to maintain the highest quality of life possible. The key to the quality of life of cancer victims is meeting their perception of quality and not necessarily the planned goals of the caregivers.

Emotional Response to Aging Physical Conditions

How the active aging respond to changes and limitations with signs and symptoms of aging is very individual. People do not change a great deal as they age. Their traditions, values, and coping mechanisms stay much the same. Some people will will struggle with aging as they did with their youth. Others will adapt with each passage of events in life.

Often there is an increased level of fear and anxiety in the elderly. In some individuals the increased anxiety is noted by family members as a change in behavior, a new expression of fear, or the repeated need for verifying information. Some aging persons are very deliberate in masking these new fears. For example, an alert elderly man who cannot see or hear well may be hesitant to attempt to manage a new environment alone. He may be capable of asking and understanding directions. However, if his compromised vision and hearing prevent him from following the directions, he will feel lost.

Depression in the elderly is common and can be very serious. Multiple losses including diminished physical abilities or the inability to cope with change may precipitate the depression.

Alcohol Abuse and Misuse in the Elderly

In the older independent adult, alcoholism can result as a continuation of habits of younger years. It can also occur as a result of loneliness after retirement and the loss of a job. Other losses that may lead to alcohol misuse or abuse include the loss of a spouse, friends, or other meaningful relationships, or the inability to cope with declining health.

The use of alcohol by the aging population may exacerbate chronic conditions or interfere with the treatment of a disease. Alcohol, also considered a drug, may interact with medications. Its use can precipitate dementia seen in the elderly. In younger years, alcohol ingestion often makes the person sleepy; in later years insomnia may be experienced. Poor nutrition may be a result of increased alcohol use.

Nurses need to be aware of the possibility of alcohol use as a contributing factor to many physical conditions experienced by the elderly. They can have many reasons for weight loss or complaints of sleeplessness. If a person demonstrates signs of frequent falls, when having a history of relatively safe activity, you should investigate the possible use of alcohol. Other changes such as signs of self neglect are clues.

Summary

All people should be supported, perhaps nurtured, through aging changes of life. This is now true during aging changes of growth and development, from birth through adolescence. We support the toddler taking his first steps, his management of body functions, and his ability to learn activities of daily living: feeding himself, bathing, dressing, and grooming. Decades later, at the completion of the life cycle, someone may be assisting him with those same activities.

Why should we support people during aging changes, during middle age, and into active aging? Perhaps, because people need information, direction, and support through all phases of development and change. This unit discussed some of the physical conditions experienced during middle age and beginning changes of the active aging years. These changes most often relate to early sensory changes in vision and hearing, and difficulties in joint mobility. Other changes related to decreased hormonal activity result in physical and emotional concerns. Nurses and other health care professionals need to be supportive during this phase of life.

The active aging, 65 years and older, may experience several chronic conditions. All systems are involved in the aging process, some to a greater degree than others. Because of the process of aging, and the development of the related conditions, a person may not perceive these conditions as problems. Making adjustments and adaptations to continue independence is also a part of the aging process. When a sign or symptom demonstrates a sudden onset, the problem may be related more to an acute disease than aging.

Nurses in all settings of practice must be aware of the importance of including the results of normal aging in patient care plans, and patient teaching for self care. In the neighborhood and community, nurses are advocates for aging and the aged. Reinforcing the directions of physicians, physical therapists, and other health professionals provides emotional support and encouragement in assisting an aging population.

For Discussion

- Discuss aging with family members, neighbors, or friends. Visit with someone who is middle aged and someone who is an active aging person.
  - What aging symptoms have they experienced?
  - Have these aging changes altered their life style?
  - Do they project any future problems related to health and aging?
- Interview an individual who has had surgery for cataracts, a joint replacement for osteoarthritis, or other aggressive treatment for a condition related to aging.
  - How had the condition changed daily activities prior to treatment?
  - What were the hopes for the future following surgery or treatment?
  - Were these expectations met?

Questions for Review

1. What are the two aging changes many people experience during middle age years?
2. What is the most common aging condition in the musculoskeletal system?
3. Why are the elderly so vulnerable to respiratory conditions?
4. How do aging changes in the cardiovascular system affect every system in the body? Give examples.
5. What are patient teaching measures to prevent urinary tract infections in the elderly?
6. What are examples of emotional responses to aging symptoms?

Unit 5
Who Are the Active Aging?

Objectives

After reading this unit you should be able to:

- Describe the active aging individual.
- Identify social issues concerning the active aging population.
- Discuss aging concerns related to retirement, health, fianances, family, leisure, and community activities.
- Discuss the nurses's role in understanding patients' concerns in social issues of aging.

Who are the active aging? What characteristics describe the active aging individual? Should there be an age, a birthday, tied to this description? Aging is very individual; some people become dependent during early aging years while others are active and independent into their 90s.

For the purposes of this discussion, age 65 will be used as a chronological point of beginning active aging. Many private agencies, retailers, and others use this age demarcation in providing services, or offering discounts for senior citizens.

An active aging older adult is at least 65 years of age and retired or semi-retired from full-time employment. This change in work status means some alteration in daily activities and schedules. Most active aging will have a living spouse, and continue to live in the same home environment. This person will have some minor physical limitations due to the normal aging process. The person will adapt to continue completing home maintenance projects and engage in other activities of choice. The greatest change in early active aging will be the additional available time that was once devoted to a job.

There are phases or stages in the active aging years that often are not easy to identify. When interviewing a family, the adult son may reflect, "I suppose the first time Dad needed me to help paint the house was the beginning of a dependency; I can't remember the exact year." During the young old years, ages 65 to 74, there may be little noticeable change in physical activity from years prior to age 65. Gradually, the aging process sets some limits on activity. In the marriage partnership, each member compensates for the aging loss of the other. One may have decreased strength and the other decreased vision. Together they can complete a home maintenance project of washing windows.

This unit will present some of the major issues and concerns of the active aging population. The first issue is retirement; the planning and managing of a major change in life. Next, and accompanying retirement, are issues of health and finances. These are two of the greatest concerns of the active aging population. Family involvement with active aging persons can play either a minor or very major role. Finally, the opportunities available for leisure activities and community participation will be discussed.

How do these issues and social concerns of the active aging population affect nursing practice? During nursing interviews in acute care admissions, office appointments, or home care visits, the nurse needs to watch and listen for clues that indicate concerns of patients. These concerns will reflect on the health and health care of the patient.

The following are two examples of social concerns of the active aging that can influence your patients and, in turn, your nursing practice. An active aging retiree demonstrates an elevated blood pressure during several office visits. In listening to Mr. Willians, you learn that his former employer is changing the retirement health benefits. Mr Williams is concerned about paying for his health care. Another patient, Mr. Mason, excited about his retirement six months ago, seems more despondent with each clinic visit to monitor his diabetes. He shares with you that he now realizes his work was really his life. No, he has not become involved in any neighborhood, church, or community organizations.

Nurses are not expected to be therapists, or solve the problems of their patients, but they are expected to be good data collectors. Sometimes, as a knowledgeable resource person, you can offer suggestions to patients to contact com-munity agencies or other helpful resources. Many times the data you collect needs to be reported to the physician, your nursing supervisor, a social worker, or other designated health professionals in your place of employment.

Retirement

Retirement is a time of loss and a time of opportunity, figure 5-1. In our society, *retirement* usually means a withdrawal from work because of age. It is a relatively new idea simply because, until recently, no one lived long enough to retire. In this country retirement has been a difficult concept because of the relationship of productivity and personal value.

Most people consider the economic loss with retirement, but do not think about other issues that are equally important and stressful. These include loss of: (1) status, (2) identity, (3) meaningful work, (4) a support group with similar inter-

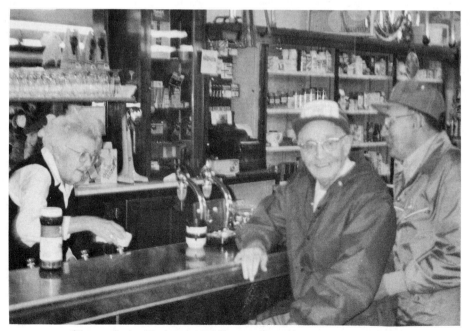

Figure 5–1 Retirement offers a time of new opportunities.

ests, (5) a daily schedule, and (6) experiences of meeting new people and learning new ideas.

Every job has an identity and a status within the work place. There are undefined expectations and job ranking by co-workers as well as the formal job descriptions and a management tree outlined by the employer. Individuals tend to describe themselves by the type of work they do. The public also has a perception of what a particular job involves. With retirement there is some degree of self-esteem lost because of the respect and value that has been placed on the job by the employer, public, and self, figure 5–2.

Completing meaningful activity is tied to our self-worth. Part of that self-worth is our own inner survival, and part is external. Society equates productivity with self-worth. The loss becomes more harsh when a retired individual realizes he will be replaced, and someone else can do his job. A second career or volunteer work can replace this meaningful activity when a person makes a healthy adjustment to retirement.

The support group in the workplace may be the workers on a particular assembly line, a secretarial pool, or nurses in a small hospital. They often support each other through personal problems as well as work-related difficulties. Friendships that develop seem like they will last forever. But the unity of the support group is tied to the work. Often this friendship or bond vanishes following retirement. The loss can be particularly devastating if the retiree did not have friends or support persons outside of the workplace.

Work schedules provide a daily routine or structure to our lives. They establish a framework to organize our time and activities. Most people are not self-directed to the point that they could randomly attack activities with minimal planning and goal setting and still be successful. We often confront a retired individual, "Why are you still getting up at 5 a.m. when you don't have to go to work?" Sometimes maintaining a previous schedule helps in finding and adjusting to a new schedule.

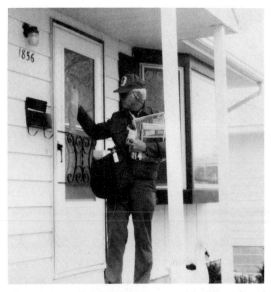

Figure 5–2   Retirement removes identity related to job.

The "fringes" of a job, such as meeting new people and learning new ideas about people and the world, are very meaningful in enriching the work experience. This loss at retirement makes the individual feel "out of the mainstream," a sense of forced disengagement from work and the world.

An additional loss in the social and emotional aspects of retirement is a possibility of role change in a household. Examples are when a husband retires and the wife continues to work, or when both retire and they decide to "reassign" household tasks, figure 5–3.

Why people retire has a great influence on their attitudes and adjustments to losses and opportunities in retirement. Mandatory retirement is now illegal, but employers sometimes offer early retirement incentive benefit packages. The objective may be to reduce costs, numbers of employees, or both. Some active aging welcome the early retirement, and others resent it. Another reason for retirement is health. There may be a deterioration of general health, or a specific condition that begins to prevent a person from physically completing their job.

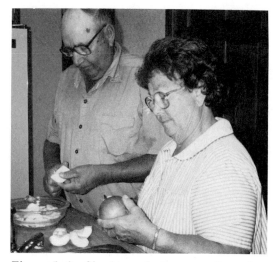

Figure 5–3   Sharing tasks is a part of reassigning roles.

Being able to complete some planning assists with the adjustment to retirement. An unforeseen event, such as a stroke, that forces immediate retirement compounds problems of health, retirement, and finances.

The opportunities of retirement are not always foreseeable, or perhaps accepted, until after a period of adjustment to losses. The success of retirement may depend on the kind of work that was done and the degree of job satisfaction. Attitudes regarding retirement, hobbies, leisure time, and time with family and friends that were in place before retirement will make a difference. Positive retirement means that, after a period of adjustment, the active aging person can focus on opportunity rather than loss. figure 5–4 summarizes concerns related to retirement.

Health and Finances

Health

Health issues that concern the active aging relate primarily to: (1) the ability to continue doing the activities they have done in the past,

PERSONAL LOSSES WITH RETIREMENT

STATUS AND IDENTITY
- expectations and ranking perceived by co-workers
- expectations by employer
- expectations of self; self-esteem
- value of position identified by self, employer, public

MEANINGFUL WORK
- self-worth related to inner survival
- self-worth related to work ethic

SUPPORT GROUP WITH CO-WORKERS
- common bond with work-related difficulties
- individual support with personal problems

DAILY SCHEDULE
- provided a structure to daily life
- provided a framework to organize time

GROWTH EXPERIENCES
- learned new ideas about people and the world
- enriched and motivated work experience

Figure 5–4   Retirement concerns of active aging

(2) the hopeful prevention of a catastrophic health crisis, and (3) the ability to pay for health care. As people add more years to their active aging, the two major concerns that emerge are health and finances. When asking the elderly which one is of primary concern, the answer is most often health. Many feel that if their health is poor, having extra sums of money for travel, or other activities, is irrelevant. When discussing losses, elderly people are frequently heard to say, "Well, at least we have our health."

How a person perceives their own health has a great impact on their active aging years.

For some, the absence of acute illness is health. The goal of participating in a church bake sale or attending a baseball game continues to be achieved. Over the years, these goals become increasingly difficult; it takes more time and effort to achieve a goal. Those with a positive outlook will continue to adapt to keep active and attempt to achieve their goals.

Other active aging individuals are not so involved. This is because their perception of health is declining function and perhaps fear of disability or death. Taking care of their health is their entire focus; they will not consider other activities. This may be a result of fear, an excuse not to participate, or a preoccupation with an illness or disability. This prevents them from participating in family or other activities.

The three primary concerns the elderly have regarding their health determine the status of their future. This future is unknown and uncertain. However, they can make some projections. Some active aging individuals can reflect on their family history and observe how their parents aged. The wellness practices that have been included in any part of their lives will also assist in projecting risk factors.

The threat of catastrophic illness makes many active aging fearful. For example, a friend who was mowing his lawn one day became hospitalized with a stroke the next day. Seeing friends face a debilitating illness with resulting life style changes is difficult. Many accept that aging carries the risk of catastrophic illness.

The concern regarding paying for health care is ongoing because of continual changes in the health care delivery system. There is a great deal of uncertainty for the active aging. This "cash and carry" generation that may not have had health benefits as employees now realize they must purchase health insurance. Those who did have health plans as employees are uncertain whether benefits will continue in retirement. Health concerns of the active aging are summarized in figure 5–5.

When receiving health care, the paperwork is confusing and frustrating to the active aging.

HEALTH CONCERNS OF THE ACTIVE AGING

ABILITY TO CONTINUE USUAL ACTIVITIES
- influenced by perception of own health
- influenced by chronic conditions that limit activity
- influenced by heredity and own wellness practices

PREVENTION OF CATASTROPHIC HEALTH CRISIS
- realized through acute health crisis of friends
- accept increased risk with aging and disease

ABILITY TO PAY FOR HEALTH CARE
- influenced by changes in retirement health benefits
- influenced by changes in government health care funding
- influenced by fixed income and increased out-of-pocket costs

Figure 5–5   Concerns of the active aging regarding own health

Where forms are sent and how payments are made may vary between government and private payers. Hospitals, clinics, and other health care settings are not uniform in billing procedures. The actual cost of insurance and the additional out-of-pocket costs are major concerns of the elderly. When the elderly are confronted with acute illnesses, they do not recover as quickly and use more hospital days in an extended time of recuperation. Paying for health care becomes burdensome and many elderly will pay off the bill with their savings. They may eliminate leisure activities, house repairs, and even adequate food to pay the bill.

Finances
Planning is the key ingredient for the active aging, especially with retirement and

finances. The unknowns of the future cannot be anticipated, but there can be a plan to guide needed changes. Couples or individuals can gather information and devise a plan for the active aging years, figure 5-6. Community or adult education provides pre-retirement planning. Today, many corporations and industries provide preretirement classes with information for their employees. Planning gives people some choices and helps them make decisions.

Retirement planning begins with gathering information about assets and personal interests. People will have to set goals with this information in mind. It is suggested that the plan be in writing so individuals can see the facts and figures. Later they can review or update the plan accordingly.

Preretirement planning involves legal aspects which include wills and contracts. This is especially important for those with second marriages or businesses. Estate planning is a part of the legal aspect and the plan will be updated when there is a move, remarriage, or other situation that indicates a major change.

Other issues included in preretirement planning are housing, leisure time, changing roles, and health. These issues all relate directly to finances. People examine the costs of living in their current home and how they will afford those costs in their aging years. Most people manage the costs and needed maintenance until a health concern forces them to consider alternative housing. They may choose to move because their home is now too large, the floor plan has become inconvenient, or they need to be nearer public transportation. Finances involved in selling a home, moving, and purchasing or renting another home or apartment will have to be considered.

How leisure time is used and financed is part of planning for active aging years. Many

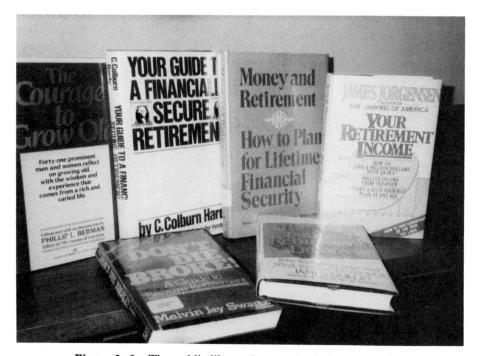

Figure 5-6 The public library is one source for gathering information about preretirement planning.

people have planned and saved for years to travel or make a hobby a new full-time job. Others look forward to gardening, volunteer work, or spending more time with family and friends. New learning opportunities are available in every community. Limitations of health and finances would determine whether a person could learn about native African animals on a safari or at the local zoo.

Finances include the management of known chronic conditions with treatment and medication. Paying for medigap health care insurance and the out-of-pocket costs for acute illnesses is a budget concern in financial planning. Despite ongoing changes, the government still falls short in paying for health care of senior citizens. At the same time, this population depends on the government for health and pension benefits.

Planning looks at the possibility of changing roles. The roles may be work related. In this country we have moved from a one career or lifetime job, to an average of three careers. This is because of the longer life expectancy and the rapid change in technology. Retirement from the primary job in the active aging years may mean the beginning of a new job with a new identity and status. Military personnel often experience this transition during middle age when they retire from a military career and begin a new job in the community.

A major concern of the active aging, and a part of preretirement planning, is establishing financial security. This is determining a source of income for retirement. The usual sources are (1) social security benefits, (2) retirement benefits or pensions from employers, (3) personal retirement funds such as Individual Retirement Accounts (IRAs) or interest on other monies, and (4) earnings from part-time work or a second career.

More than 25 percent of the elderly live entirely on social security payments. This has created a crisis because it is not an adequate income for most for food, clothing, and shelter. Also, the older the retiree the smaller the pay-

ment because wages were considerably lower during his years of working.

Planning for the active aging years includes budgeting available income to meet costs of housing, health, and daily activities. Although most people do not begin to think about this planning until they are in their 50s, financial planners suggest young people today begin planning and saving for their aging years. Figure 5–7 summarizes issues in pre-retirement planning.

Family

The family unit is the major stronghold of the active aging population. Their perception of the family unit and the roles of its members are based on values established early in the twentieth century. Men were the head of often large households. Women and mothers had responsi-

FINANCES AND THE ACTIVE AGING

- Preretirement planning allows for choices:
  - Begins with determining financial assets and personal interests
  - Involves legal activities, including wills
  - Focuses on housing, leisure time, and changing roles
  - Projects needs related to health concerns
- Preretirement planning avoids quick decisions
- Preretirement planning focuses on sources of income:
  - Social Security benefits
  - Retirement benefits
  - Personal retirement funds
  - Earnings from part-time work or second career

Figure 5–7 Issues involved in preretirement planning

bilities directly related to raising children and homemaking tasks. All goals revolved around family activities and survival. Grown children that left home stayed in the community; the family unit grew and remained together.

Today's elderly, who are healthier and living longer because of technology, also see their families separated because of the same technology. Adult children may live in all corners of the United States, or the world. Still, most elderly have regular visits with their families. For some, it continues to be the weekly Sunday dinner when the family gathers. For others, travel is planned to see children and grandchildren, figure 5–8.

In the past the elderly, particularly the dependent elderly, lived with adult children. Today, these children are not as involved in supporting their active aging parents physically or financially. In turn, these parents do not expect this support from their children. They also do not influence their children's decisions in life as

parents did in the past. However, this does not mean that adult children abandon their parents.

The remarriage of an active aging adult initiates a major change in the family unit. Previous interactions in the family, and the stability of the family unit, will influence the acceptance of this marriage by adult children and other family members. Also, the nature of the loss of the natural parent who is being replaced reflects on the response of the family. Separation of natural parents by divorce, accidental death, or terminal illness are examples of this loss. The length of time since the marital separation of natural parents and the age of the parents and children at the time of separation influence the acceptance of the new marriage. Whatever the specific factors, there are emotional adjustments for all members of the family unit. Several family units are now involved and long-time traditions, such as holiday gatherings, have to be renegotiated. Other concerns involve dispersion of belongings and memen-

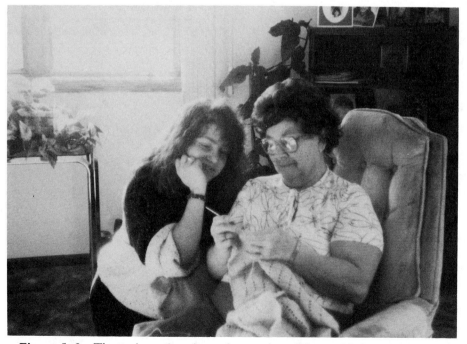

Figure 5–8   The active aging share time and traditions with grandchildren.

toes, and the issue of new wills. Families that have adapted and changed together over the years will be able to weather this major change with aging family members.

Today, there are more transitions in the family unit that relate to life style choices than life cycle changes. People are continuing their education or returning to school at all stages of life. Divorce, or loss of a job, may bring adult children back to the home of their active aging parents. Grandparents may become involved in the child care for their grandchildren. These are just a few examples of the changing household. The independence, dependence, and interdependence of the family unit is a major influence on active aging adults. *Interdependence* refers to a dependence on each member within a group. This also may be reflected in elderly couples: mutal support keeps them independent as a couple. Family issues concerning active aging adults are summarized in figure 5–9.

THE FAMILY AND THE ACTIVE AGING

- Family unit is major stronghold of the active aging.
- Elderly's perception of family unit is based on early twentieth century values.
- Twentieth century technology separates families geographically.
- Twenty-first century children may not be directly involved in life/care of elderly parent; parents not as influential in children's decisions.
- Remarriage of active aging initiates major changes in family units.
  - Nature of loss of natural parent influences family response to remarriage.
- Life style choices influence transitions in the family.

Figure 5–9 Family influences during active aging years

Leisure Activities and Community Participation

Becoming more involved in leisure and community activities is one of the opportunities of retirement and active aging. Most people have been involved in these activities during younger years. Others, through friends and members of interest groups, begin to participate by replacing job related hours with a recreation group or volunteer activity. Some elderly are motivated to search independently and join a group. However, it is more common for individuals to become involved in an activity because there was a one-to-one invitation by another person.

Activities are available in many areas of interest. Religious and volunteer group associations are the most common interactions the active aging have with the community. There are hundreds of associations that have religious, fraternal, recreational, cultural, ethnic, business, or educational focuses.

For the active aging it will be a personal preference whether a peer group or an intergenerational group is chosen. For example, a retired man may choose to stay with his bowling group as they age together. Another retiree may prefer to join a group that includes young people as well as those who are middle-aged. He enjoys the interactions of an intergenerational group.

Activities with volunteer associations can absorb a considerable amount of the elderly's time. These groups are organized to achieve a charitable goal or pursue a common interest. They satisfy the active aging's need to be involved in useful work or activity. The American Red Cross, The American Lung Association, The American Heart Association, and the American Cancer Society are examples of organizations that assist with health concerns and welcome volunteers. Active aging persons may become involved with one of these groups because they or a family member have experienced a condition that is assisted by the association.

Membership and participation in a fraternal organization may be continued. Each association demonstrates a common interest or mutual identity. They may offer members social and economic benefits such as group insurance policies. Retired individuals may continue to participate in the business, professional, or union groups that they were involved in during their years of employment. Some of these groups have specific associations for retired individuals such as the Retired Army Nurse Corps Association, which was founded to preserve the history of the United States Army Nurse Corps.

Service Corps of Retired Executives (SCORE) members are retired business persons who volunteer the expertise of their work experience. They may assist individuals wanting to start a business, or help small business owners with management problems. A retired nurse was involved in a SCORE project that assisted a medical business. The Retired Senior Volunteer Program (RSVP) involves the active aging in volunteer work in the community. Often they assist in schools, libraries, day care centers, and long term care facilities.

Older adults who have been active in politics often continue with this activity. Some become lobbyists for organizations. Their knowledge and expertise from previous work experience is valuable to many interest groups. Other active aging people work for political candidates by stuffing envelopes and making phone calls.

Some active aging adults become involved in activist groups that take positive action toward needs of their elderly peers. The Gray Panthers is a political activist group founded by Maggie Kuhn in 1971. This group has an intergenerational focus in desiring to combat ageism. The National Council for Senior Citizens has state and local groups within the organization that are politically active in voicing the views of older adults.

Many associations focus on the older population in their membership and services.

An example is the American Association of Retired Persons (AARP). With over 30 million members, it is a large and well-known organization. This organization provides services including pre-retirement planning, group health insurance, and many educational programs. These associations have lobbyists that inform policymakers about concerns of older Americans. Most organizations keep members informed through newsletters.

Education is another opportunity for the active aging. There was a time, in the past, when education was considered only for the young, work was for the middle-aged and leisure was for the old. Today, all ages are involved in these activites throughout their lives.

Elderhostel is a program that offers people over 60 educational opportunities in colleges and universities. Academic courses are offered during summer months when campuses are less populated. These lower cost programs do not include homework or tests! Some colleges offer credit courses tuition-free in "space available" classes to senior citizens. Other educational opportunities are available in adult education in community settings.

Leisure activites also mean working on hobbies, travel, and recreation or sports. Most often the individual has devoted some time to these interests during busy working years, figure 5–10. Figure 5–11 summarizes leisure activities of the active aging.

Disadvantaged Elderly

The active aging also include those who do not have access by location, information, finances, or other situations to many of the opportunities of active aging. They experience the losses of aging and many times can not achieve many of the successes and opportunities.

Homeless elderly are among the most unfortunate elderly in this country. They are a part of the active aging population; their activity involves day-to-day survival. The percentage of

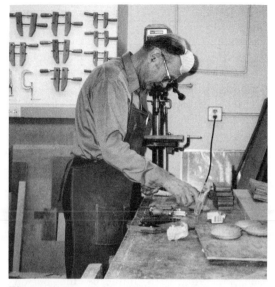

Figure 5-10   Retirement may offer more time for hobbies.

ACTIVE AGING AND LEISURE ACTIVITIES

- Religious and volunteer associations demonstrate the greatest involvement by the active aging.
  - Most achieve a charitable goal or meet a common interest.
  - Fraternal, cultural, ethnic, or recreational organizations are other choices of older adults.
  - Professional and business organizations include retired, but active members.
  - Educational opportunities include Elderhostel and community adult education.
- Hobbies, travel, recreation, and sports interests can have additional hours of leisure time during retirement years.

Figure 5-11   Opportunities of retirement and active aging

homeless elderly compared to the total population of this age group is much less because of a high mortality rate in the homeless population. The peril of being old and homeless is devastating partly because having a home gives one identity, self-worth, and independence.

Those who are homeless suffer from several physical and social disorders such as mental handicaps, chemical abuse (especially chronic alcoholism), and other situational crises. These homeless have lost jobs and homes, and many have become victims of a slow-moving social welfare system.

Health problems of the elderly homeless are exacerbated by lack of food or poor nutrition. They also suffer from inadequate medical and social services. When these services are in place, they may not be utilized by this group. This is because they are not informed of the availability, or they refuse the services. There is a general fear and lack of trust of the health care delivery system as well as fear of physical harm from the younger homeless population.

Nurses join social workers and others in attempting to support this aging population.

Homeless elderly need to be directed to health and social services and be encouraged to use them in monitoring chronic health conditions. Churches and other social institutions support shelters that provide hot meals, or bathing and sleeping facilities. Nurses may be involved in providing health screening in these settings. With the increase in the elderly population, it is likely that in this country, particularly the metropolitan areas, we will see more homeless elderly. This is another social issue the United States will be facing in the next century.

Minority aging persons may not have a decision regarding retirement. Because of financial oppression, they may be forced to work as long as possible. They may change jobs because of declining health and functional ability. Poor health in younger years that is related to limited access to health care may precipitate early retirement from a long time job.

The proximity of adult children is very important to the active aging minority family.

Participation in church, neighborhood, or community activities will be more prevalent within minority subgroups. There is more emotional comfort in remaining in the community. Many fraternal groups and other associations have objectives, services, and membership directed toward minority groups. However, aging minority individuals who have been in business and professions may have a greater interest in these associations. Concerns of disadvantaged active aging are summarized in figure 5–12.

DISADVANTAGED ELDERLY CONCERNS

Homeless Elderly
- Experience losses of aging: home, work, and other identities related to self-worth.
- No opportunities of successes with aging.
- Suffer from physical and social disorders.
- Health problems are exacerbated: poor nutrition, inadequate medical and social services.
- Lack trust in health care delivery system.
- Victims of slow-moving social welfare system.

Minority Elderly
- Financial oppression forces continued employment.
- Retirement often not an option.
- Lifelong poor health may precipitate unwanted retirement.
- Children may not live in community to be a support or part of an extended family.
- Limited income not adequate to meet health and social needs.

Figure 5–12 Concerns of disadvantages active aging

Summary

Aging is very individual socially as well as biologically. As we age, we do not change a great deal: our habits and values become seasoned from experience. However, the elderly as a population group are also individually different from one another. Each person adapts and adjusts to retirement and other social events in a different way.

An active aging adult is described as a person at least 65 years of age that has had life style changes brought about by retirement or semi-retirement. Major issues related to the active aging population include retirement, health and finances, family, and leisure activities and community participation. How these concerns affect each individual will influence the person's health and the delivery of his health care.

Retirement in our society has meant withdrawal from active employment because of age. Historically, this has been difficult because of the work ethic and relationship of productivity and personal worth. There are losses and opportunities that result due to retirement. Some of the losses are income, personal status and identity, meaningful work, a support group, a daily schedule, and new experiences.

Why people retire is a major factor influencing attitudes and adjustments to losses and opportunities in retirement. Attitudes regarding retirement that were in place earlier will make a difference in accepting the changes. Preplanning, however, will assist in the adjustment.

Health issues are those that affect the ability to continue participating in usual activities. How people perceive their their health will affect their participation in the opportunities of active aging. Those with a positive outlook will adapt and keep active.

Finances are managed best by the active aging when there has been preretirement planning. Employers, community education programs, and others offer courses to assist individuals and couples to gather information about their assets and organize to meet costs. Paying for health care is a concern and continuing uncertainty because of today's changing health care delivery system. Also, many elderly live entirely on Social Security benefits. Sources of income following retirement are usually pensions from employers, personal retirement funds, and earnings from part-time work. Regardless of the source, the income requires budgeting to manage costs.

The family unit continues to be the major source of support for the active aging population. Family members assume responsibility of aging parents. Remarriage of an aging parent initiates many emotional responses in adult children. Issues that influence responses include the nature of the loss of the natural parent, previous family traditions, dispersement of family belongings, and changes in wills.

The active aging population often continues participation in leisure and community activites that have been enjoyed for many years. There are hundreds of volunteer opportunities in service, social, fraternal, and religious organizations. Some retirees continue in business related organizations, or join groups that are exclusively senior citizen groups.

Education is a growing opportunity for the active aging. Colleges and universities offer elderhostel programs. Community adult education offers classes in crafts, finances, or recreational activities.

The active aging also include the disadvantaged elderly. One group is the homeless elderly. Their health is in jeopardy because of poor nutrition, inadequate shelter, and poor access to medical and social services. They suffer the losses in aging with virtually no opportunities.

The minority elderly are a potentially disadvantaged group. A low socioeconomic status is the major influence on plans and adjustments of retirement and aging. Financial oppression may mean that a minority older adult has to continue in the work force as long as possible. Families and the church are very important in the activities of the active aging minorities.

Nurses need to be aware of the concerns and interests of the active aging population. The patient's adjustment to retirement, financial status, and participation in social activities will influence health. These factors will influence patient teaching and the development of care plans.

For Discussion

- Interview an active aging person who has been retired five or more years.
  - Identify formal or informal pre-retirement planning.
  - Ask the individual to compare preretirement interests and perceptions with actual current situations.
- Invite a financial planner to meet with you and friends or classmates.
  - What advice do they give to the elderly today?
  - What advice would they give to you and your cohorts regarding planning today for your aging?
- Visit with a nurse practicing in a clinic or in home care.
  - How does data collected regarding the patient's concerns with retirement, finances, family, or leisure activities fit in patient teaching or patient care plans?
  - What interviewing techniques are most helpful in collecting data and assisting patients?

Questions for Review

1. What are the losses attached to retirement?
2. What event assists in adjusting to retirement?
3. Why are the active aging adults fearful of catastrophic illness?
4. What are some of the dilemmas involved with the elderly paying for health care?
5. What topics are frequently included in preretirement planning information or classes?
6. What types of activities can the active aging be involved with after retirement?
7. Why do the elderly homeless avoid available health services?

Unit 6
Community Services
for the Aging

Objectives

After reading this unit you should be able to:

- Discuss the federal government laws and monies that provide programs for the aging.
- Identify government supported programs that are offered to older adults in a community.
- Describe types of services provided in programs for the aging.
- Discuss services provided by private businesses and community organizations.
- Identify the nurse's role in community services provided for the aging.

What if? — What if your elderly neighbor's husband dies and she has no one to help her understand changes in pension benefits and transfer of deeds? What if your friend's mother is not eating well because she lost interest in cooking for herself? What if you think your grandfather's out-of-pocket expenses for his recent hospitalization are unreasonable? What if your patient has no transportation to his next appointment at the clinic?

There are many questions — they surface every minute of the day. When the questions are answered they help the active aging to remain independent. Help comes in a wide variety of services. They reach every aspect of biological, sociological, and psychological aging. They include direct services, education regarding services or self help, and support groups.

For those not knowing where to look for help, telephone services such as "Helpline" or "First Call For Help" can be good first resources. Other resources are newspapers, television, radio, churches, and Area Agencies on Aging. Community programs often place pamphlets explaining their services in drug stores, community centers, and other central areas in the neighborhood. Newsletters explain changes in Medicare

funding and news about available services, as well as senior citizen activities in the community.

Funds that are appropriated through the Older Americans Act provide funding for nutrition, transportation, and other social services. Hospitals, as a result of the changing health care delivery system, have begun to offer more community outreach programs. Large corporations and foundations, through their philanthropic programs, include funds for services for the elderly. Fraternal organizations and volunteer groups are creative in methods used to develop services that keep the active aging independent.

This unit will provide an overview of the structure of government services for our rapidly aging population. Samples of programs, and what they offer the older adult, will be presented.

The elderly, like most people, feel that nurses are their friends. Nurses are considered resource persons when the aging or their families are looking for help. You may be the first person your friend calls when she is frustrated because her mother's poor eating habits are resulting in inadequate nutrition.

Nurses are directly involved in many of the services and programs designed for the elderly.

Some nurses are aides to legislators. They provide insight into health or elderly issues during the development of government sponsored programs. Nurses are speakers at meetings of support groups for those with arthritis, figure 6–1, families of Alzheimer's victims, or respite caregivers. Your opportunities for being an advocate for America's aging are endless! Just look around you!

Legislation for America's Aging

The Social Security Act of 1935, providing government pension funds for people 65 years and older, was the first legislation directed toward America's older population. Thirty years later there were two major pieces of legislation for the elderly that would influence their lives for decades. First, the Social Security Act was amended to provide government sponsored health care (Medicare) for people 65 years and older. The second major legislation in 1965 for the elderly was the Older Americans Act. These legislative responses were part of the social reform included in President Lyndon Johnson's "Great Society" programs in the 1960s.

The Older Americans Act established the Administration on Aging (AoA), which grew out of the 1961 White House Conference on Aging. There had not been much focus on older Americans since the passage of the Social Security Act. Only a few states had developed plans for the aging. With the passage of the Older Americans Act, all states were required to implement state units on aging.

The *Older Americans Act* created a federal government program to meet the social service

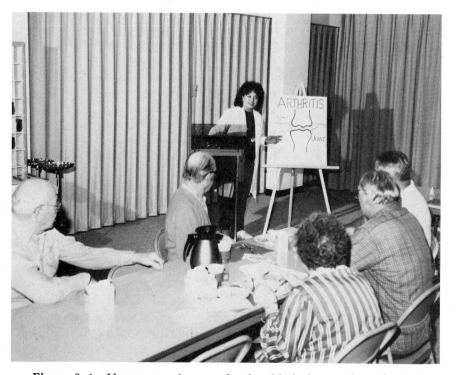

Figure 6–1   Nurses are advocates for the elderly in a variety of roles (From Ringsven and Jorenby/*Basic Community and Home Care Nursing,* copyright 1988 by Delmar Publishers Inc.)

needs of older Americans. The goal was to develop and deliver community-based services to the aging population group. It was intended that the programs would improve the lives of the elderly by providing services and meaningful activity. The historical development of the Older Americans Act is summarized in figure 6-2.

Funds appropriated provide grant monies to service needs in social and health related pro-

1965	Older Americans Act — passed
1969	Retired Senior Volunteer Program (RSVP) Foster Grandparent Program
1972	Nutrition Programs: Congregate Dining
1973	Area Agencies on Aging (AAA) mandated for all states Senior Centers and Multipurpose Centers created Federal Council on the Aging created Training and research, Community Employment Service Titles added
1975	Transportation and Home Services Legal and Counseling Services Residential repair and renovation programs
1978	Advocacy Programs Long Term Care Ombudsman
1984	Direct reporting between Commissioner on Aging and Secretary of Health and Human Services Health and nutrition education services
1988	Elder abuse prevention

Figure 6-2 Historical development of the Older Americans Act

grams. A majority of the funds are spent in this area on programs such as nutrition and transportation services. Other funds are designated for education and training, research and development, and other special projects related to gerontology. An overview of the structure and provisions of the act are listed in figure 6-3.

Community-based programs are implemented through the federal, state, and community government network. The United States Department of Health and Human Services houses the Administration on Aging (AoA). Throughout the United States there are 10 regional offices on aging. Each state has a State Unit on Aging (SUA). For some states, the division of the network ends here, and the planning of service areas begins. Other states are divided into state regions and Area Agencies on Aging (AAA). Figure 6-4 illustrates how the network of agencies that are developed from the Older Americans Act will work for an individual.

State Units on Aging

The goal of the *State Units on Aging* is to provide services and opportunities for older adults to help them remain in their own homes and communities. These State Units on Aging are the focal points in making the system work to provide services directly to older Americans. Over half of the states have independent agencies which are referred to as "Board," "Commission," "Office," "Department," or "Bureau" on Aging. Some states house the aging programs within other departments such as social services or human resources. Part of implementing the goal is the state's active participation in planning, coordinating, organizing, funding, and evaluating the programs funded by the Older Americans Act; they are advocates for all older persons.

Area Agencies on Aging

Area Agencies on Aging are public or non-profit private agencies designated to implement

TITLE I	*Policy Goals*	
	Improve the lives of older Americans: income, health, housing, employment, retirement, other community services	
TITLE II	*Legislative Directive*	
	Create U.S. Administration of Aging (AoA)	
	Directed by Department of Health and Human Services	
	Establish Federal Council on Aging	
TITLE III	*Programs to Assist Older Americans*	
	Congregate and home delivered meals	
	Services to access other services: outreach, transportation, information, and referral	
	Legal assistance, Advocacy, Support Services, Senior Centers	
TITLE IV	*Research and Training*	
	Provide support of training, research, and demonstration projects in gerontology	
TITLE V	*Employment Programs*	
	Develop employment programs in community services for those 55 and older	
TITLE VI	*Indian Tribes*	
	Provide social and nutritional services to Indians 60 years and older	
TITLE VII	*Training Programs for Older Americans*	
	Develop programs of health education; implement in senior center facilities	

Figure 6–3 Structure of the Older Americans Act

the Older Americans Act in regions or smaller areas of a state. There are over 600 of these agencies in the United States where services are coordinated, funded, and implemented.

One of the functions of an Area Agency on Aging is the development of direct services to the aging population. After specific needs and appropriate services have been identified, the complex process of implementing a service program begins. Existing community resources are utilized; a vacated retail store or former armory may become a senior center, figure 6–5. Additional funds for operating programs are often secured through private or volunteer groups, business and industry, or foundations.

Today, even a very small rural community may have a senior center where the active aging can meet, socialize, and benefit from Older Americans Act programs. The elderly themselves may have fundraisers to support their activities. Community pancake breakfasts and craft sales are two examples. Sometimes a corporation or foundation may provide funds for equipment that is part of an ongoing project. Examples are commercial popcorn or donut-making machines. A senior citizen group will sell popcorn or donuts at a community summer festival. Proceeds purchase furnishings and supplies for the center, or rent a bus to go to a large shopping center or attend a baseball game.

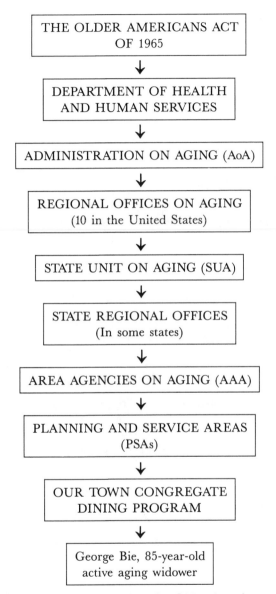

```
┌─────────────────────────┐
│ THE OLDER AMERICANS ACT  │
│         OF 1965          │
└─────────────────────────┘
            ↓
┌─────────────────────────┐
│  DEPARTMENT OF HEALTH    │
│   AND HUMAN SERVICES     │
└─────────────────────────┘
            ↓
┌─────────────────────────┐
│ ADMINISTRATION ON AGING (AoA) │
└─────────────────────────┘
            ↓
┌─────────────────────────┐
│ REGIONAL OFFICES ON AGING │
│  (10 in the United States) │
└─────────────────────────┘
            ↓
┌─────────────────────────┐
│ STATE UNIT ON AGING (SUA) │
└─────────────────────────┘
            ↓
┌─────────────────────────┐
│  STATE REGIONAL OFFICES   │
│     (In some states)      │
└─────────────────────────┘
            ↓
┌─────────────────────────┐
│ AREA AGENCIES ON AGING (AAA) │
└─────────────────────────┘
            ↓
┌─────────────────────────┐
│ PLANNING AND SERVICE AREAS │
│          (PSAs)           │
└─────────────────────────┘
            ↓
┌─────────────────────────┐
│  OUR TOWN CONGREGATE      │
│    DINING PROGRAM         │
└─────────────────────────┘
            ↓
┌─────────────────────────┐
│ George Bie, 85-year-old   │
│  active aging widower     │
└─────────────────────────┘
```

Figure 6–4 Networking the Older Americans Act

Nurses are advocates for the elderly and are resource persons knowledgable about services available in the community. You may make the difference in the independence and quality of life of a senior citizen by helping him become aware of programs that meet his specific needs.

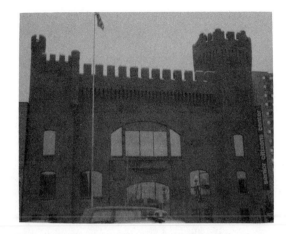

Figure 6–5 An old armory becomes a senior citizen center.

Community-based Programs for the Active Aging

Services that are provided to the aging population through the Older Americans Act assist the active aging to continue interacting with their friends and neighbors, and also bring services into their homes. Figure 6–6 identifies community-based services funded by the Older Americans Act. There are four service areas: (1) facilitating access to services, (2) providing services in the community at large, (3) providing services in the home, and (4) providing services to elderly in health care facilities.

Often the development and funding of services is a cooperative effort within public and private sectors of the community or neighborhood. Businesses, churches, foundations, clubs or organizations, and individuals join public utility companies or transportation departments to implement services for elderly citizens. A combination of volunteer and salaried workers provides services funded in a sometimes complex blending of public and private monies.

States vary in how funds are appropriated and what departments implement or oversee a project. The variables are influenced by monies

COMMUNITY BASED SERVICES

SERVICES TO FACILITATE ACCESS

- Transportation
- Outreach
- Information and referral
- Client assessment and case management

SERVICES PROVIDED IN THE COMMUNITY

- Congregate meals
- Multipurpose senior centers
- Casework, counseling, emergency services
- Legal assistance and financial counseling
- Adult day care, protective services, health screening
- Housing, residential repair and renovation
- Physical fitness and recreation
- Preretirement and second-career counseling
- Employment
- Crime prevention and victim assistance
- Volunteer services
- Health and nutrition education
- Transportation

SERVICES PROVIDED IN THE HOME

- Home health, homemaker, home repairs
- Home-delivered meals and nutrition education
- Chore maintenance, visiting, shopping, letter writing, escort, and reader services
- Telephone reassurance
- Supportive services for families of elderly victims of Alzheimer's disease and similar disorders

SERVICES TO RESIDENTS OF CARE-PROVIDING FACILITIES

- Casework, counseling, placement and relocation assistance
- Group services, complaint and grievance resolution
- Visiting; escort services
- State long-term care ombudsman program
- Other community services, as available

Figure 6–6 Older Americans Act community-based services

available, demographics of their elderly, structure of services, private and volunteer preferences, and of course politics. You can learn more about how programs are implemented in your state by contacting your board, commission, or office on aging, or the state department that is responsible for implementing the Older Americans Act.

The following discussion presents a sampling of community-based services. In any community the services offered should reflect the needs of its senior citizens.

Facilitating Access to Services

Major programs have been instituted to assist older adults in utilizing a broad menu of services including transportation, outreach, information and referral, and assessment and case management. These areas of service connect senior citizens to other programs that help in preventing early dependence.

Transportation. The transportation services provide an important link between the active aging and the community. They foster independence, figure 6–7. Area Agencies on Aging provide buses or vans to transport the elderly to physician appointments, congregate dining, adult day care, or other destinations in the community. The vehicles are handicap accessible with motorized wheelchair lifts and other equipment. Arrangements are usually made a day in advance to assure a ride at the right time.

Churches and service organizations are two additional groups that include transportation for the elderly as a part of their community outreach. Some hospitals and clinics are beginning to offer special senior programs that include free transportation to their patient's appointments.

Outreach and Information and Referral. Examples of outreach programs are those where nurses, social workers, or other professionals are staff members of a senior citizen's center. They are available to identify problems and connect individuals with appropriate services. The senior center may be a more comfortable neutral ground for some active aging to seek help.

Facilitating access to services through information and referral is often accomplished through "help" telephone services. Another method is the development of a resource directory that explains services and provides telephone numbers.

Assessment and Case Management. *Case Management* is a process of identifying the

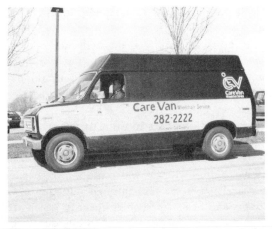

Figure 6–7 The active aging are more independent with special transportation services.

specific needs of a person, the resources to meet the needs, personalizing a plan, and monitoring and evaluating the services and results. Extensive interviewing of the individual, family, and other support persons is started by the *case manager.* This person is often a nurse or social worker, and may be titled a case coordinator. Public health agencies, home health agencies, hospitals, and other health related organizations may have staff employed in the role of case manager. Some nurse entrepreneurs have started private case management services.

Part of case management services is to determine the older adult's physical and mental abilities and limitations. This includes the safety of his environment and his ability to independently meet activities of daily living. After determining what activities require some assistance, the case manager identifies resources that can help this person remain at home with maximum independence. Resources include family, neighbors, friends, and others, in addition to public and private programs, funds, and services.

Pre-admission screening (PAS) is another service of a case manager. Most states require this screening before admission to a long term care facility. This assessment will assist in determining if the individual could remain in his home with alternative services, or if placement in a long term care facility is the best choice. *Alternative Care/Services* refers to health care and other support services given outside the traditional settings of hospital, nursing home, or clinic.

Providing Services in the Community

Numerous programs within the public and private sectors of the community assist the active aging with a wide variety of needs. Physical needs are met through nutrition programs and health screening. Security needs are met through housing services, adult day care, crime prevention, and legal services. Social needs are met through senior centers and volunteer services.

Congregate Meals.   Nutritional services are well known to the elderly, nurses, and others in the community. One of the programs is home delivered meals, often called "Meals-on-Wheels," designed for homebound people. The other program is congregate dining which is offered in senior centers, churches, schools, or other community settings for the ambulatory aging. The dining areas are located on the ground floor. They are selected to accomodate even those with minor mobility problems related to aging, figure 6–8.

The largest amount of money in a state unit on aging budget is usually appropriated for nutritional services. State nutrition program funds are added to federal dollars. Senior citizens participating in the nutrition program

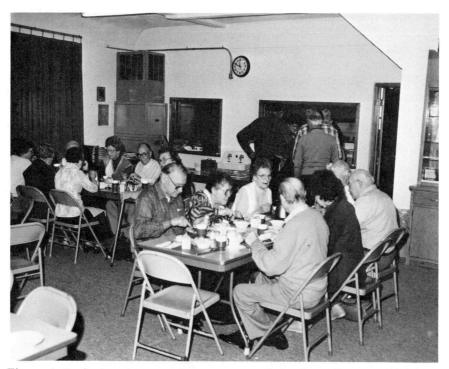

Figure 6–8   Senior citizens enjoy congregate dining in easily accessible sites. (From Ringsven and Jorenby/*Basic Community and Home Care Nursing*, copyright 1988 by Delmar Publishers Inc.)

are encouraged, but not required, to make a donation toward the cost of the meal. Those who enjoy these meals are often people who live alone and look forward to the socializing which is part of congregate dining.

Dietitians plan menus at the state or area level of administration. Each meal is to have one third of the Required Daily Amounts (RDAs) of essential nutrients. The site managers — those responsible for implementing the nutrition program in the community setting — are directed by the dietitian and other program planners. Menus are posted at the dining site, and may indicate calories in each serving. Participants requiring diabetic, low sodium, or other special diets may arrange for for these therapeutic diets.

Senior Centers. Multipurpose senior centers are a popular gathering place for the active aging. For many it is a replacement for a social or fraternal organization membership enjoyed during earlier years. Others experiencing time on their hands and loneliness find companionship. They can reminisce, share a hobby, participate in an exercise class, or join a bus tour to a museum, figure 6–9.

Programs vary according to location and membership interest. Some are service oriented while others are primarily social and recreational. Senior centers are often housed in empty classrooms in a public school (reflecting shifting demographics in a community), in part of a church, in an abandoned town hall, in a vacated inner city store, or in another central location.

Middle and lower income elderly comprise the majority of active aging who are interested in senior centers. Enrichment programs and recreational activities are first choices of the middle income older adults. The lower income elderly prefer programs that are designed to help them cope and remain healthy and independent. Transportation, despite many public and private services, remains an obstacle for

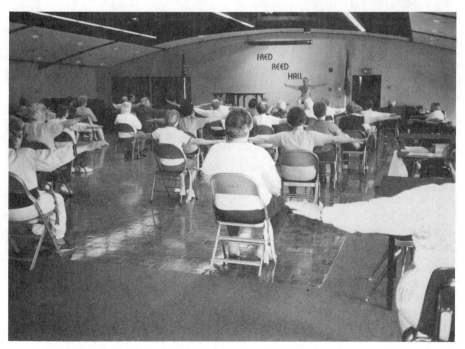

Figure 6–9   Exercise classes are a popular senior citizen activity.

many active aging. Volunteer drivers are not affordable for some centers because of insurance costs. Rural centers often must depend on neighbors and the families of participants to assist with transportation.

Counseling Services

A number of counseling services are available for the active aging through Area Agencies on Aging, hospitals, clinics, community action agencies, and other organizations. Many elderly experience loneliness; even couples remaining in their own home may be lonely. This may be because one partner has physical or mental limitations that keep both persons homebound. For most elderly, there has been a stigma attached to the use of mental health services. The willingness to share emotional problems and accept community assistance is fairly recent in our society. Health professionals need to be keen observers in order to develop strong helping relationships with the elderly. This will assure more success in making referrals to mental health services.

Peer counselors assist their active aging cohorts in working through losses or changes in their lives. These counselors are not therapists, but are volunteers who are good listeners. Through seminars or discussion groups, nurses, physicians, social workers, clergy, and other professionals present the counselors with information about loneliness, grief, and chemical dependency.

Legal Services.

Free legal services are offered to senior citizens through programs funded by the Older Americans Act and other agencies. Sometimes lawyers donate hours to these services, which may be offered in a senior center. They assist with problems related to Social Security, and Medicare and Medicaid benefits. Additional areas where senior citizens may need advice include veteran's benefits, age discrimination concerns, utility shutoffs, or mortgage foreclosure. As states pass Living Will legislation, lawyers will receive more questions about this issue.

Adult Day Care.

Like the hospice concept of care, adult day care services began in England. The services started there in the late 1950s and caught on in the United States in the 1970s. The concept has become more popular in recent years with cost containment in health care. It is another approach to help keep the elderly out of the higher cost health institutions. The major objective, however, continues to be to assist the elderly to maintain their independence by providing some physical health services and promote emotional health through social contacts, figure 6–10.

Elderly with a physical disability such as a stroke-related deficit, or a person with a dementia such as Alzheimer's, are examples of older adults in day care centers. They can manage at home with the assistance of family, but can not manage independently even for a few hours. Services at the center may include: (1) social and recreational activities such as crafts and games; (2) health services such as assistance with medications or monitoring of chronic conditions; (3) exercise programs to promote health; (4) social services such as counseling, support groups, or information and referral;

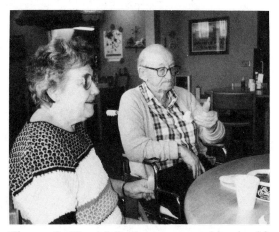

Figure 6–10 Adult day care provides health monitoring and social stimulation.

(5) nutrition counseling; and (6) transportation services. Families having to meet work schedules are particularly interested in transportation services to and from the center.

Adult day care centers may be located in long term care facilities, churches, community centers, or other sites that offer some elderly services. Costs are usually about 50 percent of daily nursing home costs. Some centers charge additional fees for specialized therapies and hygiene procedures. Funding for these services continues to be a dilemma. At the close of the 1980s, Medicare provided no funds for adult day care. Some states have Alternative Care Grant programs that assist with funding. Private insurers pay a very small amount; health maintenance policies are beginning to provide some coverage. Many families are paying all of the fees out-of-pocket.

Housing Services. For those active aging choosing to remain in their homes, there are chore and maintenance services to assist when physical limitations keep them from completing tasks. Often a network of public utilities, volunteers, and private businesses provide these much needed services. In the Minneapolis and St. Paul area, a "Metropolitan Paint-a-Thon" is held annually to paint, in one day, the homes of 300 elderly and low-income residents. Organized by the Greater Minneapolis Council of Churches, teams of volunteers from radio and television stations and business offices apply donated paint to the homes.

In the past, when the elderly could no longer live in their homes because of safety or health reasons, it meant moving to the home of an adult child or other relatives, or entering a nursing home. Today, because of a greater focus on the needs of the elderly, many other options are emerging.

Alternative living arrangements may include purchasing another, perhaps smaller, home or a home with a more convenient floor plan. Congregate housing, sometimes called "senior apart-ments" or "senior highrises," offers apartment living. Federally funded congregate housing offers subsidized rent for low-income elderly. One or more meals a day, offered in a common dining area, may be part of a program to assist in promoting adequate nutrition and social contacts. Other services related to housekeeping or personal health may be offered.

Shared or community housing provides a home for several unrelated elderly. Each person has his or her own bedroom in a house or small apartment complex. Sometimes abilities are matched to provide maximum independence for a group having individual limitations. Public health nurses or other health care personnel may have a group of clients in the same home or apartment. In some communities the term shared housing is used in reference to a person who remains in her own home and shares it with another, usually a young person.

Board and care homes provide housing for a small group of older adults. A resident receives meals and housekeeping along with a room and bathroom accommodations. These homes are not considered health care facilities; however, nurses are sometimes employed and monitor the health of residents.

Continuing care or life care communities are designed to provide a wide range of services for the changing needs of residents. The purchase agreement includes arrangements for lifetime housing. A couple may be very active and independent when moving into an apartment. However, there is also a long term care facility and health services on the campus should they require those services in the future.

Communities may have other creative housing services to meet the needs of their elderly. We will probably see more of these options in the next century.

Providing Services in the Home

The rapid acceleration of health care costs initiated programs to assist active and dependent aging recover from acute illnesses and to manage chronic conditions in their homes. Monies saved are actually in the room charges, not in the cost of delivering a therapy. The growth of home health care and related services mushroomed after the implementation of the 1983 Medicare changes, which reimbursed by diagnosis rather than hospital charges.

Home Health, Homemaker, Home Repairs.

These three basic types of services provide a broad range of assistance to the elderly who are temporarily homebound with an acute illness or more permananently with a chronic condition. Home health services are implemented by nurses, figure 6-11, and home health aides. Physical therapists, dietitians, and others may also be a part of home delivered care. Treatment and care continues to be under the direction of a physician because of the reim-

bursement system. Medicare pays only a small portion of home health services, and the person must be homebound to qualify. Some insurance companies are beginning to pay for some home care services.

Homemaker services meet another segment of managing the life of a dependent person in his home. Light housekeeping, laundry, and meal preparation are examples of tasks. A homemaker-home health aide may be employed to complete both personal care and homemaking responsibilities.

Home repairs, chore maintenance, and other services keep the home environment safe for the elderly. Through information and referral or a case manager, services may be contracted or volunteers arranged to complete necesssary repairs.

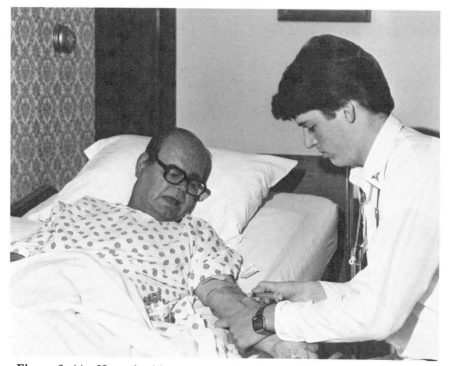

Figure 6–11 Home health nurses provide a variety of services in the home. (From Ringsven and Jorenby/*Basic Community and Home Care Nursing*, copyright 1988 by Delmar Publishers Inc.)

Home-Delivered Meals. The example of Meals-on-Wheels, the delivery of a hot noon meal, has been used several times in previous discussions. On weekdays, members of social organizations, churches, or other volunteer groups deliver the meals to the homebound. Many of the volunteer drivers and delivery persons are the active aging themselves. Those who benefit from this nutritional service include people recovering from acute illness; they may be too weak to prepare meals. The frail elderly who are managing at home with home health care and other community-based services also may receive these meals.

Additional Services. Telephone reassurance may be provided by agencies or volunteers. Planned telephone calls at scheduled times tend to reduce social isolation as well as meet the objective of assuring personal safety.

Respite care is a vital service for family caregivers as well as the frail elderly. *Respite* is defined as an interval of temporary rest. In health care it means appropriate persons or professionals to relieve the usual caregiver. The respite time may be a few hours for an appointment or errands, a weekend, or several days for a vacation. The person providing the respite could be a senior companion who visits with the individual and answers the telephone, or a nurse who monitors a respirator.

Support groups help families and other caregivers manage often difficult and lengthy illnesses and chronic conditions. Members develop a mutual bond and offer suggestions. This often helps in preventing caregiver burnout.

Providing Services to Elderly in Health Care Facilities

The Administration on Aging through the Older Americans Act continues to provide programs for older adults living in long term care facilities. One of the services is an Ombudsman Program, figure 6-12. *Ombudsman* is the advocacy role of state agencies; it works with all concerned persons with the goal of quality of care and quality of life.

In 1987, Minnesota was the first state to pass a law that would provide acute care ombudsman services for its older citizens. It

Office of Ombudsman for Older Minnesotans

The Ombudsman works with consumers, concerned citizens, nursing homes, hospitals, home care agencies, and public agencies to enhance the quality of care and quality of life of older individuals receiving health care services or supportive services at home.

THE OMBUDSMAN:
- **Investigates Concerns** from consumers or others on their behalf relating to their rights, services and benefits.
- **Mediates Disputes** between consumers and hospitals, nursing homes, boarding care homes, adult foster care, home care agencies, individual staff and public agencies.
- **Advocates for Consumers** when their rights have been violated or they are not receiving the proper care or assistance.
- **Provides Information and Educational Programs** to consumers, families, volunteers, staff and concerned citizens about consumers' rights, laws and regulations of health care or home care services, services to consumers and current issues.
- **Advocates for Reforms** in the health care and the social services system to better meet consumer needs.

Figure 6-12   Ombudsman programs help protect rights of older adults. (Courtesy Minnesota Board on Aging)

was designed to support the elderly having problems with access to health care or premature discharge from acute care hospitals. Other states are reviewing additional advocacy roles such as ombudsman programs for elderly receiving home health care.

Many elderly living in a health care facility benefit from companion services because they no longer have family and friends to visit. Two programs developed by Area Agencies on Aging are the Retired Senior Volunteer Program (RSVP), and the Senior Companion Program. They are an asset to both the active and dependent aging. The senior companions are compensated with a stipend and meet special needs for companionship in one-to-one services. Figure 6–13 identifies the community's responsibility in providing services to senior citizens.

State and Local Services for the Aging

It is difficult to separate services into neat little packages funded and implemented by specific groups for special needs of older individuals. The network is complex. It is to the benefit of the aging that public and private programs collaborate to meet needs. It may also be confusing due to the duplication of services offered by public, private, and volunteer organizations. It may be disappointing for the elderly, when they learn about services from the media, to discover that they are not available to them. Often this is due to geographical gaps in services. Many times there is no single authorative source of information for persons seeking services for the aging. It will be a challenge for all sectors to fine tune the delivery of services to the rapidly growing aging population.

Programs that are in place to assist citizens with physical and mental limitations are available to all age groups. Examples are state programs for the blind and visually impaired, the deaf and hearing impaired, and mental health programs. In many states, people who are legally blind can receive a number of services at no cost to them. Some services include: (1) talking radio over which newspapers, magazines, and other written materials are read; (2) talking books, a library of current and classic titles; (3) assistance with completing forms; (4) large print playing cards; (5) magnifiying glasses, and (6) tips on folding money to identify digits. These services also provide continued activity for the active aging with limited vision, figure 6–14.

TO FACILITATE ACCESS TO COMMUNITY SERVICES, THE COMMUNITY MUST:

- Provide information of services, schedules, fees if required; make available through extensive communication in newspapers, radio announcements, public bulletin boards, church newsletters and bulletins, and service groups.
- Provide a location to house the service.
- Contribute funds to add to federal and state monies.
- Provide volunteers to coordinate and organize a program.
- Seek professionals for salaried or volunteer staff to provide expertise for developing goals.
- Provide transportation to increase accessibility to services and programs.
- Seek community pride and commitment in ongoing services.

Figure 6–13 Community responsibilities in providing community-based services for the elderly population

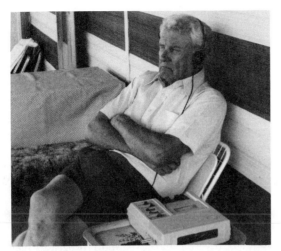

Figure 6–14 "Talking books" absorb the time and attention of the legally blind.

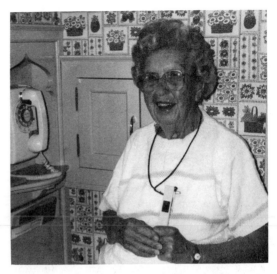

Figure 6–15 A small transmitter is the emergency link for a 96-year-old woman who lives alone.

Emergency response systems are designed more for the active aging who live alone. These systems are often sponsored by hospitals or community fire departments. Locally they may be known as "Lifeline" or "Rescue Line." A programmed unit is attached to the home telephone; the system also includes a transmitter that is worn as a wristband or necklace, figure 6–15. Whenever the person needs emergency help for events such as a fall resulting in injury or problems with breathing, the button on the transmitter is pressed. This activates the home telephone to call or connect into the emergency response center. In most programs, the center attempts first to contact the individual by telephone, while other programs immediately activate "911" or the emergency medical system.

There are methods of organizing health related information in the home for use by police, paramedics, or others who respond in an emergency medical system. One example is "Vial of Life." Information is placed in a glass tube and stored in the refrigerator. A sticker, identifying the vial of life, is placed on the refrigerator door where it can be quickly spotted by emergency personnel.

Community, Commercial, and Organizational Services

Small businesses, large corporations, service organizations, churches, and others are becoming more involved in human service projects for the elderly population. Examples of services to the elderly include reduced service charges at banks, reduced bus fares during nonpeak rider hours, a percentage reduction on meals with a "membership" card, and a specific day of the week when senior citizens are given reduced prices at grocery stores and other businesses.

One way that businesses and agencies are becoming involved is by being informal gatekeepers. These *gatekeepers* recognize and report signs of vulnerability. Persons employed as meter readers for utility companies are examples of gatekeepers. They have regular routes in neighborhoods and know the usual activities. When a sign of vulnerability is noticed, such as a change in a person's behavior or the home environment, the meter reader calls the utility office which notifies a social service agency or other designated department.

Organizations are developing programs to improve the driving skills of the active aging. These courses are offered by driving schools, community colleges, and state safety councils. The American Automobile Association (AAA) offers a Senior Driver Improvement Program and the American Association of Retired Persons offers their 55 Alive/Mature Driving course for those over 55 years of age. Some states have enacted laws that require insurance companies to give reduced rates to those who take a defensive driving/accident prevention course.

Classes in driving are new to this population group. There were no driver education classes when they were younger. They purchased a driver's license through the mail or paid a quarter for one at a local store. Today, the "classroom-only" courses review rules and regulations of the roadways and also address the aging process as it relates to driving. Problems with reaction time and headlight glare are identified. Purchasing cars that are more manageable with bold numbers and large gauges are discussed.

Nurses' Role in Community Services for the Aging

Nurses in formal and informal roles have an important and growing role in advocacy for the aging. The more formal roles are obvious in employment as hospital discharge planners, case managers, and home health nurses. Nurses in every work place need to be alert to physical and social needs of older patients and the community services that will assist with those needs.

Informally, every nurse is a gatekeeper for older family members, neighbors, and friends. Nurses do not need to be employed by a health care facility to be advocates for aging members of our society. It is important that you become knowledgeable about key agencies in your com-

munity that will assist older adults into the community services system. At all times, you are an information and referral resource!

Summary

An aging population is a new experience for the United States. Therefore, legislation and programs to meet the elderly population are even newer. If these services are considered to be in their infancy, then perhaps we can see why there are problems with access to services, duplication of services, or gaps in services. However, thousands of senior citizens in every state are involved in one or more programs that keep them independent during their active aging years.

The first legislation directed specifically toward the elderly was the Social Security Act in 1935. It provided pension funds for people 65 years and older. Thirty years later the act was amended to provide health insurance for this population group. During the 1960s, an era of social revolt and reform, the elderly also benefited with the beginning of programs and services to meet health and social needs. Many of these programs were developed through the Older Americans Act of 1965.

The network for providing services to an aging population is not only new, it is complex. Services are provided through federal, state, and local public funds as well as private monies from businesses, corporations, religious communities, service organizations, and many volunteers. Often a service is funded and implemented through a cooperative effort of many sources. Sometimes several groups provide the same service; this may be a duplication of effort. A community needs to evaluate if they are each meeting a unique population group, or providing similar services while other needs are overlooked.

The Older Americans Act established the Administration on Aging which appropriates funds through regional, state, and area agencies on aging. The funds are directed toward health and social services in community-based programs.

Communities, businesses, utility companies, and neighborhoods are beginning to develop creative responses to assisting their elderly citizens. Businesses are providing some services more conveniently or at reduced costs. Other commercial organizations as well as neighborhoods provide gatekeeping types of services for the potentially vulnerable elderly. It is exciting to follow the development of each new program and observe how a creative design or the recapture of old traditions plays a part.

Nurses have expanding and new opportunities to be advocates for the active aging in formal and informal roles. The formal roles, those in employment, can provide referral information to assist patients when discharged from the hospital. Other examples include assisting with outpatient therapies or providing support for a patient's family when they need respite.

All nurses, whether in active or inactive practice, are information sources for the active aging. It is important for nurses to continue gathering information about health and social services for the elderly. The elderly have lived nearly a lifetime in a more simple health care delivery system. Now the system is more complicated and the services are expanding as the numbers of elderly grow. Nurses must assist the aging by putting them in touch with the programs and services that will keep them independent. Remember, some day they will be you!

For Discussion

- In a small group discussion identify services in your community that are specifically for active aging citizens.
- Invite a person from a public agency, business, or organization in order to learn about programs they implement for the elderly in the neighborhood or community.
- Visit several senior citizens or invite a group to your class. What programs are they involved in and what are their views on services for the aging?
- Visit a senior center, accompany a Meals-on-Wheels volunteer, or ride on a special senior transportation van to experience a service.
- Invite a home health nurse to share how community-based services assist the agency's clients.

Questions for Review

1. What were the objectives of the Social Security Act in 1935 and the Admendment in 1965?
2. What are two nutrition programs funded by the Older Americans Act?
3. What are situations that prevent elderly from getting services when they are needed?
4. What are four examples of services the older adult may get in the community? In the home?
5. What are the nurses' primary roles in community services that are provided for the elderly?

Unit 7
Patient Care Teaching for the Active Aging

Objectives

After reading this unit you should be able to:

- Recall concepts of patient teaching.
- Describe adaptations of patient teaching for the aging population.
- Discuss basic functional assessment of the active aging.
- Discuss approaches to promoting wellness in the active aging.
- Identify safety concerns in teaching active aging self care.

Headlines during the closing years of the 1980s:

SELF-NEGLECT IS GROWING PROBLEM FOR SENIORS

ELDERLY AMERICANS DO WELL LIVING ALONE

MORE DEMAND PREDICTED FOR CARE OF ELDERLY

ELDERLY DISMISSED QUICKER AND SICKER

AGING BABY BOOMERS STIR CONTROVERSY

GERONTOLOGY GROWING FAST AS A CAREER OF THE FUTURE

The issues, contradictions, and changing solutions bubbled over into nearly every newspaper, periodical, and television news and documentary program. Everyone learned about this new aging population, but not everyone was certain what the future held.

For nursing, the future projections hold some certainty; nurses will be assisting and taking care of more elderly in whatever practice setting is chosen. The changes in the health care delivery system in the last decade indicate that patients, including the elderly, will be responsible for more of their health care and receive more care and treatment outside the hospital. This concept dramatically increases the amount of patient teaching to be completed by nurses. In the past, nurses independently completed the cycle of the nursing process; some subjective data was obtained in assessment and evaluation. Now, and in the future, patients will be completing all stages of this process. Nurses will be teaching information and skills to assist in the process and monitor patient progress, figure 7-1.

This unit will review some of the fundamentals of patient teaching and focus on special considerations related to teaching the active aging population. These considerations include designing methods of teaching that focus on physical changes with aging, especially sensory deprivation. Language and communication barriers are important with all elderly, but especially with refugees and others who have come to the United States during their adult years.

Promoting wellness and the highest level of function requires a functional assessment by the nurse. This assists in determining how well a

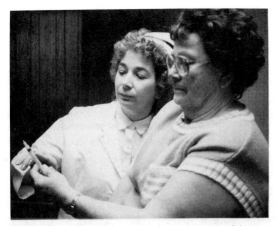

Figure 7–1 Nurses are doing more teaching as patients become more responsible for their own care.

person is able to manage day-to-day in his present environment. Teaching will emphasize and strengthen the patient's existing abilities; attitudes and motivation are keys in any patient teaching. Determining what the active aging want and need to know will assist in maintaining the desired wellness and compliance with new therapies.

Safety is paramount in all patient teaching. For the active aging, teaching safety in taking medications is extremely important. The 12 percent of the population over 65 years of age consumes 25 percent of the prescription drugs and numerous over-the-counter medications. Adequate nutrition and exercise are important in maintaining wellness and independence. Safety in patient teaching also includes encouraging the well elderly to have chronic conditions, as well as acute diseases, monitored by physicians, nurses, and other health professionals.

The myth that an elderly person cannot learn needs to be dispelled before discussing patient teaching for the active aging. There is no research that proves that the elderly become less intelligent or cannot learn new information. Due to the normal physical changes with aging, it may take some older adults more time to pro-

cess and respond to new information. Their slower reaction time may cause those who are uninformed about normal aging to believe the elderly cannot learn. Decreased blood flow to the brain, resulting in slower brain metabolism, and vision and hearing changes contribute to the slower or sometimes inaccurate, responses. Figure 7–2 identifies some myths about older people and learning.

Previous education and experience may influence elderly learning abilities. If a person had limited formal education and has not used reading skills to a great extent, reading and understanding some information may be difficult. Current popular methods of presenting information include computer software and video presentations. The elderly may have difficulty with these methods because they are not familiar with computers and VCRs. Could you explain or demonstrate the use of a butter churn, wringer washing machine, crank start automobile, or the application of a mustard plaster? We are products of our environment, experiences, and time on earth.

Chronic health problems may affect the elderly's ability to manage new information.

- All older people are fragile and weak.
- Older people gradually lose the functions necessary to perform most skills.
- Older people live in the past and have no interest in the present or the future.
- Older people need to have their decisions made for them.
- Older people cannot do anything for themselves.
- Older people cannot learn because they are set in their ways.
- Why should older people learn new things? Their productive years are over anyway!

Figure 7–2 Myths about older people and learning

Oxygen deprivation, related to chronic obstructive lung disease or cardiovascular problems are examples of conditions that result in continual fatigue and difficulty in concentrating, and present other obstacles to learning.

Some of the roadblocks to learning that the active aging experience will also be discussed. The elderly can, and most of the time want to, learn new information. They are especially motivated when it means continued independence.

For nurses, patient teaching can be challenging and exciting. You can see the results of your teaching and the efforts of your patients in their expression of accomplishment. Patient teaching can be one of the most rewarding parts of your nursing practice.

Review of Patient Teaching Concepts

Patient teaching has always been a part of basic patient care. It includes explanations of why and how procedures are done. Perhaps you have explained to a patient that the catheterization for residual urine will determine if she is emptying her bladder when voiding. Then you explained some basic steps of the procedure, the approximate time involved, and that you needed her cooperation. Other examples could be teaching a patient how to measure his intake and output, accurately read a scale to monitor diuretic therapy, or maintain aseptic technique when changing a bandage at home.

Patient teaching in recent years has incorporated more formal models and methods. Increased technology, advancement of medical and nursing specialties, and reduced inpatient days have been part of the reason for growth of patient teaching tools and nurses employed specifically for positions as patient educators. These nurses may have responsibilities for only diabetic, hypertensive, or ostomy patient teaching. Still, the bedside nurse, nurse generalist, clinic nurse, and others in positions of direct patient care are responsible for, and involved in, much basic patient teaching. They also collect data for the nurses involved in more formal patient education, and reinforce their teaching.

A safety factor for nurses, related to patient teaching, is the reality that you must know what you are talking about. For some situations, such as aseptic technique and hygiene measures, the principles are firmly planted in the nurse's daily activites. Nurses cannot expect to be current on every topic. Sometimes you may feel "rusty" on anatomy and physiology of a system, or a disease process. Before initiating patient teaching, consult references and other professionals to be certain you know the subject.

Principles of Learning

Principles of learning are important to review in recalling concepts related to patient teaching. In your nursing education you have focused on specific knowledge, skills, and attitudes. Patient teaching involves these same concepts in (1) presenting information, (2) determining task ability, and (3) determining the patient's ownership of the task or process. The key concept is the ability to complete a task. However, the patient also needs to have enough information and a willingness to comply to be successful in completing the task.

Patients need some information, but do not need to be experts! For example, they need to know about principles of handwashing and where to touch bandages in learning about aseptic technique. They do not need to know the history of germ theory or the names and characteristics of specific pathogens.

The ability of the patient to complete a task is important in patient teaching. However, unlike nursing education, the patient does not need to achieve a degree of efficiency. In some situations, accuracy or prioritizing steps is also not important. An example is a family member learning how to make an occupied bed. If the safety and comfort objectives are met, the time to complete the task is not important. The corners do not need to be mitered, or the linen assembled in a particular order.

Task ability also includes the person's physical abilities or limitations. The requirements of a task need to be analyzed to determine what specific physical attributes are needed. This may include strength, dexterity, endurance, or visual acuity, figure 7–3.

The patient's willingness to take an ownership in part of his care and comply with treatment may require some "detective work" by the nurse. In nursing education this principle of learning is identified as attitude and is developed through a study of professional etiquette and ethics, combined with personal attributes. For the patient this ownership of care may be short term and welcomed or rejected.

For one patient, the desire to take care of himself and to be independent is the motivation for learning. Another person may not want to learn about her disease or may believe she can not learn. Accepting information about her condition or successfully completing a part of the task, such as drawing insulin into a syringe,

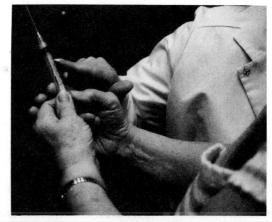

Figure 7–3 The nurse evaluates the patient's finger dexterity and visual acuity to manage injections.

may be the first step of ownership.

Table 7–1 compares principles of learning related to nursing practice and patient teaching. In "turning over" to patients tasks previously owned by nurses, one must realize that patients do not need to have the degree of skill and commitment that nurses have.

NURSE	PATIENT
KNOWLEDGE Theory: Studying underlying principles of several subjects to practice nursing	**INFORMATION** Most important facts: Learning adequate pieces of information to safely and successfully complete self care
SKILLS Performance: Practicing skills to an identified degree of accuracy and efficiency; includes multiple concurrent observations and tasks	**TASK ABILITY** Performance: Strength and skill to complete self care or simple procedure to meet basic objective; considers physical and psychosocial limitations
ATTITUDE Role model of nursing: Ownership of practice; dependable and responsible; behavior reflects ethics and etiquette of profession	**OWNERSHIP OF TASK** Compliance with care/therapy: Motivation to learn and complete self care; often short term effort and commitment; may require family support

TABLE 7–1 Comparing Principles of Learning in Nursing Practice to Patient Teaching

Steps of Patient Teaching

The Nursing Process is a helpful problem-solving tool in patient teaching as well as in other aspects of patient care. When there is appropriate individualized assessment and planning for patient teaching, the implementation should be smooth, and the evaluation an ongoing monitoring of progress. Good preparation helps you avoid "spinning your wheels" which would be a poor use of time for you and your patient. Patient teaching goals would not be met.

Assessment and planning include three steps that summarize concepts of beginning patient teaching. Step 1 — data collection related to the person as an individual — and Step 2 — data collection related to the person and his learning needs — are part of the nursing assessment. Planning includes Step 3 — individualizing patient teaching.

Step 1: Data Collection; The Patient as an Individual.

Nurses collect patient data in formal and informal ways. A formal method is collecting patient data for a hospital or outpatient admission form. During patient care, objective and subjective data are collected informally through conversation, direct questions, and verbal and nonverbal clues. This activity also plays an important part in patient teaching as you are "establishing rapport" and "developing a trust relationship." This relationship, in part, helps reduce anxiety and fear for future self care as well as current care and treatment.

Learning about some of the person's basic **values** and **priorities** helps determine where patient teaching may fit. Has personal health been a major lifetime concern? Is it a major concern now, or do family, work, finances, and other values have a higher ranking? The influence of health in values and priorities has developed as a result of previous experience with illness. This could include the course of an illness, results of therapy, or experiences with physicians, nurses, health care facilities, and other health care personnel.

The nurse utilizes listening and other therapeutic communication skills to obtain clues that will assist in developing productive successful patient teaching for each person. Part of the success is adapting to an individual's life style — how he approaches his environment and the world.

Step 2: Data Collection; The Patient and His Learning Needs.

The first piece of data collected needs to be what does the patient want to know or learn? There can be a conflict between nurse goals and patient goals in patient teaching. The nurse, for example, may have patient teaching focused on reinforcing a low salt diet and antihypertensives to lower blood pressure to prevent a stroke. The patient's focus is, "How am I going to pay for these expensive pills and get to the store to buy different food?" The nurse identifies the patient's need first, then networks community resources to assist with payment and transportation. Now the patient will be more willing to listen to nursing and medical goals.

The individual's **readiness to learn** is a second important piece of information. There are many potential blocks to a patient being able to learn, and then remember, information on how to complete a self care task. For example, a clue indicating that readiness to learn was not evaluated is a patient who can not recall or repeat information, or perform a return demonstration of a skill.

The person's anxiety or fear related to his condition, the learning environment, his ability to complete self care, or a number of other concerns can interfere with his learning. Depression or a stage of grieving, such as denial or anger, block the patient's ability to process information.

Readiness to learn is also inhibited by the health care delivery system of the past. The patient role has been passive for people seeking health care. It was like taking the car to the mechanic for repairs; people took their bodies to the doctor and hospital to be fixed. Most people do not get actively involved in car repairs, but ask general questions about problems and pay the bill. They did the same with health problems. Today, patients sometimes need to be told that they are responsbile for learning to take care of themselves in wellness and illness. For the elderly this may be a special concern because they were part of that passive system for many years.

The patient's current knowledge of his condition is important baseline data for specific patient teaching. His knowledge may be very limited and he may require some basic information about the anatomy and physiology of an organ or system, what happens with the disease process, and what is the usual care and treatment. For example, the patient may need to be given some basic information about her circulatory system before teaching her how to change a bandage on a stasis ulcer, figure 7-4.

For some people with chronic conditions, a change in health status or a new treatment method may involve learning new information or skills. When a person with diabetes is admitted to the hospital, the nurse collects data to determine the patient's level of knowledge and degree of self care. Some diabetics have been noncompliant for years, others keep well informed and are motivated to continue learning. For the informed patient, the new learning may relate to the use of a blood glucose monitoring device.

Limitations that may interfere with learning are often related to acquiring information or completing a task. Literacy, the ability to read and write, varies considerably within population groups in the United States. Factors that contribute to difficulties with these skills are also varied. They include access to education, level of education completed, ongoing use of literacy skills, primary language, and other influences. People are often embarrassed to admit that their reading and writing skills are weak, or that they cannot read. Nurses need to have the patient assist in determining what

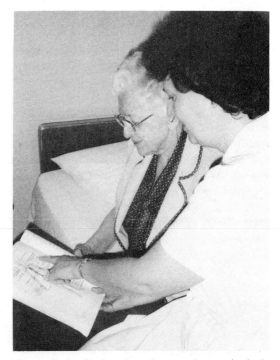

Figure 7-4   Patient learning needs may include information about anatomy and physiology.

teaching method would be most helpful, such as a video demonstration, a nurse demonstration, audio tapes, a series of pictures and drawings, or other methods.

Physical limitations may inhibit the ability to complete tasks. For example, a patient may be able to verbalize the steps and reasons for self administration of insulin. However, if arthritic joints make it difficult to manipulate the syringe or impaired vision prevents her from determining the correct dose, she cannot complete the task. Patient teaching must then include a family member or other support person in a team effort.

Data collection must include identifying support persons, such as family members, friends, neighbors, and others, who may be direct caregivers or be able to assist when needed. This is particularly important for persons living alone.

Step 3: Planning; Individualizing Patient Teaching. The first part of the plan is to **set realistic goals**. Goals need to identified by both the patient and nurse and be achievable within a reasonable time frame. Short-term objectives can meet long-term goals. All the items discussed in steps 1 and 2 need to be considered.

Prioritizing considers what the patient feels is important and what the nurse believes should be first. Many times the nurse and patient have to compromise. Two guides are helpful in this process. One is the use of Maslow's Hierarchy of basic human needs. If the patient is struggling to meet needs in the first physiological level, little if any teaching can be accomplished. The patient having difficulty breathing has no other concern. Information should be limited to a few basic facts. As people have more basic needs met, their readiness to learn also increases.

The second guide is to determine what the patient needs to know to complete a task. Often nurses are tempted to add many "nice to know" items of information. At some point in time a person may want this information, but when learning new information the extra data leads to confusion and frustration.

Information should be specific and presented in short time frames; a building block approach to learning. You need to repeat information either verbally or with a second teaching method. Ask for feedback to verify learning. Review important points. The time required for the patient to receive, absorb, sort out, and comprehend the information in his style will vary. It may depend on the severity of his illness, any physical limitations, and other influences.

Planning includes deciding what methods or ways of teaching information should be used. Utilizing more than one method is suggested. A combination of booklets to read, a demonstration by the nurse, and an audio tape provides a variety. It also stimulates interest, reinforces information, and avoids errors when one of the methods is not comprehended. For example, a

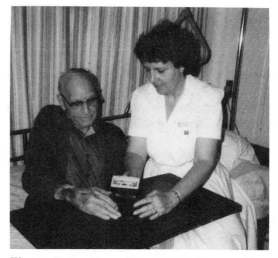

Figure 7-5 An audio tape of the procedure assists the patient with self care at home.

patient is dismissed from the hospital and will need to continue intravenous antibiotic therapy at home. He will be assisted by family members and receive periodic monitoring by a home health nurse. The patient and family are given information to read that explains the purpose and steps of the procedure. Later, the nurse answers questions related to the information, and demonstrates administering a dose of the medication and the heparin flush that keeps the needle patent. The patient practices the procedure in the hospital with nurse supervision; he is given an audio tape of the procedure when dismissed. The audio tape is the back-up plan for the first days when the patient may not feel very self-confident, figure 7-5.

Programs or packages of patient teaching tools have been developed for specific conditions such as diabetes, Crohn's Disease, hypertension, and many others. They are developed by foundations, pharmaceutical companies, insurance companies, and support groups. Hospitals, clinics, and other health care settings often develop information sheets that are designed to meet their protocol. Nurses are creative and often improvise in developing individualized patient teaching tools.

"Ordinary language" needs to be used both in written and verbal instructions. If medical terminology is required, the specific words or phrases should be explained simply and clearly. Nurses become adept at incorporating ordinary language and medical terminology into practice. The nurse questions the patient, "Have you urinated since you finished your test?" On the chart the nurse documents, "States voided following intravenous pyelogram." When the patient will be continuing self care at home, it is important to verify that all teaching methods were clear and comprehended by the patient.

Explaining the meaning of test results or medication directions is important. What is the meaning of positive and negative? Is negative good, bad, or no results? Taking a medication t.i.d. with meals does not mean 10 a.m., 1 p.m., and 8 p.m. A diuretic ordered for b.i.d. does not mean in the morning and before bedtime.

Planning a learning environment is important to promote successful patient teaching and learning. Sights and sounds that are disruptive are obstacles to learning. You also need to consider the method of teaching in assessing the environment. Adequate lighting is needed for reading information or visualizing markings on a syringe or container. A large open floor area near the bed is required to demonstrate wheelchair transfers. Privacy is a consideration in teaching ostomy care or how to change a mastectomy dressing. Table 7-2 summarizes the beginning steps of patient teaching.

Documenting Patient Teaching. All patient teaching must have ongoing documentation for safe and efficient care. Insurance companies, government agencies, and others also require it. Many health care facilities have flow charts or other tools to document patient teaching. You need to follow documentation guidelines learned in nursing courses and where you are employed. Figure 7-6 is one method of documenting patient teaching.

BEGINNING STEPS OF PATIENT TEACHING	
Step	**Objectives**
1. Data Collection: The Patient as an Individual	• Establish rapport and trust relationship. • Assess the person's values and priorities. • Identify previous experiences with illness.
2. Data Collection: The Patient and his Learning Needs	• Identify what the patient wants to know and learn. • Assess readiness to learn. • Identify current knowledge of condition and treatment. • Identify limitations that may be obstacles to learning. • Identify support persons who may assist patient.
3. Planning: Individualizing Patient Teaching	• Set realistic goals. • Set priorities with patient. • Identify what patient NEEDS to know. • Identify appropriate teaching methods. • Establish a learning environment.

TABLE 7-2 Summary of Patient Learning Steps

REGINA MEMORIAL HOSPITAL
PATIENT TEACHING FLOW SHEET

TEACHING AREA	DETERMINES BACKGROUND KNOWLEDGE	EXPLANATION (INSTRUCTIONS)	NURSES DEMONSTRATION	PAMPHLET	OTHER TEACHING METHOD	RETURN DEMONSTRATION BY PATIENT	PATIENT RESPONSE
			INITIAL AND DATE				
Diagnostic Test (List)							
Diet							
Intake and Output							
Ambulation							
Pain Medications							
TCH/Inspirometer							
TENS Unit							
Surgical Procedure							
Dressing/Incision							
Vital Signs							
Foley Catheter							
PROM/AROM							
Medications							
Drainage Tubes							
Oxygen Therapy							

#52G4   PATIENT TEACHING FLOW SHEET

Figure 7-6   Sample documentation tool for patient teaching
(Courtesy of Regina Medical Complex, Hastings, MN)

REGINA MEMORIAL HOSPITAL
PATIENT TEACHING FLOW SHEET

TEACHING AREA	DETERMINES BACKGROUND KNOWLEDGE	EXPLANATION (INSTRUCTIONS)	NURSES DEMONSTRATION	PAMPHLET	OTHER TEACHING METHOD	RETURN DEMONSTRATION BY PATIENT	PATIENT RESPONSE
	INITIAL AND DATE						
Continuous Irrigations							
PROM/AROM							
Medications							
Drainage Tubes							
Oxygen Therapy							
Ostomy Care							
Hickman Catheter							
Hyperalimentation							
Home IV Therapy							

#5204

PATIENT TEACHING FLOW SHEET

Figure 7–6   (Continued)

Adult Learning

Adults have a different focus on learning than children. They want the learning to be practical and meet the need of some personal, work, or social role. Learning for children is subject oriented; the information is often totally new. Their learning is a part of biological and social development. In the problem-solving approach to learning, adults relate information to previous experiences and want to compare new and old experiences.

Nurses should consider the focus of adult learning when planning patient teaching. The information has to be relevant to the patient. Methods also have to be practical, not boring, and must consider problem-solving needs. Memorizing insignificant data would not be a successful approach to adult patient teaching.

Designing Patient Teaching for the Active Aging

Patient teaching is customized to meet individual patient needs. Although people in a cohort may be more different than alike, general conclusions are made for baseline information. This is true when developing patient teaching for the elderly. It is based on what is considered to be the normal aging process.

There are physical changes and psychosocial factors that influence learning in the older adult. Physical changes that may challenge new learning include sensory deprivation, joint changes, a slowed nervous system, and cardiovascular changes that result in diminished endurance.

Aging Physical Changes Influence Patient Teaching

Impaired sensory perception, in vision or hearing, make learning more difficult for the older adult. Limited vision, for whatever reason, makes reading information difficult. Corrective lenses in some situations help if the elderly have had regular eye examinations and the prescription is current. Large print materials and adequate lighting with reduced glare are helpful, figure 7-7. If vision is severely limited, audio teaching tapes may be the best teaching tool.

Hearing loss is common — the higher pitched frequencies are more difficult for the older adult to hear. To assist this person to hear information, the nurse must assure that environmental noise is minimized, and remember to face the patient and speak in lower tones. It may be helpful to use hand gestures and pictures or other items to help with explanations. Family members and other support persons should be coached on behaviors that will assist the elderly to hear more clearly.

Dysarthria is difficulty in articulating sounds, which results in unclear pronunciation of words. It is related to aging changes in facial muscles and joints. Using therapeutic communication skills will help the nurse to verify the elderly's questions and comments. A combination of sensory limitations make conversations and social interactions particularly difficult for the very old elderly.

Sensory changes in taste and touch will probably not influence your methods of patient

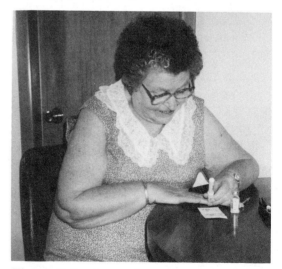

Figure 7-7 Assess the environment to meet learning needs of those with impaired sensory perception.

teaching. The diminished sensation of touch may play a role if you want to have the patient manipulate levers or buttons on equipment. The difficulty in distinguishing textures or surfaces, combined with decreased visual acuity, may lead to errors in operation of equipment. Teaching adaptations for the aging sensory system are summarized in table 7-3.

SENSORY CHANGES IN THE ELDERLY		
Change	Result	Teaching Adaptation
The EYE: muscles weaken lens flattens	decreased visual acuity presbyopia	Avoid small print Determine if reading glasses or corrective lenses are used and effective Use large print materials if more effective
lens becomes yellow, opaque	difficult to distinguish color differences, especially blues and greens	Use yellow or orange for teaching materials Use contrasting materials Avoid high gloss paper, laminated or shiny coverings Avoid colors that merge: white paper, supplies on white table top
iris becomes rigid	slower accommodation to light	Avoid glare, use adequate indirect lighting Allow adjustment time from dark to light area
retina blood supply is reduced	loss of center vision	Position to use peripheral vision Provide magnifying glass if effective Provide audio teaching tapes
The EARS: cerumen impacted tympanic membrane sclerosed	conduction hearing loss: sound transmission	Speak clearly, face person, facilitate lip reading
inner ear blood supply diminished: auditory nerve impairment	perception hearing loss: high frequency sounds; difficulty discriminating between words	Lower pitch of voice Reduce background noise Provide written as well as verbal instructions Assess audio sounds of video teaching tapes Assess use, condition, and effectiveness of hearing aid

TABLE 7-3   Teaching Adaptations for the Aging Sensory System

Generalized stiffening of joints, resulting in slower and sometimes more difficult movement, indicates that patient teaching for the elderly needs to progress at a slower pace. The combination of reduced cardiac output and central nervous system aging changes results in reduced psychomotor ability. Response time is increased and endurance time is decreased.

These musculoskeletal and cardiovascular changes suggest several adaptations in patient teaching for the elderly. Teaching sessions should be shorter in length than with younger persons. Each session should have a small number of specific key tasks or goals. Practice times, as well as teaching times, should be shorter and slower paced. Enough practice time should be allowed for the person to master the skill and promote a feeling of success and readiness to go on with additional learning, figure 7–8. Verbalizing each step as the task is completed helps the patient to concentrate and have more control over what is being done.

Praise and applause are always appropriate responses by the nurse assisting the elderly with patient teaching. They have also been caught in the myth that they can not learn. Step-by-step, most elderly can successfully achieve skills to maintain their independence. Table 7–4 summarizes teaching adaptations for the aging musculoskeletal and nervous systems.

Aging Psychosocial Factors Influencing Patient Teaching

Self image as a learner is a factor for everyone; it affects self-confidence. The elderly may not have been challenged with learning new skills for years. Many of today's elderly did not have more than an eighth or tenth grade formal education. Aging minority populations have had less formal education than many of their cohorts. Many elderly feel they do not have the learning ability to manage new skills. Most rely on problem-solving skills they have used during their lifetime. For example, someone may feel the need to write down everything you say, even if it is information described in a

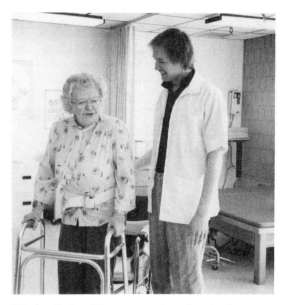

Figure 7–8 Allow more time for psychomotor tasks.

booklet. This preferred method of learning for them should be incorporated in the patient teaching plan. Figure 7–9 identifies some psychosocial factors that impede learning in the elderly.

Part of this use of previous learning styles is the ability to retrieve long-term memory more easily than short-term. Building on past experiences will help in learning new information and tasks. Learning for the elderly may also be affected by their many losses.

Loss of socially valued roles affect self-worth and in turn the ability to learn. Loss of personal and economic resources result in the elderly questioning the affordability of care and the value of learning new skills for self care. Long-term conditions such as chronic obstructive lung disease and diabetes require ongoing medications, supplies, and equipment. This indicates the need for community resources and patient teaching to manage the condition.

A primary language other than English makes new learning difficult for the elderly. Some elderly, during their youth, attended

MUSCULOSKELETAL/PSYCHOMOTOR CHANGES IN THE ELDERLY		
Change	**Result**	**Teaching Adaptation**
MUSCLES/TISSUES: Muscle mass is reduced, muscles weaken	Strength is reduced Endurance is shortened	Pace activities Plan short teaching sessions
Tissue elasticity lost; includes heart, blood vessels, other tissue	Reduced cardiac output: fatigues more quickly	Allow adequate practice time and sessions. Use aids with lifting to compensate strength
BONES/JOINTS: Bone density decreases	Pathological fractures occur	Evaluate learning activity
Cartilage erodes	Rib cage less mobile: exertional dyspnea increased	Pace teaching sessions, allow rest periods
Joints degenerate	Joints: stiff, painful	Provide comfortable seating/positioning Consider need for joint dexterity
NERVOUS SYSTEM: Neurons decrease in number	Difficulty in integrating functions	Consider need for fine motor movements
Cerebral vessels narrow	Blood flow reduced: forgetfulness	Use multiple teaching tools, reminders
Myelin sheath degenerates	Transmission time reduced: reaction time, reflexes allowed	Plan more time for tasks

TABLE 7–4   Teaching Adaptations for Aging Musculoskeletal and Nervous Systems

- Retirement or loss of a socially valued role
- Low self-esteem and lack of self-confidence
- Living on low and fixed income
- Having a primary language other than English
- Family and friends are not readily available
- Reduced ability to remember recently acquired information
- Losses, such as loved ones, friends, health, or sense of self-worth
- Long established habits, such as dietary patterns
- Low motivation; the task seems too overwhelming to handle
- Previous education and experience may be very different from today
- Unfamiliar with current teaching methods, such as computers and VCRs

Figure 7–9   Aging psychosocial factors that are obstacles to learning

schools that combined English and ethnic languages. Others came as immigrants and learned enough English to manage work and social roles. The elderly refugees arriving in the United States during the last two decades have had many adjustments to encounter. They experienced a new culture, a new language, and new expectations regarding the elderly.

The principles of adult learning apply to the elderly refugees as they do to other members of their cohort. They want the information to be practical and useful for everyday living to maintain their independence. The learning barrier for these elderly is not having the language skills to acquire and understand information about the health care delivery system. They are unable to learn about personal rights and safety. Many of their cohorts depend on life experiences to assist them with new learning. Elderly refugees have not mastered new cultural experiences and expectations to apply to adult learning and problem solving.

To facilitate patient teaching for elderly refugees and other ethnic populations, more bicultural and bilingual staff are needed in senior and community centers, clinics, and other health care facilities. Services need to be culture sensitive as these elderly prefer to maintain their culture and combine their traditional medicine with the medicine commonly practiced in the United States. Psychosocial influences in patient teaching for the elderly are summarized in table 7-5.

Nurses and Active Aging Patient Teaching

Nurses need to be sensitive to patient needs whatever the age or the situation. In the rapid pace of health care today, it takes a special effort to slow your pace to meet the learning needs of aging patients. Despite the time crunches, nurses must be advocates for the elderly, having a willingness to invest extra time and effort to assist older patients in maintaining independence.

Interviewing the Aging Patient

Techniques in interviewing patients require practice and an alertness to the special needs of an individual. The aging, as a population group, have unique characteristics to consider during an interview or time of data collection.

Data collection is an ongoing process of collecting information about a patient. A patient interview is also data collection, but is usually a planned time with a specific goal, and may include a special data collection tool. For example, at the time of hospital admission the nurse interview and assessment collects a wide variety of information to assist in the care of a patient during his stay. The discharge planning nurse interviews a patient to determine the resources needed to assist the patient at home, figure 7-10. A patient's first visit to a clinic or consulting physician will involve more interview time by the nurse. The case manager will have a lengthy interview or perhaps multiple interviewing sessions to complete a functional assessment and determine if the person can manage at home.

It is helpful, and perhaps more successful, to interview the elderly early in the day. There is a higher level of alertness, particularly in those beginning to have memory deficits or some degree of dependency. Also, events of the day which could be potentially stressful will not interfere with concentration. When arranging the interview, or prior to the first questioning, it is helpful to explain to the elderly patient what types of questions you will be asking, and why you are asking them. He also needs to understand that he has the right to not answer a question.

The environment needs to be considered for an interview just as it is during patient teaching. Assure comfort by carefully choosing the type of chair or other furniture. Discomfort experienced with arthritis or other physical conditions should be minimized as much as possi-

PSYCHOSOCIAL CHANGES IN THE ELDERLY		
Change	**Result**	**Teaching Adaptation**
Short-term memory deficit	Can remember things from the past in detail. Recent events may be absent or the individual covers up what he does not remember.	— Small reminiscence groups stimulate memory and offer peer communication. — Build on past experiences to help learn new information and perform new tasks. — Provide materials to take notes even though all information may be in booklets or pamphlets. — Repeat information. Demonstrate several times, and repeat again at a later time. Plan patient return demonstration.
Losses	Retirement may severely limit what the person can afford. Loss of social roles and of health may affect motivation to learn, self worth, and self-confidence.	— Use economic and community resources. — Teach the patient how to access resources. — Use group sessions or specific support groups to facilitate learning and to assist in learning that others have problems as well. — Allow time to grieve and heal as well as time to process new information. — Assess for signs of depression or fatigue and take appropriate action.
Primary language other than English	This makes new learning difficult because culture and expectations are different.	— Evaluate all new information and be certain it is practical and useful. — Bicultural and bilingual staff are needed to help facilitate teaching. Encourage those in the area to assist. — Services need to be culture sensitive.
Methods of teaching are different	Education and experience may be very different from today.	— Select the teaching method that is most appropriate for the individual. — VCR tapes or computers may be used if the person has used them in the past. — Incorporate past experiences; be aware of the individual's educational level.

TABLE 7–5   Teaching Adaptations Related to Psychosocial Changes in the Elderly

ASSESSMENT GUIDE FOR HOME HEALTH CARE SERVICES

Questions hospital nurses should consider before discharging their patients.

- **PREVIOUS HISTORY**
  - Was the patient receiving home health services or help from a caregiver prior to this hospitalization?
  - If yes, why were they receiving services, and does that reason still exist?
- **CURRENT STATE OF HEALTH**
  - Does the patient need a periodic assessment of a body system (such as edema, BP, wound healing)?
  - Is the patient on new medications or have significant changes in current medications occurred that could require assessment of side effects or response?
  - Does the patient require a skilled procedure such as a sterile dressing change?
  - Has the patient experienced a major change in body image (such as amputation, colostomy, paralysis, cancer diagnosis)?
  - Does the patient or family need more teaching of a procedure, new diet, or new diagnosis like diabetes?
- **ACTIVITIES OF DAILY LIVING**
  - Does the patient need help to perform personal care activities such as bathing, dressing, toileting, eating?
  - Does the patient need assistance of another person with ambulation?
  - Does the patient have some functional limitations that require assistance?
- **SOCIAL SUPPORT SYSTEMS**
  - Does the patient live alone?
  - If yes, does the patient have family or friends available to help when needed?
- **ENVIRONMENTAL**
  - Will the patient need help in managing the home surroundings, for example cooking and housekeeping, in their current physical condition?
  - Are there stairs, upstairs bathrooms or bedrooms or other obstacles which they are currently unable to manage?
- **MENTAL**
  - Does the patient have periods of confusion or extensive forgetfulness?
  - Does the patient seem anxious about the discharge or being able to manage at home?
  - Has the patient had problems coping with this hospitalization?
  - Does the patient have a history of emotional problems or treatment for depression?

If You Answered YES to Any of These Questions Discuss Home Care With Your Patient, the Physician, Discharge Planner, and a Home Health Care Agency.

Home Health Agencies Offer Skilled Nursing, Home Health Aides, Companions, Physical Therapy, Occupational Therapy, Speech Pathologists, Equipment, and Supplies.

Services May Be Round the Clock or One Hour Visits Planned to Meet the Needs of the Patient.

Figure 7–10 Sample assessment guide to determine a patient's abilities and limitations (Courtesy of Shamrock In-Home Nursing Care, Inc., Rochester, MN)

ble. Other environmental considerations include adequate lighting, temperature, reducing noise, and placement of chairs to facilitate communication. Three to four feet is usually a comfortable distance to promote trust and meaningful dialogue. Be sure you are at eye level with the patient. This also promotes emotional comfort as well as enhancing verbal communication; the patient may need to lip-read to understand.

It is wise to carefully utilize therapeutic communication techniques. Open-ended questions, such as, "Tell me how you manage to wash up and get dressed every morning," promote more lengthy responses. When you want more direct answers, ask the question differently, such as, "What hours of the day do you take your water pill?" Be alert to how you are framing your questions so you avoid "providing an answer" or "passing judgement" during the interview. Examples are, "Do you have sharp stomach pains after every meal?", or "Are you really taking all that antacid?" Also note how patients ask questions and frame their comments. It may provide you with clues regarding their understanding of medications, if their support system is strong, and other valuable data.

There are advantages and disadvantages to having a family member or other persons present during a patient interview, figure 7–11. One advantage is accuracy of information when you question the reliability of the patient's answers or comments. Perhaps the patient experienced a stroke and cannot recall events prior to a fall. The family member is a witness who can describe the events. One disadvantage is that the elderly person may allow the family member to "talk for him." You will be obtaining the family member's perception of the patient's problems or needs. The interview could become patronizing or dehumanizing, with the patient only indirectly involved.

Attitudes toward aging by the nurse interviewer and the elderly patient influence the interview and the outcomes. The elderly are sensitive to reactions of others. Nurses need to have confronted their own views on aging.

Negative attitudes or stereotyping, such as "all elderly are dependent and frail," are reflected in conversation and body language. The nurse also must determine the attitudes of the patient toward his own health and aging.

Patience is a key to obtaining cooperation from the patient and having a successful interview. You need to take time to permit a narrative of their perception of events as well as some reminiscence in taking a history. However, it is important to keep the interview on track. Use therapeutic communication skills to clarify information and direct the conversation toward additional data collection.

Practicing patience with clear concise questioning is very important with telephone triage. *Telephone triage* is sorting data given over the telephone by the patient or family. The objective is to determine the urgency and type of medical attention needed. This method of interviewing is implemented primarily by clinic nurses. Home health nurses and nurses working in out-patient services may complete telephone triage when receiving calls from patients. It is especially important with the elderly to clarify and validate their comments and questions. Sometimes an emergency medical system needs

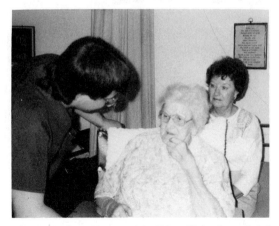

Figure 7–11 Determine if it will be beneficial for a family member to be present during an interview.

to be activated; other times the person has questions about medications or symptoms.

Establishing a mutual trust is another key to the whole process of interviewing. History taking can be lengthy if a considerable amount of data is needed from all areas of aging: biological, sociological, and psychological. A functional assessment will require information from these areas and may take more than one interview session. The initial interview will assist in determining the endurance time of the patient, and if family members or others should be present during all or parts of future interviews. A series of interviews will also allow the patient time to develop a trust relationship. Figure 7–12 summarizes the process of interviewing elderly patients.

Active Aging Functional Assessment

A *functional assessment* involves an interview and examination of a person to determine his/her ability to manage activities of daily living. For the active aging, this includes the ability to manage day-to-day activities independently in the home and community. The interview and examination includes physiological, psychological, and sociological aspects of aging.

Activities of Daily Living (ADLs) are daily self-help tasks that include hygiene activities, grooming, eating, toileting, and limited mobility. Limited mobility means getting out of bed or a chair and ambulating short distances. The persons ability to accomplish these tasks may require some assistance to remain independent.

Instrumental Activities of Daily Living (IADLs) are skills that are necessary to interact with the environment and community and require use of equipment and a degree of mobility and endurance. These tasks may include light housekeeping and laundry, preparing one's own meals, communications (telephone and mail service), and managing money. The IALDs require an ability to manage some problem solving.

- Be in touch with own views on aging
- Plan interview for early in the day
- Keep interview sessions as brief as possible
- Explain types of questions that will be asked
- Assure physical comfort: furniture, body position, room temperature
- Reduce environmental noise
- Position yourself facing the person and at eye level
- Assess appropriateness of family members participating in interview
- Practice patience; allow reminiscence
- Plan more than one session when extensive information is needed

Figure 7–12 Key points when interviewing aging patients

Nurses in hospitals, clinics, outpatient services, home care, and other settings perform functional assessments with active aging patients. They utilize formal and informal methods of assessment. Perhaps your patient, recovering from a fractured hip, tells you she is fearful of steps and does not feel she is doing well in physical therapy. Earlier, during personal care, she told you about living alone in a third floor apartment; the older building does not have an elevator. This information is part of a functional assessment. You need to document the information and report to the primary nurse or discharge planning nurse. Your patient may need to have extended recovery in a convalescent center, receive community services at home, or be provided with other services that will enable her to return to independent living.

Physical Aspects of Functional Assessment

Functional assessment focuses on the person rather than on an illness or condition. Physical assessment is part of the process. You need to evaluate the patient's ability to complete self care as well as manage therapies independently at home. This part of the assessment also determines if a physical condition might interfere with psychosocial functioning. For example, a patient states, "I don't need to think about driving the car, I'm not going out of the house." Further questioning reveals his fears of going out into the community or interacting socially because of his new ileostomy. In another example, a clinic patient states he will not give himself an afternoon dose of insulin. The problem, you discover, is not the added dosage or injection, but the possibility of having to give himself an injection in a restaurant or other public place.

Psychosocial Aspects of Functional Assessment

Data collection for a functional assessment related to psychosocial aging includes the patient's environment beyond the hospital or clinic. Important data collection includes information about the patient's home, his support system, his problem-solving ability, and his mental health status. Case managers, discharge planning nurses, home health nurses, and others interview extensively or visit patients' homes to determine patient needs, which may include additional family or community services.

Nurses in clinics and other outpatient areas also interview with a focus on potential vulnerable situations in the patient's home environment. "Soak in the bathtub for 20 minutes, 3 times a day," the clinic patient is told. Does the patient have a bathtub? Could he get in and out of a bathtub if he has one? Without following through the assessment and patient teaching, health teaching and therapies may not achieve the desired results. Perhaps the patient's apartment has only a shower. Unless reasons for treatments are explained, the patient does not have a foundation or baseline to consider them in relation to his home or life style.

Generally, a person's home needs to be considered as the environment in which daily

activities are managed. Every room and all aspects of furnishings, lighting, ventilation, safety of pathways, access to appliances, and countless other items need to be analyzed when considering the activities of a particular individual. For example, your patient has a generalized right-sided weakness following a stroke. He lives in a two-story home. Your visit with him will determine if there are railings on stairways, if grab bars should be installed in the tub/shower area, or if he can manage a dial telephone.

Nearly half of the elderly population have gait or mobility problems. This has a great impact on their ability to transport or move themselves around, even in a familiar environment. In many situations, physical limitations need to be considered in light of maintaining of a quality of life rather than rehabilitation to a previous life style, figure 7–13.

The location of this home environment is another consideration. Is it one level on the ground floor, or a walk-up with no elevator? Is this home in a neighborhood with convenient access to purchasing food, clothing, health care services, and other needs? For example, a patient is dismissed from a large metropolitan hospital following cardiovascular surgery. He is to have laboratory tests every other day for ten days, followed by weekly tests to monitor drug therapy. The laboratory facility closest to his

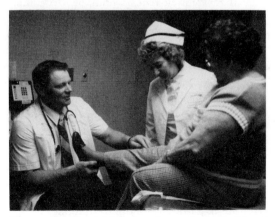

Figure 7–13 Managing her osteoarthritis at home will be a part of patient teaching.

farm home is a 30-mile drive. He cannot drive during this early convalescence and his wife never learned how to drive a car.

Another consideration in the psychosocial aspects of functional assessment is the person's support system. Even when an active elderly individual, or couple, manages independently, there must be a back-up support system. This is very important when one member of the couple is dependent and the other needs a time of respite.

The nurse determines the support persons, their roles and potential roles, and the degree of personal commitment. Many "first-line" support persons have been identifed in other discussions. They are usually a spouse, adult children, other relatives, neighbors, and friends. During the interview and functional assessment, the nurse may discover other caring individuals that are willing to assist on an interim basis or in a respite role. Some of these individuals could be former co-workers, religious or social group members, or a retired nurse who lives in the community.

Functional assessment becomes a complex evaluation because the three areas of aging are interrelated. For example, confusion in an independent active aging individual is an important part of data collection when determining his continued independent status. Is his confusion related to a physiological conditon, drug therapy, social isolation, or grieving and depression?

It is often difficult to "draw the line" between safe and unsafe situations related to confusion and vulnerability. Nursing and family judgements are utilized in the attempt to determine the elderly person's ability to remain independent and at home. The ability to remove oneself from danger becomes a concern both for physical and mental safety. Can the elderly reason and problem-solve a situation? Are they vulnerable physically or mentally? How have they managed compounded losses? Do they demonstrate signs of depression and a premature giving up? Figure 7-14 summarizes the parts of a functional assessment of the active aging.

Promoting Wellness in the Active Aging

Promoting wellness became the rally slogan of health care in the 1980s. This called for every generation to focus on lifestyle choices that promote health and longevity. Although the motivation of society should be for health alone, much of the drive was because of the cost of illness care.

Two keys to a healthy old age are exercise and good nutrition, figure 7-15. If a person has grasped these concepts during younger years, he will enter old age in a healthier state than many of his cohorts. However, initiating these habits in later years will also improve quality of life.

Moderate daily exercise improves physical and mental health. It improves cardiovascular function which in turn improves the status of all other systems. Walking is the best kind of exercise for the active aging. It does not require any special equipment. Like any other age group, the elderly should wear good fitting shoes. A physician may be consulted if there are questions regarding the need for special walking shoes. The active aging who have been involved in more active sports, such as tennis and running, can probably continue more strenuous activities well into later years.

"Good" nutrition is the second key to a healthy old age. The active aging should be guided to consume a basic four diet. Increased fiber is important for elimination problems experienced by the aging and has also been idenified as a potential factor in reducing cancer risks. Patient teaching related to nutrition includes basic information about essential nutrients, portion sizes, and how to read labels when purchasing food.

Generally, as people become older, they need fewer calories to maintain adequate body weight. With decreased activity, a 75-year-old man requires about 400 calories less per day, and a 75-year-old woman about 500 calories less per day than when they were in their 40s. Between ages 50 and 75, most can decrease

FUNCTIONAL ASSESSMENT

Goal:	Determine person's ability to independently manage day-to-day activities: personal care and interaction with environment
Data Collection:	• Activities of Daily Living (ADLs) personal hygiene grooming eating toileting ambulating short distances • Instrumental Activities of Daily Living (IALDs) preparing own meal laundering own clothes light housekeeping communication (telephone, mail) managing money
Process:	Interview with person Observation of person and environment Assess abilities and limitations Identify support persons and resources

Figure 7–14   A summary of the functional assessment process

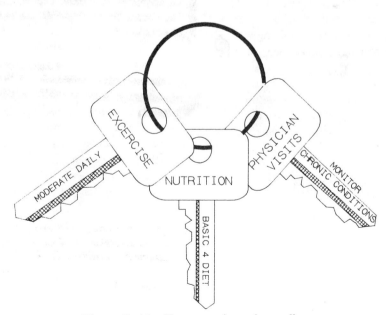

Figure 7–15   Keys to active aging wellness

their calorie intake by 200 calories per day to maintain body weight.

Adequate water intake is also part of good nutrition. The active aging are encouraged to drink 2000 to 2500 cc of fluid daily. It is important for the many medications the elderly consume and for normal body functioning. They are often reluctant to drink adequate fluids because of stress incontinence, problems with awakening at night, or other complaints. Nurses should encourage the elderly to drink fluids earlier in the day and also explain to them the function of fluids, especially water.

The elderly, as they age, tend to have more chronic health problems and are at risk for more acute illnesses. In addition to the two keys of healthy living, the active aging should be encouraged to monitor their health regularly with a family physician and comply with prescribed therapies for chronic conditions. This will assist them in maintaining their current health status. Therapeutic diets such as low sodium, low cholesterol, reduced calorie, and diabetic diets are examples of diet therapy for chronic health problems.

Teaching basic health habits related to exercise and nutrition and observing happy, healthy, older adults is part of the reward of nursing practice. Nurses reinforce the teaching of dietitians as well as the explanation of treatments by physicians. You are an information and referral person, and an advocate for the active aging. This means you will be teaching healthy life styles at the patient's bedside, in his home, and in your neighborhood.

Safety Concerns in Teaching the Active Aging

It has been identified that there may be a conflict in views between the nurse and patient in establishing goals and planning care. The nurse views safety as a primary concern, but the patient may have a different perception of a situation. The patient, for example, may feel that getting to the bathroom by himself is very important. The nurse has focused on raised side rails because the patient received a narcotic analgesic. Nurses are responsible for identifying potential safety concerns, making them known to the patient, and incorporating appropriate intervention in patient teaching.

There are several methods, or tools, you may use to organize your data. Figure 7-16 illustrates the most common methods. You are probably familiar with some of these from your nursing education. Be sure you are collecting data for psychosocial as well as physical needs. Remember, assisting the elderly to remain in an active aging status requires a focus on the whole person and his environment, not just his illness.

Medications and the Active Aging

Special consideration in patient teaching should be focused on the active aging and the medications they are taking. The elderly average two to four perscriptions per person. Two areas of concern regarding safety in administering medications to the older adult are the need for increased patient teaching, and increased awareness of effects of drugs on the elderly by health professionals.

Patient teaching should be broadened and reinforced in areas of basic information about the purpose of the medication, how it affects the body, and specific information about taking the medication. Some of the problems with compliance indicate that nurses and other health professionals must verify that the patient has received information about medications, figure 7-17. Questions should be asked, and feedback obtained, to determine that the patient's understanding is complete and accurate.

It is important for nurses and others involved in interviews with the elderly to obtain a complete medication history. Some of the problems relate to self-medication with *over-the-counter* (OTC) drugs. These are medications that can be purchased without a prescription at drug or grocery stores. The most common OTC medi-

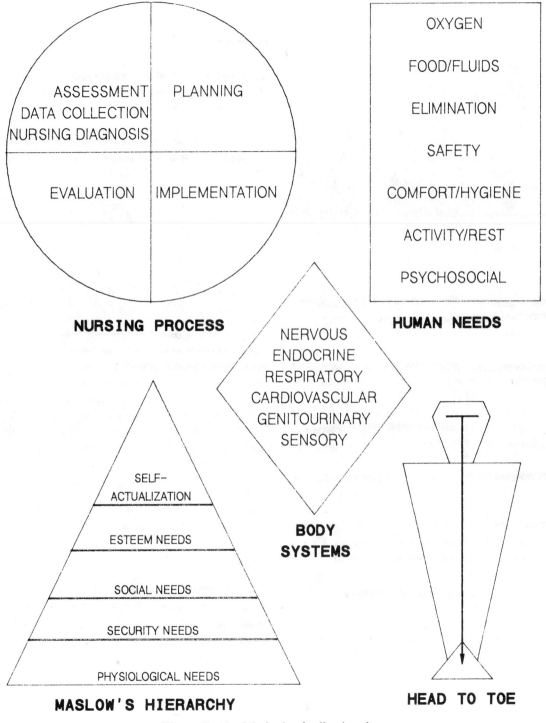

Figure 7-16   Methods of collecting data

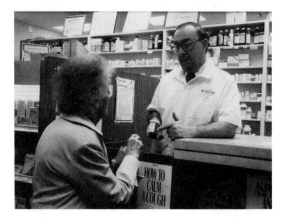

Figure 7–17 A pharmacist explains special directions for taking medications.

cations used by the elderly are laxatives, antacids, analgesics, and vitamins. Many older adults do not consider taking these drugs as taking "medications." Their perception of medication is a prescription written by their physician. Interviews need to verify prescriptions as well as OTC drugs to assess for interactions and other potential problems.

Many elderly do not understand why they are taking a medication, which may lead to noncompliance. There are some estimates that one out of five prescriptions are never filled. The cost of the medication may be a factor. However, some elderly will not have the prescription filled with a less costly generic product, even when instructed to do so. Their belief is if it costs more it must be better.

Self-medication may also mean taking another person's prescription medication. An elderly woman, for example, has her blood pressure checked at a health fair screening. The reading is high, and she admits to the nurse it has been high and she should see her doctor. She returns home and takes one of her husband's antihypertensives.

Some elderly mix several prescriptions in one bottle. They include enough for several days; they do not want to carry several bottles.

One pill bottle may be difficult to open and the medication is poured into another bottle that has a different label. Prescription medications are "saved." Often the elderly quit taking an antibiotic or other medication when they feel better and before all the medication is taken. Later, they self-medicate when a repeat episode occurs.

These behaviors do not mean that health professionals are negligent in patient teaching. It is a combination of events. Sometimes the teaching is not adequate, or not understood by the patient. Other times, the patient chooses not to comply. This underscores the need for a thorough medication history and clear concise patient teaching regarding medications. Figure 7–18 summarizes some problems with abuse and misuse of medications by the elderly.

The second concern is the need for increased awareness of the effects of medication on elderly body systems. In reviewing the normal aging process you learned that there is a decline in liver and kidney function. The rate of glomerular filtration in the kidneys begins to decline in the 40s. This means that by the 70s and older, drugs will not be eliminated as rapidly. The percentage of water in the body decreases with age and can result in a higher concentration of drugs in the system. The slowing of the metabolic process can result in an exaggerated response or a longer response time from medications. All of these possibilities indicate there is the potential for a normal adult dose of a medication to be toxic in the elderly. This is enhanced with the multiple drugs taken by this age group.

Some common side effects related to the higher concentration of "normal" doses of medications include agitation, confusion, poor appetite, and lethargy or depression. These are common behaviors of other problems, so may be overlooked. Nurses need to be alert to physical and emotional changes in their patients and document and report the observations. This assists physicians in evaluating drug therapy. Remember to consult drug references

ELDERLY'S ABUSE AND MISUSE OF MEDICATIONS

- Sharing medications
- Self-medicate
- Save medications, especially antibiotics
- Stop taking medications when feeling better
- Mix several medications in same bottle
- Place medication in another bottle having different prescription label
- Double dose:
  - generic and "trade" pills look different
  - memory problems: do not remember if pill was taken, take a second pill
- Poor storage: kitchen or other warm area
- Vague with medication history:
  - do not consider OTC purchases of medications
  - do not recall names of medications or reasons for taking
  - do not relate complaints to side effects: do not know or remember side effects
- Errors with taking multiple medications:
  - impaired vision
  - memory problems
- Other conflicts:
  - sees several physicians
  - prescriptions filled at more than one site
  - medications not monitored by single pharmacist

Figure 7–18   Some problems that occur with elderly taking medications

to review and update information on the medications your patients are taking.

Normal laboratory values are based on averages of the physiology of 20- to 40-year olds. With the elderly, it is difficult to determine if the lab test results reflect a medication, a disease process, or the influence of normal aging. When reviewing lab results, as a part of your data collection for planning care or patient teaching, remember that acceptable levels for the elderly may be different from the normals listed. Elevated levels may reflect the normal physiological changes in the aging body. However, some elevations are not acceptable because of the change in absorption, metabolism, and elimination of medications. Table 7–6 summarizes information about medications and laboratory tests and the elderly.

Patient teaching will not include as much information about laboratory and diagnostic tests because patients do not need to have an extensive involvement in the procedures. There are three items of information you need to give to the patient. The first is basic information about the test and why it was ordered. Second, pre-test instructions should be reinforced. For example, the patient should not eat or drink for eight hours prior to the test. Be sure to add the exclusion of water if it is appropriate. Some people do not think that water "counts." Finally, focus on any information that will assist the patient to be compliant with the tests and care. Explain why repeat tests may be necessary.

It is a challenge for nurses and other health care professionals to collect data related to the sometimes complex nature of elderly health care, then sort out the teaching needs to assist in maintaining independence. The rapid changes in diagnostics and almost daily changes in drug therapies add to the challenge.

DRUG THERAPY IN THE ELDERLY		
Drug	**Nursing Considerations for the Elderly**	**Laboratory**
Cardiovascular drugs: 1. Cardiac glycosides and antiarrhythmics digitoxin digoxin deslanoside atropine pronestyl quinidine *Lanoxin* *Mepitil*	— Daily maintenance dose for the elderly may be smaller than for younger adults. Efficiency of organ function is not as great in the older adult, which affects absorption rate and excretion rate. — Usual signs and symptoms of drug toxicity may be masked by other conditions and may be life threatening. Observe for signs of nausea, vomiting, decreased appetite, fatigue, visual disturbances, or other signs of toxicity. — Daily apical and radial pulse for a full minute should be monitored with significant changes reported to the physician. Instruct patient and responsible family member about drug action, dosage regimen, how to take the pulse, and what to do when signs of drug reaction take place. — Teach the patient and his family that when refilling prescriptions, one brand should not be substituted for another. — Document baseline data before beginning therapy to aide the physician in subsequent dosage adjustments	Therapeutic blood levels of digoxin range from 0.5 to 2.5 mg/ml. Calcium, potassium, and magnesium levels are monitored. EKG
2. Antianginal drugs isosorbide nifidipine nitroglycerin propranolol verapamil erythrityl tetranitrate	— Watch for signs of headache and visual disturbances. — May cause orthostatic hypotension. Advise to change positions slowly and to lie down when dizzy. Blood pressure should be monitored twice daily. — Supplies of medications should be replaced every three months to assure maximum potency. — Nitroglycerin comes in many forms. Patients need complete and detailed instructions for safe use to achieve maximum effect from the drug. — Duration of effect may be prolonged in the elderly. — Drugs in this group should be used with caution in those who have impaired liver or kidney function.	Lab values are not indicated.

TABLE 7–6 Responses of Elderly to Frequently Prescribed Medications

DRUG THERAPY IN THE ELDERLY		
Drug	**Nursing Considerations for the Elderly**	**Laboratory**
3. Antihypertensive drugs atenolol captopril hydralazine dydrocholoride methyldopa metoprolol tartrate	— Use cautiously in those who have cardiac failure or renal insufficiency. — It is important to record accurate baseline data before therapy is begun. Sitting, standing, and lying blood pressure readings will be essential as many elderly experience orthostatic hypotension without drug therapy. Side effects include hypotension and sedation. The drugs also tend to mask symptoms of shock. — Blood pressure should be measured daily. A responsible family member can be taught to take and record these readings. — The best therapeutic effect from many of these medications may be achieved by regular daily dosage in the evening in order to avoid the symptoms of drowsiness. — Patients should be taught about the disease process so that they understand the importance of taking their medications even when they are feeling well.	Monitor CBC before and during therapy to detect hemolytic anemia.
Respiratory Drugs 1. Spasmolytic drugs aminophylline theophylline *Broncho dilator*	— These drugs should be used cautiously in the elderly with congestive heart failure or other circulatory impairment. — The elderly should be warned that dizziness is a possible effect from the drug before the start of therapy. — Patients should be questioned closely and warned that the use of over-the-counter remedies combined with these drugs may result in excessive central nervous system stimulation. — Daily dosage in the elderly may need to be decreased due to slower metabolism and excretion rates. — Those who have difficulty swallowing pills or capsules should not chew time-released capsules but open the capsule and sprinkle the beads over soft foods and then swallow.	Therapeutic theophylline plasma levels are 10 to 20 mcg/ml.

TABLE 7–6   (Continued)

DRUG THERAPY IN THE ELDERLY		
Drug	**Nursing Considerations for the Elderly**	**Laboratory**

2. Antihistamine drugs
    diphenhydramine
    methdilazine
    cyproheptadine
    Seldane
	— Use with caution in those with glaucoma, peptic ulcers, hypertension, or cardiac disease.
	— May cause confusion, insomnia, and vertigo in the elderly.
	— These drugs may cause GI distress in the elderly. Advise them to take with food or milk.
	— Photosensitivity may be experienced by the elderly. They should be cautioned to avoid prolonged exposure to the sun or to be well protected during therapy.
		No laboratory tests are indicated.

Analgesic drugs
1. Nonsteroidal anti-inflammatory agents
    ibuprofen
    indomethocin
    naproxen
    phenylbutazone
    sulindac
	— These drugs should be used cautiously in those with history of cardiac decompensation, renal disease, hepatic dysfunction, or thyroid disease.
	— They should be taken with food or milk to avoid GI distress and used with great caution in those with a history of ulcer disease. Patients should be watched closely for signs of tarry stools which might indicate GI bleeding.
	— These drugs should not be used for those with nasal polyps or those who are known asthmatics.
	— The elderly should be monitored carefully for weight gain, increase in blood pressure, and peripheral edema as these drugs cause sodium retention.
	— Periodic eye exams during therapy are recommended as the drugs may cause visual disturbances.
	— Short-term therapy will usually reduce the incidence of serious side effects in the elderly.
		Hemoglobin and bleeding time and CBC to monitor for blood loss.
		
		Check renal and hepatic function during long-term therapy.

2. Narcotic drugs
    codeine
    meperidine
	— Should be used with extreme caution in all elderly as they may depress all body systems and mask many symptoms and conditions.	No laboratory tests are indicated.

TABLE 7–6 (Continued)

DRUG THERAPY IN THE ELDERLY		
Drug	**Nursing Considerations for the Elderly**	**Laboratory**
2. Narcotic drugs (continued)	— When codeine is used in cough syrups and in combination drugs for treatment of pain, the elderly should be reminded that the drug is constipating so that appropriate therapy can be instituted. — The use in elderly should be monitored very closely to avoid addiction, depression, and allergic reaction.	
Antibiotic drugs	— Many cause diarrhea, nausea, vomiting, and fungal infections. The elderly should be closely monitored for signs of dehydration. — The patient should be instructed to take the drug exactly as prescribed, even after he feels better. The entire quantity should be taken and not saved for the next illness, or shared with family or friends with similar symptoms. — Always check for allergies before beginning administration of these drugs. Then administer with caution and monitor closely for signs of allergy. — Many of these drugs can and should be taken with food to minimize the GI symptoms that are common. Pharmacy should label the bottle with a sticker to indicate whether or not to take with food. — If fever or chills develop or rash occurs, the drug should be stopped immediately and the physician called. Allergies in the elderly can be life threatening. *Anaphylactic*	Obtain cultures for sensitivity before the first dose is given.
Anticoagulant drugs	— Elderly should be monitored closely for bleeding gums, bruising, nosebleeds, hematuria, and tarry stools. They are especially sensitive to the warfarin effect and dosages need to be titrated carefully. — All aspirin products should be avoided. Encourage the patient and responsible family member to be sure to read labels on over-the-counter medications.	Regular prothrombin times. The therapeutic level is 1½ to 2 times control.

TABLE 7–6   (Continued)

DRUG THERAPY IN THE ELDERLY		
Drug	**Nursing Considerations for the Elderly**	**Laboratory**
Anticoagulant drugs (continued)	— Encourage the patient to read labels on food products. Those containing vitamin K may cause altered response to the drugs. — Encourage patients to use an electric razor for shaving to avoid nicks and to brush teeth with a soft tooth brush to avoid damaging the gums. — The drug should be taken at the same time every day to achieve the maximum effect and to help assure compliance.	
Over-the-counter drugs 1. Analgesics	— Can be very dangerous as they are used without supervision. Many cause liver, kidney, and GI problems; and blood discrasias, visual disturbances, skin rashes, tinnitus, and hearing loss with chronic use. — They can be used to treat minor aches and pains, though medical advice should be sought if symptoms persist. — Can be used to treat fever though febrile episodes can be very serious in the elderly and medical advice should be sought and the source of the fever identified. — Because of many possible drug interactions, those patients who are taking prescription medications should consult with the physician or pharmacist before taking any analgesic. — Elderly should be closely monitored for signs of bleeding from gums or GI tract or bruising when long-term therapy is used.	No laboratory indicated, except in long-term therapy, when the hemoglobin or prothrombin time are advised to detect blood loss or alteration in clotting time.
2. Antacids	— These should be used with caution in the elderly with decreased GI motility, dehydration, fluid reduction, chronic renal disease, and suspected intestinal obstruction.	No laboratory tests are indicated.

TABLE 7–6 (Continued)

DRUG THERAPY IN THE ELDERLY		
Drug	**Nursing Considerations for the Elderly**	**Laboratory**
2. Antacids (continued)	— Those containing aluminum can cause constipation and those containing magnesium can cause diarrhea. Encourage the patient or the responsible family member to read labels and be aware of either in patient and treat accordingly. — Many of the antacids prohibit the absorption of medications by binding with them. Check with the physician before taking any of these products. — Many are very high in sodium. Encourage the patient to read labels carefully to avoid problems with those who must limit sodium intake.	
3. Laxatives and stool softeners	— Rather than rely on laxatives and stool softeners, encourage the patient to increase exercise, intake of high fiber foods and cereals, and fluid, especially water. — If there are symptoms of nausea or vomiting, or abdominal pain, do not give these medications. Encourage the patient to seek medical advice. — Encourage the patient to wait for a response to the drug rather than to take more. Many become laxative dependent by expecting the bowels to move every day.	No laboratory tests are indicated.

TABLE 7–6 (Continued)

Summary

Nurses are using more time in patient teaching today and it will increase in the future. This is because the changing health care delivery system places more responsibility of health care on the patient.

Reviewing principles of learning is important preliminary information in planning patient teaching. Nurses develop a degree of knowledge, skills, and attitudes to be successful in practice. The active aging will need (1) knowledge about their condition or a task, (2) the physical and mental skills to complete a task, and (3) compliance, or an ownership of their care. Patients do not need to be experts in nursing skills. However, they do need a degree of motivation and commitment to be successful.

The Nursing Process can be utilized in planning patient teaching. Beginning steps are in the assessment and planning phases. Step 1 includes data collection about the patient as an individual. The most important part of this step for nurses is to establish rapport and develop a trust relationship. Other parts of this step include learning about the persons's values and priorities related to health, and how their lifestyle will influence learning and compliance with self-care.

Step 2 includes data collection related to the patient and his learning needs. You must determine what the patient wants to know and learn. There may need to be a compromise between patient and nurse regarding what is most important. Additional data should include the person's readiness to learn, and his current knowledge about how his body works, how his condition has affected his body functioning, and information about therapies he is receiving. Limitations that may influence learning methods or the person's ability to complete a task include physical limitations, literacy level, and primary language. It is also important to collect data about support persons. Even the most independent active aging need back-up support systems.

Step 3 is in the planning phase of the Nursing Process, and focuses on individualizing patient teaching. The ingredients of this step include setting realistic goals, prioritizing tasks, and deciding what teaching methods will be most appropriate for the individual.

Implementation of patient teaching will be smoother when there has been careful planning. Evaluation is a joint effort between the patient and nurse and usually includes ongoing monitoring by the nurse. Documentation continues to be important to assure quality of care.

Designing patient teaching for the active aging considers the normal aging process in adapting tools and methods of teaching. Sensory losses such as decreased vision and hearing are important considerations when adapting patient teaching. Psychomotor changes in the active aging may indicate that patient teaching should progress at a slower pace. Strength and endurance are often reduced and response time is slowed. The elderly are also caught in the myth that they are no longer capable of learning. Older minority patients, especially refugees, have different life experiences, cultural customs, and primary language. These may be added obstacles to learning.

Interviewing the elderly requires patience and a respect for their individuality and life experiences. Nurses must confront their own attitudes about aging to be successful in interviewing and planning patient teaching. It is helpful to interview the elderly early in the day, explain the questions that will be asked, and assure physical comfort. The nurse determines if it is appropriate to have family members participate in the interview.

A functional assessment determines the ability of an individual to manage from day-to-day in his environment. It assesses ability to meet personal needs such as hygiene, eating, and ambulating short distances. The person's ability to manage in his environment is also evaluated. This includes preparing meals, completing light housekeeping, using the telephone, managing money, and other similar activities. The functional assessment focuses on the person and not just his illness.

Today and in the future, the functional assessment is important in determining the best place for the elderly to live and manage their lives. Discharge planning nurses, home health nurses, social workers, and private case managers complete screening procedures in implementing functional assessment. All nurses contribute to functional assessments of the elderly with ongoing data collection.

Promoting wellness in the active aging involves patient teaching related to moderate exercise and good nutrition. These are important keys to health at any age. Another important part of teaching wellness is to encourage the active aging to have their health routinely monitored by their family physician.

Safety concerns are part of every phase of the Nursing Process. Nurses view safety as first and most important when prioritizing care; patients do not always have the same perception of priorities. Patient teaching involves sharing and compromising with patients.

Patient teaching related to medications becomes more important as people become more responsible for their own care. The elderly have some difficulty in complying with drug protocol. This may be because they do not have enough information about their medications.

Medication dosages and laboratory values are based on results expected in healthy 20- to 40-year olds. The normal aging process influences the absorption, metabolizing, and elimination of drugs. Nurses need to be aware of side effects and possible toxic responses to medications in the elderly.

Patient teaching. Challenging. Rewarding. You are an information and referral person. You are an advocate for the elderly. Never underestimate the value of information you are giving the active aging. It may be the piece of information that keeps them active and independent!

For Discussion

- In a small group discussion, identify difficulties you have experienced when teaching elderly patients. Explore possible reasons why these difficulties occurred.
- Identify a teaching need of an active aging patient to whom you were recently assigned. Using the Nursing Process, and basic steps of patient teaching, write a patient teaching plan.
- In a small discussion group, role play an elderly patient interview, a functional assessment of an active aging person, or patient teaching wellness for the active aging. Critique the patient information, use of therapeutic communications, and attention to the environment.
- Invite an older adult to your class to share feelings about learning new skills. Ask him/her to identify problems as well as what he/she believes would help make learning easier.

Questions for Review

1. What are three principles of learning related to patient teaching?
2. What is the most important nursing action in beginning patient teaching?
3. What are three pieces of data to collect in
   a. collecting data regarding the patient as an individual?
   b. collecting data about the patient and his learning needs?
4. What are three physical changes in normal aging that could influence patient teaching?
5. What are the adaptations in patient teaching required for changes identified in number 4?
6. What are four considerations to implement when interviewing the elderly?
7. What is a functional assessment?
8. Why is a functional assessment important in the active aging?
9. What are two wellness concepts for promoting healthy aging?
10. What are two problems related to the elderly and medications they take that makes patient teaching so important?

Section 3
The Dependent
Aging Population

Who are the dependent elderly? A clear line cannot be drawn to define this group according to age, medical problems, or other characteristics. A variety of situations and individual circumstances lead to identifying a person as dependent. *Dependent Elderly* are those persons over 65 years of age who rely on another person for assistance in completing some or all personal tasks for daily living on a long-term basis, often for the remainder of life.

Some situations that lead to dependency include the increasing debilitating effects of chronic disease as well as the exacerbations of normal physical aging. A person may have managed asthma and respiratory problems since childhood. Later, as an elderly adult, when all physical energy is directed toward breathing in end-stage emphysema, that person is dependent.

Dependency is not directed specifically toward an age group. However, the cohort over 85 rapidly becomes the most dependent of the elderly population. The 65 to 74 young old age group show little change in activity, health, and independence if they have been relatively healthy throughout their lives. More of the population begins to show some signs of dependency between the ages of 75 and 84. These may or may not significantly change the person's life style. After age 85, increasing numbers of this population group are dependent in several areas. Over 25 percent of this group are residents of long term care facilities compared to under 5 percent of the total 65 and older population.

All of us will, at some time, develop at least minor difficulties with aging symptoms or chronic disease. Our key to independence will be managing the difficulties.

Chronic diseases experienced by independent elderly are usually stable, controlled, or experience slow progression.

There are three situations that can be evaluated when attempting to establish a point or time when an individual moves from an independent to a more dependent life. Dependency seems to occur when (1) difficulties with daily personal activities cannot be managed independently, (2) chronic disease is out of control, or (3) a support system is absent or breaks down. The difficulties may be a combination of medical and functional problems.

Living alone with congestive heart failure that is out of control is an example of a dependent elderly problem. The increased dyspnea and peripheral edema begin to lead to noncompliance with therapy. This is because it becomes too exhausting to make meals, to get to the drug store for more medicine, or to the doctor for monitoring symptoms. There must be family and/or community service intervention.

When dependency occurs, there are at least three to five chronic problems, and often one problem exacerbates or compounds another. For example, a diabetic may manage at home independently for years until advanced vision problems occur and the individual can no longer see well enough to draw up insulin in the syringe. This person can continue to give himself the injection if a family member is taught how to prepare the syringe. If this is not possible, a home health nurse may set up a week's supply of syringes. It is when this arrangement is not successful, or other problems compound the difficulties, that long-term care becomes the best option.

The family is usually the major support system. However, members may not live nearby, or they may have work schedules that allow very little time to assist. Some family members are unwilling or afraid to help with personal tasks or medical treatment. The aging person may live in a rural area that has limited support services. Funding also plays a role in the decision whether a dependent person can continue to live at home. Often, a substantial amount of home care costs is out-of-pocket as government and other insurance is not yet covering many of these costs.

One situation that frequently leads to the transfer of the person and his care from the home to a long term care facility is the burnout of the family caregiver. The caregivers often continue until they suffer chronic physical or emotional fatigue. They can no longer continue, even with assistance from community services.

One problem in trying to establish the difference between independence and dependence is the variations in the normal aging process. It is gradual; changes are subtle; and the elderly learn to adapt. Life goes on, especially for those living alone, until a crisis occurs. A newspaper headline shouts, "Elderly Woman Found Unconscious with 17 Cats in Filthy Home." People gasp, how can that happen? It does. Gradually health and strength deteriorate. The person, and perhaps even a neighbor, did not realize that she could no longer adequately take care of herself, her pets, or her home.

Elderly couples, into their nineties, often continue to manage very well in their homes. They have grown dependent together, with the strengths of one compensating for the weaknesses of the other. If the more active person, for example, experiences a fall and fractures a hip, the vision and hearing dependency of the other is multiplied several times. That person probably cannot stay at home alone while the other recovers.

Many people do become frail as age and chronic conditions increase. *Frail*, meaning physically weak and vulnerable to injury or disease, is a term frequently used when describing the dependent elderly. It usually is a combination of problems with decreased mobility, strength, and endurance, plus a weight loss. This presents the picture of the frail elderly.

In many situations, people are managing their health and daily activities with long-term care services. *Long-term care* is health and/or social services required by persons with some type of functional disability. Individuals of any age often live in their homes and work in the community, but require some services to remain there.

Alternative Care or *Alternative Services* are the titles sometimes attached to the social services provided outside the traditional health care settings and in the home and community. When the term "grant" is attached to these titles, it refers to government or private monies that have been allocated to develop or implement an alternative service. In the changing health care delivery system, we will see more long-term care provided outside the traditional health care facilities.

This section will discuss some of the issues of dependent aging, especially those related to the elderly and caregivers in long term care facilities. With increasing numbers of dependent elderly, there will room for only the very frail and more ill elderly in long term care facilities. *Long term care facilities* are health care institutions that provide health care and services for activities of daily living for a long period of time, often the remainder of a person's life. Not all dependent persons in long term care facilities are elderly. Many dependent younger people live temorarily or permanently in long term care facilities. Some examples are victims of accidents who have spinal cord injuries or central nervous system trauma such as Reyes Syndrome. Meeting the many physical, emotional, and social needs of residents who are not elderly will not be discussed in this section.

Unit 8 will present some of the diseases and chronic conditions experienced by the dependent elderly. Sample situations with care plans are included; nursing diagnoses are utilized with selected resident problems.

In Unit 9, issues related to the psychosocial aspects of dependent aging will be introduced. The behaviors and needs of individuals with dementias will be discussed, including the social implications of increasing forgetfulness and confusion.

Experiencing loss will be the focus of Unit 10. The loss of independent decision making combined with loss of home and life style when entering a long term care facility are two points of discussion. Issues of depression, suicide, and dying and death related to the elderly population are other topics. Religious and spiritual issues, and the role of the nurse in supporting the dependent elderly's beliefs, will be presented.

Unit 11 raises several dilemmas facing the dependent aging and their caregivers. Examples of issues are resusitation orders, living wills, use of drugs, access to care, and dilemmas of family caregivers.

Care plans for the dependent aging will be presented in Unit 12. This will follow the nursing process in presenting assessments of the elderly and planning for activities of daily living. Implementation includes the adaptations to meet aging changes and a review of procedures related to increased technology in long term care facilities. Evaluation focuses on maintaining the highest level of functional ability in the dependent elderly.

Unit 8
Physical Conditions Experienced by the Dependent Aging

Objectives

After reading this unit you should be able to:

- Discuss symptoms of disease and aging that contribute to dependent living.
- Describe events related to conditions that transfer an individual from active to dependent aging.
- Identify interventions that are important in assisting the elderly to live with chronic diseases.
- Discuss appropriate resident care to promote the highest functional level in the dependent elderly.

The elderly do not not look forward to dependency in aging. None of us will. Perhaps it is because it seems so permanent. Acute situations are perceived as having an end time when life can go on "as usual." However, dependency in aging is considered "forever," with a progression toward increased dependency.

Aging, as stated earlier, sneaks up on us. It is a gradual process; but when dependency arrives, it seems to have happened all too quickly. The uniqueness of each individual will determine how dependency is met and accepted. Some elderly accept that it is a part of the life cycle; an event that is almost certain in old age. Others have problems coping and seem to make dependent years more difficult for themselves and their caregivers.

Dependent aging can have a quality of life that is meaningful and rich for the elderly and the people surrounding them. It can be a time to reflect on accomplishments and to guide the next generation to assume new roles. Nurses as advocates and caregivers of the dependent aging promote and contribute to the quality of life the elderly so richly deserve. These dependent elderly are the strongest members of their cohort because they survived illness and injury in their youth and adult years without the medications and medical technology we have today.

The 85 and older age group is becoming older and larger in number. At the turn of the twentieth century there were barely one thousand people 100 years or older in the United States. The number of citizens a century old is projected to be in the millions 20 years into the next century, figure 8-1.

This unit will discuss the exacerbations of disease and aging conditions that contribute to the change from active to dependent aging. Part of the discussion will explore what events lead some people to long term care facilities while others, seemingly more physically or mentally limited, continue to manage in their own homes. Mobility, endurance, and sensory deficits are major considerations in comparing active and dependent aging.

Discussion of medical and nursing intervention of chronic disease dependency will focus on the needs of residents in long term care facilities. The physician usually has been managing the condition for many years. Diagnostic tests are no longer pertinent because the disease has been identified. Laboratory tests are ordered to monitor drug therapy, an acute event such as an infection, or to comply with state or federal requirements.

Continuing Musculoskeletal Difficulties

Muscle strength continues to decrease because of reduced activity. The aches and pains related to osteoarthritis continue on in advancing age. However, the elderly manage and few become residents of long term care facilities because of this condition. Degenerative joint disease is more often a secondary diagnosis. Residents receive a number of analgesics and anti-inflammatory medications to help manage the discomfort and maintain a level of activity. Nurses monitor for side effects related to gastrointestinal irritation.

Two musculoskeletal conditions that result in dependent living are rheumatoid arthritis and hip fractures. The arthritis usually has been progressing for years and the individual anticipates the possibility of living in a health care facility at some time. Hip fractures are a sudden traumatic event and in only a few days a person may need to deal with more dependent living. Amputations of extremities also involve the musculoskeletal system, but usually are the result of complications of diabetes or peripheral vascular disease.

Rheumatoid Arthritis

Unlike osteoarthritis, rheumatoid arthritis (RA) is not a disease of normal aging; this condition may have an onset before middle age. Its etiology is unknown, but has been linked to the immune system. This systemic disease has exacerbations and remissions. Joint changes eventually result in ankylosis and deformities, figure 8–2. People who have this chronic inflammatory disease may be anemic and tend to be underweight.

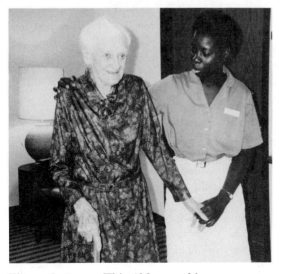

Figure 8–1 This 106-year-old woman continues to enjoy an active life.

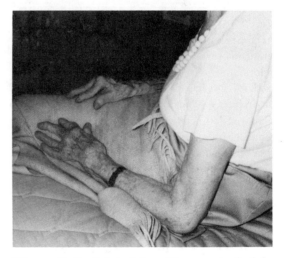

Figure 8–2 Joint deformities are typical in rheumatoid arthritis.

Events that may determine a change in living arrangements for a person with RA include (1) increased physical limitations and inability to complete self care, (2) lack of or loss of caregiver in the home, (3) complications, such as a decubitus ulcers, resulting from limited activity, or (4) the need to have drug therapies and personal safety monitored.

The focus of dependent care with rheumatoid arthritis is mananging pain and promoting comfort. Nonnarcotic analgesics such as acetaminophen, or nonsteroidal anti-inflammatory agents such as ibuprofen are often prescribed in large doses. Prednisone, a corticosteroid anti-inflammatory drug, may be prescribed for short-term therapy if the resident is experiencing a painful exacerbation. Because of the gastrointestinal irritation of these medications, a resident may receive ranitidine, cimetidine, or sucralfate.

Nursing intervention to promote comfort includes providing a firm supporting mattress, a bed cradle or other device to keep bed linens off painful joints, and sand bags or pillows to assist in positioning for comfort. Plate collars, adaptive utensils, long-handled tools for grasping, plus creative measures initiated by caregivers assist the resident in maintaining a degree of independence.

To maintain mobility and prevent contractures, physicians may prescribe physical therapy measures such as paraffin baths for the hands, intermittent splints for positioning, or range of motion exercises. Residents need to maintain social contacts; using a Hoyer lift to transfer to a supportive wheelchair can help meet this goal. The limited activity endured by these residents challenges nurses to maintain skin integrity and bowel function.

Hip Fractures

Osteoporosis is usually the predisposing cause of hip fractures in the elderly. It is generally believed that in many situations, a spontaneous fracture occurs first which results in the fall. The fracture, occuring most often at the neck of the femur, is stablized with orthopedic pins and nails by open reduction and internal fixation. Postoperative care includes pain and infection control and structured physical therapy. These elderly require much support and encouragement because of the fear and anxiety relating to the possibility of another fall.

Elderly persons experiencing this trauma can recover and have a nearly complete return to previous activity. Situations that lead to long-term care placement include: (1) the need for extended convalescence and physical therapy before returning home, (2) the inability to manage physical therapy and ambulate (the caregiver at home cannot manage increased dependency), or (3) other chronic conditions were exacerbated with this event.

Nurses in long term care facilities may be responsible for continuing post-operative nursing care if a resident is admitted within a few days of the surgical procedure. This care requires monitoring the function of all systems, observation of the incision, and supporting the prescribed physical therapy. You may be removing the sutures or staples as the resident is not usually transported to the physician's office for this procedure.

Emmaline Alt, age 84, is presented in **Care Plan 1**. She is a retired lawyer, never married, and has lived independently all her adult life. Two weeks ago Emmaline tripped on a small rug in her apartment, fell, and sustained a left hip fracture. She tolerated surgery very well, but was admitted to a long term care facility a week ago for continued physical therapy and assistance in regaining her independence. Emmaline lives on the third floor of an older apartment building that does not have an elevator. Nursing care considerations relate to her impaired mobility and a long history of constipation now complicated by the side effects of analgesics. She is somewhat familiar with her new environment as she has been a "friendly visitor" from her church. Goals of care include assisting her to return to her apartment.

RESIDENT CARE PLAN

DATE	PROBLEM	GOALS	TARGET DATE	APPROACH	RESOLVED DATE
8/8	Impaired physical mobility R/T left leg trauma, reduced strength and endurance M/B inability to transfer, ambulate or reposition self independantly.	Will exhibit ability to reposition self, transfer s̄ assistance, and ambulate 100 ft. c̄ assistance.	11/8	P.T. 5x week: gait training. Walk in hall bid c̄ assist of 1 et gait belt; advance 15 ft. per week. Teach bed positioning techniques.	
8/8	Self care deficit: bathing, grooming, toileting, dressing lower extremities R/T lower extremity trauma et weakness M/B inability to ambulate, to obtain self care supplies or to position self to tie shoes.	Demonstrate ability to complete self care to return home.	11/8	Set up bath et grooming supplies; encourage independance c̄ hygiene. Encourage self dressing; assist c̄ lower extremities.	
8/8	Alteration in bowel elimination: constipation R/T limited activity, narcotic analgesics, slowed peristalsis M/B ō daily stool per habit, reluctant to drink fluids, states feels bloated.	Maintain G.I. function, return to daily bowel elimination pattern.	9/8	Stewed prunes q a.m. (resident request) Colace 100 mgm qd Encourage fluids to 1500 cc qd. Assist to bedside commode.	

NURSING ALERT		
Full Code		

MEDICAL DIAGNOSIS:	Fracture L hip, DJD, Chronic constipation						
NAME	NUMBER	ROOM	BIRTHDATE	AGE	ADMIT DATE	PHYSICIAN	DATE	PAGE
Emmaline Alt	1468	122	2/9	84	8/5	DR. Littleton	8/8	1

Continuing Respiratory Difficulties

The elderly experience gradual exertional dyspnea as they advance in age. Most elderly learn to pace their activities. An 85-year-old joked that his rest periods were getting longer than his work time.

Pneumonia is a threat to the dependent elderly. It is a common cause of death to many elderly with chronic problems other than the respiratory system. The weakened immune system, poor cough reflex, limited activity, inability to consume adequate fluids, and general vulnerability to infections all contribute to the lung involvement. Medical treatment with intravenous antibiotics and fluids are not always successful in the frail elderly.

Emphysema

Chronic obstructive pulmonary disease (COPD) is second to cardiovascular disease as a cause of disability in the United States. Progressive chronic debilitating dyspnea is the respiratory symptom that results in dependency in the elderly.

Emphysema is characterized by destruction of the alveolar walls. It is usually the result of years of insult to the lungs from disease and environmental irritants. The destruction of the alveolar wall means there is less total alveolar surface to transport oxygen to the blood and return carbon dioxide to the lungs to be exhaled. The air gets "trapped" in the lungs. As the body tissues require more oxygen, the respiratory center in the brain signals an increased respiratory rate to no avail. The increased respiratory rate exhausts the individual; little additional oxygen is delivered to the cells.

Events that lead the elderly with emphysema to long term care facilities are related to the profound dyspnea and weakness. They use every ounce of energy to breathe. The condition may be unstable even with drug therapy and supplemental oxygen. The person can no longer care for himself and family and community services may not be available or are exhausted. Residents with emphysema are more often the young or middle old; the nature of the disease does not lend itself to longevity.

Medical treatment continues with supplemental oxygen and bronchodilaters, figure 8–3. These medications are given orally by inhaler, or nebulizer treatments. Examples of these drugs are spasmolytics such as theophylline, or adrenergics such as terbutaline sulfate or metaproternol sulfate that relax smooth muscle of the airways. Antibiotics are prescribed for acute respiratory infections, and diuretics may be given to help control edema.

The more independent patient is taught techniques to improve breathing, such as pursed lip and abdominal or diaphragmatic breathing. The postural drainage procedure may be taught to a family member. The dependent resident with emphysema usually can no longer tolerate these methods of improving respiration.

Recall that the supplemental oxygen is prescribed at low rates, such as 2 to 3 liters or

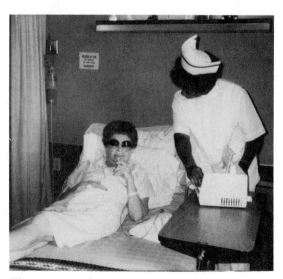

Figure 8–3   Oxygen therapy assists the elderly with chronic respiratory problems.

less per minute. It is the low level of oxygen in the blood, not the high level of carbon dioxide, that stimulates respiration in people with emphysema. This is important to remember when elderly experience a myocardial infarction. At this time, higher levels of oxygen are often prescribed to relieve pain and provide oxygen to the tissues. In emergencies, even a brief medical history is critical to avoid problems that could occur if a person with emphysema received a high level of oxygen.

There is no cure for emphysema. There can be control with (1) drug therapy, (2) improved nutrition, (3) moderate exercise for health maintenance, and (4) physician monitoring of health to avoid complications or acute illness. Dependent residents with emphysema are sometimes identified as having "end stage COPD." This means that medical treatment, even changing medications or dosages, is no longer successful in controlling the disease progression. The resident has progressive chronic dyspnea; eating a meal or answering a few questions will exhaust him. An orthopneic position does not improve breathing; he may even try to sleep in a lounge chair. You will observe a very anxious, irritable, gasping individual. He may have noisy, raspy respirations and a harsh deep cough. A "barrel chest," ruddy complexion, and diaphoresis from efforts to breath are other symptoms. Regardless of the number of years the resident has had this chronic problem, he can be in a grieving stage from multiple losses. A denial or other response to the disease will reflect his changed life style and response to limitations.

Nursing care is challenging for these individuals. Goals include reducing dyspnea and increasing physical and emotional comfort. Every activity is paced to minimize the dyspnea. Plan for the resident to participate in his care as much as possible. Avoid making him more dependent by doing everything for him. Attempt to reduce his anxiety by administering medications promptly and respecting his sched-

ule as much as possible. He needs your empathy and support; he will probably die of pneumonia or heart failure while he is a resident in a long term care facility.

Care Plan 2 presents selected problems of 80-year-old Alfred Johnson. He is a widower who had been living for the last several years in a supervised apartment for the eldery; there are no children or other known relatives. Mr. Johnson, a retired accountant, enjoys reading and has been a member of an "arm-chair" travel club; he has never been more than 40 miles from home.

Mr. Johnson perceived his health as good until his recent admission to a long term care facility. Alfred was diagnosed with emphysema 5 years ago; he has a 126 pack-year history of cigarette smoking. Recent repeated hospitalizations for respiratory infections, exacerbations of symptoms, and the need for continuous supplemental oxygen ended his smoking habit. He has developed hypertension during the last few years and is now legally blind because of untreated cataracts.

Permanent placement was the decision for Mr. Johnson due to his fears of managing the oxygen equipment, his inability to cope with his disease, and his progressive dependence.

Continuing Cardiovascular Difficulties

Exertional dyspnea in the dependent elderly is also related to decreased cardiac function. Each year of aging finds the elderly pacing their activities more because of complaints of breathlessness and decreased strength. The heart cannot pump enough blood to meet the demands of the body.

Health problems of middle age and young old years contribute to the dependent lives of the elderly. This includes hypertension, coronary artery disease, and residual effects of a heart attack. Complications of these conditions,

RESIDENT CARE PLAN

DATE	PROBLEM	GOALS	TARGET DATE	APPROACH	RESOLVED DATE
8/15	Impaired gas exchange R/T loss of lung elasticity, anxiety, history of smoking M/B exertional dyspnea and circumoral pallor.	Demonstrate effective respiratory rate and effort. Reduce anxiety.	9/15	Oxygen @ 2-4 L/mn continuously. Monitor respiratory rate et effort q shift, prn. Theodur 200 mgm bid Vanceril Inhaler π puffs qid HOB↑30°, reassure, and anticipate needs.	
8/15	Activity intolerance R/T dyspnea, fatigue M/B inability to walk more than 50 ft., takes one hour for grooming and dressing.	Continue to manage ADL's independantly.	9/15	Encourage pacing of self care activities. Rolling walker for room ambulation. W/C transport to dining room.	
8/15	Ineffective coping: Individual R/T management of disease M/B refuses to learn how to operate oxygen concentrator, inhaler.	Regulate oxygen liter flow and demonstrate correct use of inhaler.	9/15	Teach oxygen therapy @ 1-2 steps per week. Allow time to accept responsibility of tasks.	

NURSING ALERT

Legally blind

MEDICAL DIAGNOSIS: COPD, hypertension, cataracts

NAME	NUMBER	ROOM	BIRTHDATE	AGE	ADMIT DATE	PHYSICIAN	DATE	PAGE
Alfred Johnson	2418	348	6-10	80	8-11	DR. Bellows	8/15	1

such as a stroke, rather than the disease itself result in dependent living in a long term care facility. In addition, and like other chronic conditions, the disease progression, the inability to complete self care, and the loss of a support system indicates the need for a change in living arrangements.

Congestive Heart Failure

Pump failure is perhaps the most simple description of congestive heart failure. Symptoms are described as "left-sided" or "right-sided" failure. Left-sided failure demonstrates respiratory symptoms and right-sided failure produces systemic signs of edema, particularly in the lower extremities and the abdomen. Because of the nature of the circulation process, poor pumping means it will begin to "back up." The result is that one-sided failure will soon lead to failure on both sides.

A scenerio of events occurs when, for example, a person has had one or more heart attacks, which weakens the effectiveness of the myocardium. The left ventricle cannot contract efficiently to expel the blood into the aorta. Reversing the route of cardiac circulation, the next structure to have difficulty is the left auricle, followed by the pulmonary veins, and then the lung tissue. Signs observed are dyspnea, wheezing, and a productive cough that may include frothy blood-tinged sputum.

The effects of the ineffective heart pumping move to the right side of the heart and eventually general circulation. Edema in the feet and ankles is observed as well as an enlarged abdomen because of involvement of the portal circulation. The slower circulation in congestive heart failure and the engorgement of vessels leads to a seeping of fluid into the body tissues. This is observed as edema.

Drug therapy includes: (1) cardiotonics such as digitoxin that help strengthen the heart muscle contraction, (2) diuretics such as furosemide to remove the tissue fluid, and (3) vaso-

dilators such as isosorbide dinitrate that allow the vessels to accommodate larger blood volumes. In addition, limiting sodium intake and reducing or pacing activity assists in helping the heart to function more efficiently.

Nursing care for the dependent elderly who are experiencing congestive heart failure symptoms includes all measures that reduce the workload of the heart and improve circulation. The resident needs to be involved in his daily activities; nurses assist in planning and pacing the activity. Promoting venous return is important; be sure to check that the resident's feet are elevated when sitting in a chair or wheelchair. Monitor drug therapy, observing for therapeutic effect and possible side effects such as signs of hypokalemia.

Care Plan 3 identifies some problems experienced by Willie Holden. Willie, at age 99, is a veteran of World War I, and the oldest of nine siblings. He was a farmer, having lived with two single sisters. Willie was admitted to the long term care facility as a result of mild, but yet compounding, experiences of old-old aging. He never sought medical attention until age 91, when he demonstrated signs of cardiovascular aging. His medications, diet, and pacing of activities were managed by his sisters. Recently he was seen in an emergency room, having experienced dizziness. He demonstrated signs of dehydration. His care plan focuses on monitoring his cardiac status and promoting continued independence.

Peripheral Vascular Disease/Amputation

The peripheral circulation of the lower extremities is at risk for a number of reasons. Aging and disease threaten the ability of the circulatory system to supply tissues with needed oxygen. The arteriosclerosis and compromised immune system of aging, and the congestive heart failure, varicosities, and diabetic neuropathy of disease processes, are examples of problems with tissue perfusion. Wound healing

RESIDENT CARE PLAN

DATE	PROBLEM	GOALS	TARGET DATE	APPROACH	RESOLVED DATE
7/18	Actual fluid volume deficit R/T medications, reduced intracellular fluids M/B compaints of dizziness, 10 lb. weight loss in one month, poor skin turgor.	Restore fluid volume	8/18	Daily weight q a.m. B/P qd Monitor lung sounds and peripheral edema q shift. I & O Encourage fluids @ meals 200 cc between meals	
7/18	Alteration in cardiac output: decreased R/T aging changes in heart vessels: aortic stenosis, CAD, CHF, M/B chest pain and dyspnea on exertion and cyanotic nailbeds.	Reduce incidence of chest pain and dyspnea	8/18	Isordil 200 mgm qid po Dyazide ⊤ cap bid po Verapamil 240 mgm qd po Pace activities B/P and P qd Lo Na diet	
7/18	Activity intolerance: ADL's R/T dyspnea, fatigue and weakness M/B inability to complete selfcare, or ambulate 20 feet c̄ assist-ance.	Promote limited selfcare: feeding bathing upper body tolerate ambulation to bathroom s̄ dyspnea	10/18	Provide supplies for hygiene; encourage limited self care. Set-up meal tray Use walker and gait belt, assist of 1 to bathroom. Allow adequate time.	

NURSING ALERT

MEDICAL DIAGNOSIS: Aortic stenosis, CAD, CHF, benign controlled hypertension					Allergy: PCN	
NAME	NUMBER	ROOM	BIRTHDATE	AGE	ADMIT DATE	PHYSICIAN	DATE	PAGE
Willie Holden	3280	241	2/5	99	7/14	DR. Hart	7/18	1

and maintaining tissue integrity are ongoing challenges. Many residents of long term care facilities became dependent as a result of the need for an amputation.

Nursing care for a resident having an amputation may include post-operative care. The person may have been a resident because of other dependent conditions, or be admitted following surgery because new circumstances made it a necessity. Physicians may discharge the person a day or two following surgery; the observations and care follow the usual protocol of wound assessment and monitoring the recovery process. Care plans focus on existing abilities to maintain the maximum degree of independence. Many residents are not fitted with a prosthesis because of decreased physical strength and endurance related to other chronic conditions; these wheelchair residents can manage physical and social independence very well.

Care Plan 4 presents selected concerns of Emil Tinkerman, a 91-year-old diabetic. Mr. Tinkerman's diabetes was discovered at age 85 during studies following a lengthy period of "not feeling well." He had difficulty complying with new eating habits, and began to demonstrate complications of diabetes with vision changes and poor peripheral circulation. Recently, following his right below-the-knee amputation, and difficulty in healing a lesion on his left foot, his 82-year-old wife realized she could no longer assist him at home. Their children, now in their 60s, are beginning to have their own aging problems. Mr. Tinkerman's care is directed toward maintaining skin integrity and preventing infection.

Gastrointestinal Complications

Gastrointestinal problems are not usually the single reason an elderly person becomes dependent, or is admitted to a long term care facility. The exacerbation of problems related to this system are more often a complication of bedrest or a consequence of other chronic conditions.

Nutrition and hydration in the dependent elderly often is the total responsibility of the nurse or other caregivers. When the resident is physically or mentally dependent, he cannot feed himself or respond to a physiological stimulus of thirst or hunger. Residents receiving nothing by mouth, when having nasogastric or gastrostomy tube feeding, require continual assessments of nutrition and fluid balance. Regular monitoring of weight and assessment of skin turgor, mucous membranes, and dilution of urine are examples of observations.

Residents independent in eating also require ongoing nutritional monitoring. There are many obstacles to the intake of adequate nutrients. First, there are problems with missing teeth, no teeth, or dentures that no longer fit because of weight loss. Second, there can be positioning problems related to conditions such as arthritis or a stroke. Some residents may have difficulty even using adaptive utensils.

Anorexia can be a side effect of medications or respiratory secretions. Some residents just do not like the food. Remember, food habits have been well established for many years. Residents may not care for the type of food, seasonings, the therapeutic diet, or the mechanical soft diet ordered because of a denture problem. It often requires a diligent effort of the nursing and dietary departments to meet the resident's preferences and his nutritional needs within often limited menu guidelines.

Dehydration

Dehydration is serious and potentially life-threating to the frail elderly. Because intracellular fluid decreases with age, there is less total body fluid. Therefore, any fluid loss is significant in the elderly. Only a few hours of vomiting, diarrhea, fever, or other loss of fluids can result in dehydration and electrolyte imbalance. Following the evaluation of blood chemistries, intravenous fluids are the usual treatment for electrolyte replacement. The resident may

RESIDENT CARE PLAN

DATE	PROBLEM	GOALS	TARGET DATE	APPROACH	RESOLVED DATE
9/8	Potential for infection R/T hyperglycemia, aging decreased immune response M/B ulcerated area on left 5th toe, dusky foot, weak pedal pulse	Prevent infection in Lt foot	10/8	Monitor foot for changes q8h Measure ulcerated area qd Use handwashing procedures P.T. qd – whirlpool Keep left foot elevated, dry dressing Prevent bumping foot	
9/8	Impaired physical mobility R/T Rt. BKA, Lt foot neuropathy, decreased strength and endurance M/B unable to transfer or use walker independently	Ambulate to bathroom with 1 assist	11/8	Teach transfer technique Transfer, ambulate c̄ use of gait belt, walker, assist of 1. Verbalize cues Increase distance as tolerated ROM q8h	
9/8	Impairment of skin integrity R/T poor circulation, limited mobility, aging fragile skin, M/B reddened areas on coccyx, areas of purpura on arms	Maintain continuity of skin Prevent pressure ulcers	10/8	Massage around reddened areas when position changed q2h Keep skin clean, dry Apply lotion to skin with a.m. and p.m. cares Encourage fluids between meals Protien snacks	

NURSING ALERT

No aspirin	DATE 9/8

MEDICAL DIAGNOSIS: Diabetes Type II, Rt. BKA amputation, Lt. foot ischemia

NAME	NUMBER	ROOM	BIRTHDATE	AGE	ADMIT DATE	PHYSICIAN	PAGE
Emil Tinkerman	7345	255	3/9	91	9/4	DR.Claypool	1

be transferred to an acute care setting, or receive continued monitoring and treatment in the long term care facility.

The elderly can become dehydrated so quickly that it takes continual nursing surveillance of the signs and symptoms to avoid this potential threat. Nursing measures to encourage fluids are important, such as extra sips when administering medications, figure 8–4, offering preferred beverages, and using cups or containers that are easily managed by the resident.

Chronic Constipation/Impaction

Maintaining the elimination function of the gastrointestinal system is also a concern. During the active aging years, many became dependent on over-the-counter laxatives. Physical activity has continually decreased and there may be difficulties in consuming adequate fiber and fluids. Medications which have side effects of constipation are additional problems. The constipated stool becomes difficult to expel. The physical energy required to evacuate stool takes more effort than some dependent elderly can manage, especially those who are weak and become easily fatigued. Fecal impaction is a complication of infrequent defecation. The stool is usually dry, hard, and the leakage of watery fecal stained drainage around the impaction may have the appearance of diarrhea.

Treatment for chronic constipation depends on the resident's medical history. Physicians may order a bulk-forming laxative such as psyllium, or a stool softener such as docusate sodium. Enemas and suppositories may also be ordered. However, they may not be effective as reduced sphincter control makes it difficult for the elderly to retain these preparations.

Bowel and bladder programs in long term care facilities combine medical and nursing measures to promote maintenance of gastrointestinal functioning. The medical staff may approve facility-wide use of unprocessed bran, prune juice, or other measures to be given as needed. Nurses administer these preparations to

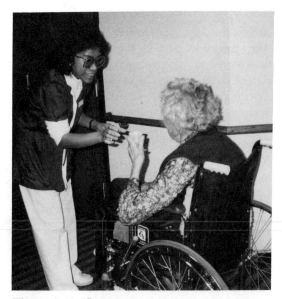

Figure 8–4 Long-term care nurses are responsible for the hydration of residents.

residents experiencing problems with bowel elimination patterns. Caregivers assist residents to the bathroom or portable commode approximately every two hours.

Genitourinary Complications

The continued loss of muscle tone contributes to difficulty with bladder control. Urinary incontinence becomes more likely the older the elderly become, and the more other conditions make them dependent. Central nervous system problems such as paralysis related to a stroke or other trauma result in incontinence. When confused, the resident may not remember to go to the bathroom.

Urinary Incontinence

Complications of urinary incontinence make it difficult for a caregiver to manage an elderly family member at home. The situations that may make long-term care placement necessary include frequent urinary tract infections and unmanageable skin breakdown.

Bowel and bladder programs in the facility include assisting the resident to the bathroom every two hours. Some confused residents ask to be assisted too frequently, for example, every fifteen minutes. This is a behavior dilemma. Assisting the resident to the bathroom frequently does not promote adequate bladder tone and misses the objective of the program. Incontinence may be difficult to manage when the resident receives diuretics. Caregivers are most successful with bowel and bladder programs when they become acquainted with the resident's voiding habits and behavior patterns.

Sometimes a dependent resident can no longer participate in a bowel and bladder program because of physical or mental limitations. Incontinence management is usually then cloth or or disposable liners for undergarments, or the placement of an indwelling catheter. Choosing a method involves the physician, nursing department, resident's family, and the resident if he is able to make decisions. Issues in the decision include: (1) the resident's physical condition and limitations, (2) maintaining skin integrity, (3) preventing urinary tract infections, and (4) supporting the resident's dignity. If the indwelling catheter is the choice, it is changed on a periodic basis and is usually permanent.

Renal Failure

Chronic renal failure will eventually occur in residents having congestive heart failure, diabetes, or other conditions that may be toxic to the kidneys. It is more often the cause of complications of chronic disease than a primary kidney disease.

Treatment for renal failure in elderly residents is usually conservative; symptomatic comfort care is implemented. Fluid intake is monitored and the characteristics of urine noted. Skin care is especially important with these residents. It is unlikely that the dependent elderly would be considered candidates for dialysis because of other chronic conditions and the generalized debilitation of systems.

Chronic Nervous System Events

Degenerative changes in brain tissue continue to occur. The results can range from benign mental dullness to major confusion behaviors. Neurologic problems that occur in the elderly and result in dependent aging are debilitating deficits of a cerebral vascular accident (CVA, stroke) and Parkinsonism.

Parkinsonism

Parkinsonism is a group of neurological symptoms that progress slowly. It begins with faint tremors that gradually become more pronounced; skeletal muscles become rigid and weakness develops. The individual demonstrates a shuffling gait, poor balance, and a masklike appearance. Speech becomes slowed and slurred, and there is difficulty with drooling and swallowing.

Medical treatment includes physical therapy to maintain joint mobility, and the medication levodopa to help decrease the symptoms. Nursing care supports ambulation and range-of-motion activities practiced in physical therapy. Allowing the resident time to complete self care tasks promotes the continuation of his highest functional level.

Long-term care residents may have lived with Parkinsonism for many years. The disease progression and level of dependency, combined with lack of available support systems, will signal the need for long term care facility placement.

Cerebrovascular Accident (CVA, Stroke)

The incapacitating nature of a severe stroke can make an individual dependent literally "overnight." Strokes are the third leading cause of death in the elderly population. Most incidents in this age group are a result of cerebral thrombosis.

Labeling a stroke mild to severe usually focuses on the degree of physical deficit and prognosis of long-term residual effects. Impairment of communication may be dysphasia or total aphasia. Hemiplegia may be evident in weakness or paralysis. There are sensory deficits in alteration of visual field and alteration in sense of touch.

Treatment following an emergency acute phase of a recent stroke includes physical therapy, occupational therapy, and perhaps speech therapy. If a thrombus is the cause of the event, anticoagulant therapy is usually planned to help avoid future strokes. Other drug therapy will focus on predisposing causes such as hypertension. It is often a long rehabilitative period and requires patience by the elderly victim, the family, and all health professionals. There is much frustration expressed by the patient; the family requires support because of the sudden, shocking nature of a stroke. Post-stroke depression is difficult for the family to manage. The elderly, for example, may spontaneously weep when seeing a friend, or may not seem excited over progress in physical therapy.

The elderly victims of a stroke become residents of long term care facilities because of the nature of their deficits and the need for services such as physical therapy. They may have other chronic conditions that were exacerbated by the stroke. The spouse cannot manage and other family members and community services cannot meet their needs.

Residents in long term care facilities receive a functional assessment to evaluate abilities or limitations related to aging and other chronic conditions as well as the deficits of a stroke. Nursing care supports areas of mobility, communication, and self-care needs. Goals include: (1) retain joint mobility and prevent contractures, (2) establish a method of communication in remembering the resident understands you even if he cannot talk, (3) plan personal care to promote the highest level of independence, and (4) prevent complications related to skin integrity, incontinence, and loss of self image.

The elderly who are residents of long term care facilities because of other dependent conditions may suffer strokes as this is a high-risk population for this event. Nurses must be alert to symptoms. These frequently are a change in general appearance, behavior, or difficulty with speech.

Care Plan 5 includes selected problems of Margaret Sprong, an 81-year-old who recently experienced a stroke. Limitations related to communication and self care precipitated admission to a long term care facility. Her health had been relatively stable, with a history of hypertension and aging cardiovascular symptoms. She lived in the same home she and her husband moved into early in their marriage. Mrs. Sprong's 60-year-old son lives in the same community. Pre-admission screening concluded the son would not be able to assist his mother. She could not receive intermittent home care because of her aphasia. Goals of care include promoting self-care and preventing social isolation.

Continuing Sensory Difficulties

All abilities related to sensory stimulus continue to decline, particularly when there were more pronounced changes during active aging. Blindness or deafness alone do not indicate the need for long term care placement; people of all ages manage these limitations in an active life. For the elderly, placement is precipitated by other chronic conditions or exacerbation of disease. The aged may also become blind while a resident of a health care facility.

Eye observation and care are important for all residents. Caregivers need to remember eyeglasses are a part of grooming in personal care. Nurses assess the effectiveness of corrective lenses; they discuss with the resident and family the need for an eye examination. Because of decreased secretions, the eye is vulnerable to infection. The aged may have artificial tear solutions ordered to help ease eye discomfort due to decreased tear production.

RESIDENT CARE PLAN

DATE	PROBLEM	GOALS	TARGET DATE	APPROACH	RESOLVED DATE
4/30	Impaired verbal communication R/T expressive aphasia M/B difficulty in expressing needs, frustration c̄ stating inappropriate words.	Able to communicate needs to caregivers	5/30	Allow time to attempt verbalization Use "flash cards" for frequently used phrases Encourage hand signals Ask questions requiring yes/no answer Talk to Margaret and expect a response	
4/30	Self-care deficit: ADL's R/T Rt. sided weakness M/B life-long right-handedness, inability to manage eating utensils, dress self.	Margaret will be able to complete ADL's with minimal assistance	7/30	Use adaptive utensils, plate collar, bent spoon or fork, built up handle O.T. teach self dressing/grooming techniques Allow time to complete self-care Praise all efforts and build on successes	
4/30	Fear R/T nature of disabilities in speech and movement M/B uses words "can't", "won't", and facial expressions of fear and frustration	Increase feelings of emotional comfort and self-confidance	5/30	Reduce environmental fears maintain same self-care schedule/caregivers Promote decision making in self-care Use simple directions Praise accomplishments	

NURSING ALERT

Allergy: Iodine

MEDICAL DIAGNOSIS: CVA: Rt hemiparesis, Expressive aphasia

NAME	NUMBER	ROOM	BIRTHDATE	AGE	ADMIT DATE	PHYSICIAN	DATE	PAGE
Margaret Sprong	4891	186	7/14	81	4/25	DR. Parlance	4/30	1

Blindness

Limited vision, or blindness, in residents is usually the result of untreated cataracts, glaucoma, diabetic retinopathy, or macular degeneration, figure 8-5. Residents may be receiving medical treatment including timolol maleate eye drops, or oral acetazolamide sodium to help reduce the intraocular pressure of glaucoma.

Care plans for residents with limited vision will focus on existing abilities and limitations. Some residents will benefit from state services for the blind such as talking books. Other

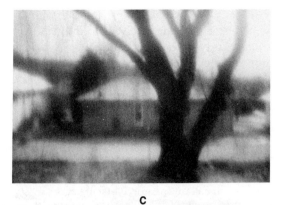

C

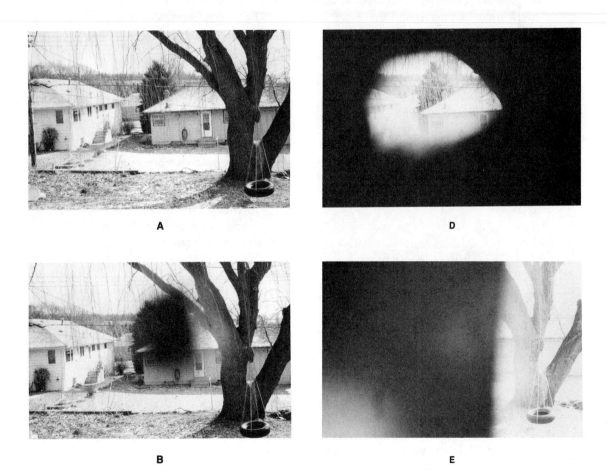

A

B

D

E

Figure 8–5   Several visual deficits may lead to blindness. (a) normal vision; (b) macular degeneration: note the area of absent central vision; (c) cataract: note blurring of vision over entire field; (d) glaucoma: note only very central portion of vision remains; (e) hemianopsia: note left half of visual field is absent. May occur in either side of field or in the upper or lower half.

residents may be confused or have other limitations that impede the involvement in these programs. For all residents with limited vision, nurses and other caregivers must remember the courtesies of communication. These include introducing yourself, announcing when entering or leaving the room, and including the time of day in your conversation. Personal care is organized to promote self care. Total feeding and bathing should be avoided unless the resident is completely dependent.

In **Care Plan 6**, Katie Rinkenberger's safety and social needs are identified. At age 84, Katie needed to move to a long term care facility because the family support system could no longer help her. Katie, widowed at age 70, devoted her life to her family; she was proud of her homemaking abilities. Osteoarthritis caused her continual discomfort, but it was blindness related to her glaucoma that led to her dependency. Her children live in the city, but have health and financial problems that prohibit them from helping her. Turning the stove gas burner on high, rather than off, resulted in a minor fire in her home. Katie needed other living arrangements.

Deafness

Most residents have experienced some gradual hearing loss. Problems related to limited hearing usually result in decreased social interaction. This may lead to withdrawal from the environment and a progressive total functional decline.

To maintain functional ability in the hearing impaired, routine ear inspections need to be a part of data collection. Residents have multiple limitations and a decreased response is often acknowledged by caregivers as an exacerbation of another chronic condition. Impacted cerumen may compound hearing loss, and be the reason for reduced responses. Some physicians have nurses irrigate resident's ears on an as-needed basis. Ear drops three or four days prior to the irrigation procedure may be ordered to help emulsify the cerumen.

Nursing care for the hearing impaired resident includes implementing communication techniques and providing hearing aid care. Long term care facilities often store a hearing aid near the resident's medications during the night, or other times when it is not being worn. These devices are very small and could easily be misplaced or damaged. It is the responsibility of the nurse to check the batteries and take care of the appliance. Inserting the hearing aid is a part of personal care or grooming.

Decubitus Ulcers

The impairment of circulation and skin integrity can result in decubitus ulcers, despite diligent nursing measures. There are several factors that make the dependent elderly high-risk for this complication of limited activity. Aging skin is fragile and easily damaged; "skin tears" result from the slightest pressure. It is like rubbing a fresh peach with your thumb. A poor nutritional state, bony prominences, reduced sensations of pain and pressure, and the inability of the elderly to reposition themselves contribute to the skin vulnerability.

Preventing skin breakdown from developing is a problem, but prevention is also the best treatment. One reason is that it takes much longer for the ulcers to heal in the elderly. Use nursing measures of frequent repositioning, massaging around boney prominences, and good skin care.

Endocrine Changes

Complications of diabetes lead to dependency in the elderly. These complications relate to the long-term effects of diabetes on the small blood vessels and nerves. Diabetic neuropathy is the broad term used to describe these results. Perhaps the disease has affected the peripheral vessels and the need for an amputation occurs. Retinopathy may lead to dependency in the elderly diabetic or the kidneys may go into failure and other systems become involved.

RESIDENT CARE PLAN

DATE	PROBLEM	GOALS	TARGET DATE	APPROACH	RESOLVED DATE
2/23	Potential for injury R/T limited vision, hearing, limited movement M/B can only see outline of large objects, needs to have speaker at close range, walks short distances with assistance.	Environment will remain safe; accidents and injury prevented.	5/23	Orientate to any new environment Verbalize actions/steps Keep side rails up, call light in place Speak slowly and clearly	
2/23	Potential social isolation R/T sensory impairment M/B difficulty in communication c̄ roommate, caregivers.	Participate in two facility events per week.	4/23	Verbalize facility events to Katie Include in musical events Assess events that are enjoyed, meaningful Encourage family to visit; read mail	
2/23	Alteration in comfort: Chronic pain R/T joint stiffness, swelling M/B states "I can't move in the morning until I get my pain pills," complaints of hip and knee pain when ambulating.	Reduce joint discomfort.	3/23	Ibuprofen 200-400 mgm q4h prn for discomfort po Tylenol ᷒ tabs q4h prn for pain po Plan activity for 30 min. after analgesia Assist c̄ positioning for comfort	

NURSING ALERT

Allergy: PCN

MEDICAL DIAGNOSIS:	Blindness 2° glaucoma, osteoarthritis						
NAME	NUMBER	ROOM	BIRTHDATE	AGE	ADMIT DATE	PHYSICIAN	DATE	PAGE
Katie Rinkenberger	6821	342	12/3	84	2/19	DR. Bright	2/23	1

Diabetes diagnosis and management was not as sophisticated when today's elderly were young. They did not have the benefit of this new technology, or may not have been compliant with the treatment available. Whatever event brought the individual to the long term care facility, the care needed will require alert nursing assessment and action.

Elderly diabetics do not always demonstrate the symptoms as expected in younger persons. Recall that the "polys" such as polyurina are not as pronounced in the elderly. Diagnosis is often made when investigating other problems such as infections. Demonstrating atypical symptoms is also evident in hypoglycemia. It may be more common for the elderly to exhibit behavior changes such as disorientation, slurred speech, poor sleep patterns, or convulsions, Table 8–1.

Very few diabetic dependent elderly are actively involved in their diabetes management. Nurses are responsible for the blood glucose monitoring, administering insulin, and observing for symptoms of hypoglycemia or hyperglycemia. Not all insulin dependent elderly diabetics are controlled, despite the fact that dietary meal planning and physical activity

polydipsia & polyphagia

	DIABETIC ACIDOSIS	INSULIN REACTION
Cause	Low or non functioning pancreas: not enough insulin Activity is decreased with no dietary adjustment Other diseases or conditions tax available insulin Infection Emotional stress Dietary excess	Pancrease is hyperactive: too much insulin is produced Physical activity is increased without reducing insulin dosage or adjusting dietary intake Dietary insufficiency
Symptoms	Gradual decrease of appetite Incessant thirst Nausea and vomiting Skin flushed and dry Headache Sweet, fruity breath Decreased blood pressure Rapid, thready pulse Weak, stumbly gait	Excess hunger Lethargic, somnolent Sluggish physical response Skin is cold, clammy, moisit Extremities may tremble Irritability Confused Garbled speech Generalized weakness
Blood sugar	Usually in excess of 300mgm/dl	Usually less than 60 mgm/dl
Urine sugar	Usually positive, but not always	Negative
Progression	Gradual	Rapid
Intervention	Regular insulin and fluids	Small amounts of orange juice with sugar dissolved or other carbohydrate that is easily swallowed, such as soft candy. Glucagon

TABLE 8–1   Characteristics of Diabetic Ketoacidosis and Insulin Reaction in the Elderly

seem stable. Loss of appetite, acute illness, and other factors dictate continued monitoring by nurses.

Nursing care for diabetic residents includes ongoing attention to the functioning of all body systems. These elderly have a higher risk for problems in every system. Because of the decreased peripheral sensations, the potential for injury increases. Caregivers watch for possible thermal injuries in providing adequate clothing when the resident is going outside, or checking the temperature of a warm solution. Pressure areas on the feet are noted and shoes checked for correct fit.

Dependent elderly diabetics are not like the elderly with a hip fracture or stroke, where there is the possibility of rehabilitation and improvement. This elderly person experiences ongoing degenerative changes. In addition to alert nursing intervention for the disease process, the nurse provides psychosocial support to the elderly person experiencing the threat of new losses such as vision or a part of an extremity.

Cancer and the Dependent Elderly

Residents in long term care facilities may have had experience with cancer treatment in younger years. They may have been declared "cured," and it was not the condition to precipitate admission to the facility. Like their active aging cohorts, regular monitoring of the involved system will continue. Additional assessments keep nurses alert for potential symptoms of recurrence or metastasis. Nurses usually perform the monthly breast examinations on dependent female residents as a part of periodic nursing assessment.

Dependent elderly who come to the long term care facility because of their cancer are usually in terminal stages of the disease. Hospice care may not be available in the home and alternative plans of care are not manageable by the family or community.

The major concern following admission is pain control in keeping the resident as comfortable as possible. Other goals include attempting adequate nutrition and hydration, and maintaining skin integrity. Daily priorities are cooperatively established by the resident and nurse as many activities identified on a care plan often cannot be tolerated. In addition to analgesia, comfort measures such as oral care and positioning contribute to pain management.

Residents may be receiving cancer treatments such as radiation therapy in a hospital or clinic outpatient setting, or chemotherapy administered by facility nurses. Side effects to be monitored include gastrointestinal disturbances, bleeding tendencies, and risks of infection.

Nursing measures to meet psychosocial needs of terminal cancer residents include arranging time and space for the family and other persons important to the resident. Often a visit by the parish priest or other community clergy is requested by the resident and family. The facility chaplain, social service, or nursing service can assist with arranging requests. Privacy is provided which sometimes takes creative planning. Frequently two residents share a room which limits space for family members. A chapel area or meeting room can provide a private area if the resident is able to be in a wheelchair.

Emotional Response to Declining Health

The elderly resident's response to becoming more dependent on the assistance of others usually reflects his lifelong adaptations. A person's coping mechanisms remain relatively constant. Perhaps you have heard a family visitor remark, "Dad always kept everything inside. I don't think he's going to let us know what's bothering him." You will see a variety of responses to dependency. Some residents will be very quiet and others will be quite vocal. The variety of facility activities may interest some, while others prefer or impose their own social isolation.

In long-term care nursing there is the opportunity of observing and learning about changes over weeks and months. You will develop a long-term trust and helping relationship with the residents. The elderly are a treasury of knowledge and life experiences.

Summary

Dependency in aging is an accumulation of physical and mental limitations rather than a specific disease or condition. Limitations in mobility and thought processes are the two major functional deficits that introduce dependency. Impaired physical mobility which involves the musculoskeletal system, and activity intolerance which involves the respiratory and cardiovascular systems, set the limitations. When an elderly person is capable of completing personal hygiene, but has difficulty in getting supplies or does not have the endurance to complete the task, he has a self-care deficit.

Problems with confusion interfere with independence. For example, an elderly person may be very mobile, but if he no longer has the problem solving ability to complete tasks, he will be dependent in most activities of daily living.

Living with limitations does not mean the elderly need to live in a long term care facility. It is the absence or breakdown of support services that transfer the dependent elderly into a long term care facility. The support system includes the family; often there is burnout of the caregiver.

Chronic conditions contribute to dependency. The older the elderly, particularly after age 85, the more chronic conditions the person experiences. Most are progressive and gradually place more limitations on the aged.

How a resident responds to dependent aging will depend on his lifelong approach to change. Most of us use the same coping methods throughout life. Some residents are accepting and live fully their quality of life. Others may withdraw in a social isolation, or be resentful. Nursing practice in a long term care facility can be rewarding. You have the opportunity to observe and participate in continuity of care for weeks and months. The long-term trust relationship developed with the residents provides you with a unique insite into aging America.

For Discussion

- Visit with a dependent elderly resident in a long term care facility.
  - Assess his functional abilities and limitations.
  - Interview the resident to assess his perception of his limitations now and at the time of his admission.
- Review the medical history and nursing interview of several elderly patients or residents where you are assigned. Share the information about aging and dependency in a small group discussion.
  - Identify the types and numbers of chronic conditions and the older age groups they represent.
  - Identify the condition or situation that indicates some dependency.
  - Identify nursing measures that assist these patients in maintaining their highest functional level.

Questions for Review

1. What are three symptoms expressed by the elderly that are signs of dependent aging?
2. What are two situations that may result in a dependent elderly person being admitted to a long term care facility?
3. What are two chronic conditions that lead to dependency in the elderly? Identify the symptoms that cause the dependency.
4. What are two complications of limited activity that confront the elderly?
5. What are nursing measures to prevent the complications identified in the preceding question?

1. mobility — endurance — sensory deficits.

2. Stroke — Hip fracture

3. — Emphysema — SOB, deaphoreesis ruddy complexion, Barrel chest

— Older elderly — diabetic
any impairment of musculoskeletal respiratory, cardeovascular that isn't able to be cared for by family member

4. Constipation — Skin intergrity

5. nutrition
ROM
Cleanness of skin
turning

Unit 9
Psychosocial Aspects
of Dependent Aging

Objectives

After reading this unit you should be able to:

- Differentiate between mental illness and organic brain disorders.
- Discuss delirium or acute brain syndrome.
- Discuss dementias or chronic brain syndromes.
- Describe nursing intervention for behaviors demonstrated by residents with dementias.
- Discuss social implications of dependent aging.

Control! That is what all of us want in our own lives. To have control of our lives means that we have the authority and ability to direct and regulate our activities. We want to be a part of the decision-making process. When this control is removed we feel threatened. We all have, in some way, experienced this feeling of uncertainty or danger. During school years, we did not have the authority to control some parts of our lives. At the time of an acute illness perhaps we did not have the ability to make decisions for ourselves.

The elderly, in most situations, have the authority to control their lives, but begin to lose the ability. Previous units have discussed physical limitations that may lead to dependency and the loss of control of physical or functional activities. This unit will focus more on the mental limitations that precipitate dependency and the loss of decision-making control over personal activities.

The discussion of the normal aging process and related diseases or conditions tends to focus on the change in body structure and the effects on system functioning. When discussing the difficulties of mental impairment related to aging, the focus is directed more toward the person's

behavior than changes in the brain. This unit will identify some of those behaviors.

Mental illnesses usually begin during younger years. Some of the symptoms demonstrated in these illnesses, such as hallucinations, may be observed in elderly people who are victims of aging brain syndromes. However, the elderly usually demonstrate the behavior as a result of aging factors and the deterioration of brain cells.

Psychiatric nursing intervention will not be discussed in this unit. The objective is to focus on changes in the aging brain and other chronic conditions that alter mental functioning in the elderly population. You may wish to use psychiatric nursing references for further review of functional disorders.

In the past, some degree of confusion, with accompanying dependency, was expected in the elderly. It was considered only a matter of time until a person was labeled "senile," and little effort was made to determine a cause. Today, there is ongoing research, new therapies, and nursing interventions to address a variety of conditions related to mental impairment in the aging population.

Brain syndromes in the elderly are basically manifested in an acute or chronic nature in symptoms and progression. Like other aging conditions you have studied, acute conditions have a more rapid onset, are more illness or disease oriented, and may be curable. Chronic conditions tend to have an insidious onset, progress slowly, are manageable with therapies, and are with the person for the remainder of life.

The active aging population may experience acute mental impairment with (1) an episode of illness, (2) an adverse medication response, (3) dehydration or other metabolic imbalance, or (4) other short-term conditions. Nurses in hospitals and other acute care settings are alert to changes in behavior that signal these complications. Remember, the elderly will develop these acute symptoms more quickly than younger adults.

In long term care facilities, nurses observe more chronic brain disorders that precipitate dependency. These elderly may also experience an acute episode in addition to the chronic impairment. Making these additional assess-ments can be challenging to nurses, especially when the resident is very confused and not able to present complaints.

Nurses and other caregivers often spend more time and effort in managing behavior problems in confused elderly than in implementing personal care, figure 9-1. Results of the behavior changes affect the resident and his family. This includes social isolation for the resident, and a sense of helplessness and frustration in family members.

Psychosocial aspects of nursing care with the dependent elderly can be challenging, frustrating, and rewarding. Often the rewards are seen only in the expression of comfort and peace in the eyes of the resident. Look for it!

Aging and Mental Health Disorders

The mind is a fascinating and mysterious thing! Researchers have learned so much, but do they have only a small part of the potential

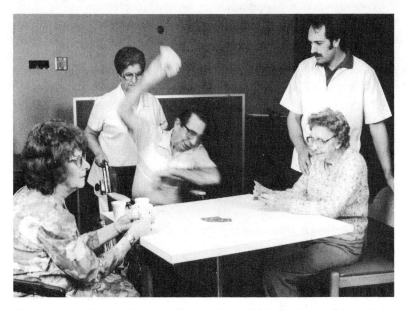

Figure 9-1 Nurses often spend more time with behavior problems than personal care. (From Hegner and Caldwell/*Assisting in Long-Term Care,* copyright 1988 by Delmar Publishers Inc.)

information? In the past, mental health or psychiatric disorders have been aligned with personality development. Childhood experiences during developmental stages determine, to a great extent, the adult personality. Difficulties occur when a person develops abnormal coping mechanisms and demonstrates dysfunctional behavior. Today, we know that biochemical imbalances can result in mental health disorders. This includes the influence of alcohol and illegal drugs.

For the purpose of this brief discussion, mental health disorders will be viewed as psychotic maladjustments that are not results of aging organic changes in the brain cells. A psychosis is characterized by personality disintegration and loss of contact with reality. Examples of these illnesses include: paranoia, manic-depression, schizophrenia, and obsessive-compulsive disorders.

Behaviors demonstrated in people having psychological disorders include: bizarre delusions and hallucinations, severe mood disturbances, phobias, hyperactivity, and inappropriate speech patterns or use of words, such as rhyming. The disorders exhibit problems in relating to others, anger or aggression, disruption in thought process, and anxiety or depression. Many of these people cannot lead functional lives, while others manage very well with psychotherapy and medications.

The history of mental health treatment in the United States is interesting and disturbing. The trend today is to center care for the population with mental handicaps and mental health problems in community group homes. There is not a clear picture of the aging with mental health disorders. People who have been marginally dysfunctional have remained at home. Family members structured their activities and everyone coped.

Some physicians have noted that behaviors associated with diagnosed mental illness tend to "burn out" during old age. If the behavior is still present, it is usually much less active. For example, a paranoia may still be demonstrated

in a statement indicating a particular food is poison; the resident will not eat the food.

As this person ages there may be other chronic problems, such as emphysema, that contribute to a dependency. Nurses in long term care facilities may see residents with a secondary diagnosis indicating a history of mental health illness. Recent changes in admission guidelines do not permit persons with a primary diagnosis of a mental health disorder to enter a long term care facility. Group homes are the residences of choice.

Some of the elderly with mental health disorders are among the homeless. Perhaps they were institutionalized in their younger years. These "state hospitals" began to close during the last three decades. The goal was to service former patients with community social programs. Some became residents of a small number of group homes, others managed to adapt and "make it" independently in the community. Still others "fell through the cracks" of the social welfare system. They became part of the street people population.

Because this population has other chronic health problems that are not monitored, their life expectancy is not the length of the average aging population. We have yet to see how the elderly population of the next century will be affected by mental health disorders. Will improved treatment modalities result in group homes for elderly with functional disorders? What impact will today's social ills have on the mental health of the future's aging population?

Acute Organic Brain Disorders in Aging

Confusion is frustrating even when you are quite certain you are not confused! Have you ever been awakened suddenly from a deep sleep by the sound of a telephone? Did you find yourself grasping for mental clues of day, time, or where you were? Perhaps you did not yet have it "together" before you answered the telephone and you responded, "Who?", to your best friend or neighbor! How did you feel during that brief time of confusion? *Confusion* is a state of mental disorder with the inability to distinguish between things. We become embarrassed during a short-term episode, and anxious if we suspect it may recur or be progressive.

An acute organic brain disorder or *delirium* is a short-term episode of an altered state of consciousness. The person is confused and usually described as disoriented and unable to cooperate or follow directions. Confusion may so mild, or subtle, that caregivers may question whether there is a problem. However, the level of consciousness may also deteriorate to a near coma state, where only repeated or painful stimuli initiates a response.

The cause is most often related to a toxic condition in the body resulting in altered brain functioning. Examples of toxic conditions that interfere with brain functioning are fever, dehydration, malnutrition, electrolyte imbalance, and adverse reactions to medications, including anesthesia. Hypoxia will cause temporary disorientation. Head trauma or brain tumors can result in a delirious state. When collecting data regarding previous acute illnesses, a patient may refer to an episode of delirium as being "out of my head." Examples of predisposing causes of acute organic brain syndrome are summarized in table 9–1.

Nurses must assess for signs of the person's inability to maintain control over thought processes and behavior. In addition to disorientation and uncooperative behavior, the patient may give inappropriate answers to questions, and demonstrate restlessness, agitation, and anxiety. This patient cannot change his behavior. It will improve when the toxic problem is eliminated and symptoms disappear.

CONDITION	PREDISPOSING CAUSE
Hypoxia	Advanced Congestive Heart Failure Advanced Chronic Obstructive Pulmonary Disease Myocardial Infarction
Metabolic Alterations	Dehydration Hypoglycemia Malnutrition Drug Therapy Organ Function Failure
Toxic Responses	Kidney Failure Alcohol Drugs Anesthesia
Trauma	Brain Tumors Cerebrovascular Accidents Blow to the Head
Fever	Infection Dehydation

TABLE 9–1 Cause of Acute Organic Brain Syndrome in the Elderly

You may have observed mild or short-term confusion in an elderly patient who seemed "fine" yesterday. For example, a stubborn elderly man is recuperating in a circle bed. He refuses to eat or drink because, "I never ate laying down and I'm not going to start now." In two days he suddenly becomes disoriented. Laboratory findings demonstrate electrolyte imbalances. Another example is a 75-year-old woman hospitalized for a transient ischemia attack, accompanied by a hypertensive crisis. Having no previous history of hypertension, she is given a thiazide diuretic. Within 12 hours she is extremely agitated and confused. It is discovered she is sensitive to the diuretic as her serum sodium is 116 mEq. Following a restricted fluid intake, the sodium level increased, and she became alert again.

In acute or long-term care, nursing intervention during a time of confusion includes assuming all safety responsibilities until the person is alert again and able to manage himself and his environment. If he is agitated, restless, or hyperactive, it may indicate the need for physical restraints to prevent self-inflicted injury. Restraints may increase the agitation, so therefore should be applied with caution. Someone should remain with the patient at all times. Caregivers must remain calm, be reassuring to the patient and family, and move at a quiet unhurried pace. The number of people in the room should be limited, and noise and other environmental stimuli controlled and minimized. This calm and stable environment supports the confused person during the time his thought processes are out of control, figure 9–2.

Part of the ongoing assessment is to determine if the patient is oriented. Does he know the time, where he is, who he is, and other pertinent data relevant to the situation? Even if he is wrong, reassure him and provide the correct information. However, do not overload his sensory intake by giving him unnecessary information or explanations.

Independence is promoted by allowing the confused person to complete self care if he is

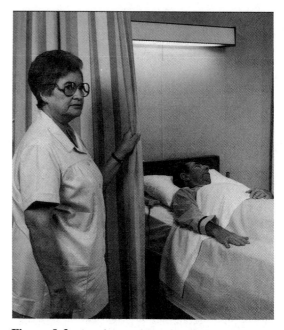

Figure 9-2 A calm, stable environment supports the patient experiencing delirium. (From Hegner and Caldwell/*Assisting in Long-Term Care*, copyright 1988 by Delmar Publishers Inc.)

able. Ongoing assessments determine changes in behavior and thought processes and the ability to complete tasks such as feeding, grooming, and hygiene. Physicians may order antipsychotic and antianxiety drugs to help the person through this uncomfortable time.

Nurses need to be alert to predisposing causes and clues from patient histories that may indicate acute organic brain syndrome. When a frail, acutely ill, confused elderly person is admitted to the hospital, it should not be assumed that confusion is normal for this patient. Care plans and goals should address the confusion as well as physical problems. The psychosocial care is as challenging as the physical care. Family members may need more support and assistance than the patient during this difficult period. They are anxious and fearful about the outcome of the illness. They may grieve the temporary "loss" of the parent or spouse who does not recognize them at this time.

Chronic Organic Brain Syndrome

The fear of "losing my mind" is very real to the older population. They see friends "slip away" when they cannot function socially. They confront themselves with their own memory problems; they have difficulty recalling names and dates. Nurses must reassure the elderly that temporary memory lapses are common in the aging process.

Dementia is the broad term used to describe chronic brain syndromes that demonstrate gradual progressive loss of intellectual abilities. *Senility* is an outdated term that is still heard, but primarily from persons outside health related professions. The word itself just means old. Its use is in stereotyping behaviors that can result from the normal aging process such as forgetfulness, memory lapses, and slow reactions in communication or motor responses.

Dementia is characterized by the loss of cognitive ability. *Cognition* is the ability to process information; it is the process of knowing and thinking. Losses, to a varying degree, in dementia include intellect, memory, orientation, and judgement. Those suspected of having developed a dementia demonstrate a loss of recent memory. They have difficulty in concentrating, in completing simple calculations, and in learning new information or tasks. Signs of fluctuating mood changes may also be exhibited. Residents, especially those who perceive some situation as a threat, or feel anxious in any way, may also demonstrate signs of psychotic symptoms such as delusions. Family members may identify a potential problem when an aging parent has increasing difficulties with usual household tasks and routines. Nurses validate the potential problem when attempting patient teaching.

It is estimated that more than 5 percent of the elderly are victims of dementia and perhaps half of this number have the Alzheimer type. There are many probable causes of this old age loss of mental functioning. Altered sensory perception can contribute to the impairment. In many situations, the cause is eventually related to inadequate supply of oxygen to the brain, or other insults that interfere with brain functioning. Table 9-2 differentiates characteristics of confusion in the elderly.

Multi-Infarct Dementia

Multi-infarct dementia occurs following repeated strokes or transient ischemia attacks that have destroyed small areas of brain tissue. Often these events affect speech, memory, and coordination. There may be long periods of stable functioning and even periods where there seems to be improvement. The association with hypertensive disease indicates that the vessels are vulnerable to many problems. This person is at risk for a major stroke.

Treatment for multi-infarct dementia includes managing hypertension and preventing further strokes. Sometimes this is effective and the dementia is stablized; the person maintains a functional level. Other times the dementia continues to progress. Many of these people eventually become residents of a long term care facility.

Chronic Organic Brain Syndrome

Chronic organic brain syndrome (COBS) as identified on a resident's chart is a dementia that is of uncertain cause and onset. Often it refers to the probability of cerebral arteriosclerosis. The vessels deteriorate and no longer bring nutrients to the brain cells. The tissue withers and is not functional. It is slow, progressive, and irreversible. Unlike the multi-infarct dementias, these residents do not demonstrate periods of stable activity or even possible improvement.

In early dementia, the person attempts to "cover up" or compensate for the memory loss. Excuses are manufactured and lists made for routine or daily activities. Memory loss progresses until family members become aware of

CLASSIFICATION	CHARACTERISTICS	OUTCOME	TREATMENT
Multi-infarct dementia	Results from emboli and infarct in brain tissue. Sudden onset.	Irreversible though not progressive unless further infarct occurs.	Prevent further dementia by treating hypertension or other causative factors.
Senile dementia organic brain syndrome	Develops slowly. Progressive. Of uncertain onset.	Irreversible. Progresses unpredictably though usually slowly.	No treatment.
Alzheimer's disease	Characteristic pattern of deficit evolves.	Irreversible. Progresses more or less predictably and rapidly.	No treatment.
Depression	Many causative factors, such as loss of mate, economic status, disease, or aging. Gradual or situational onset.	Reversible if recognized and treated.	Drug therapy. Psychotherapy. Treat causative factor.
Drug or disease induced confusion	Abrupt, rapid onset. Often associated with other neurological signs.	Reversible if cause is recognized and treated promptly.	Remove problem drug from regimen. Treat disease that is causing confusion.

TABLE 9–2 Differentiating Confusion in the Elderly

the problem. Then they often attempt to conceal the problem from friends and other social contacts. Higher brain functions may be affected in later stages and the person will have difficulties in walking and speaking.

There is no treatment for this irreversible loss of mental functioning. Each elderly confused resident needs individual, and ongoing, assessment to determine what activities will be most helpful to promote a continued quality of life. In early dementia, occupational therapy, activity groups, or other expressive therapy may be helpful to maintain a level of function. Most drug treatment is prescribed to manage symptoms. For example, the physician may order a sedative for difficulties with sleep, or a psychotropic for severe agitation.

Nursing intervention for elderly residents with dementias is individualized according to the person's abilities and limitations. Goals include maintaining the resident's dignity and quality of life. Routines are established to promote a level of independence and minimize further confusion. The independence may be implemented in allowing limited choices in dress, jewelry, foods, or ambulation exercises. The resident is still exercising the freedom of choice.

Safety is always a high priority for nurses. The resident's care plan is revised periodically to meet changing concerns. As dementia progresses, more personal and environmental safety concerns are addressed. The losses in dementia mirror the development in early childhood; the abilities lost demonstrate reverse order of early accomplishment, figure 9-3. At some time nonedible items, such as shampoo, must be stored in locked cupboards. Wandering is common. Like a toddler, the resident must be continually watched. He needs frequent remind-

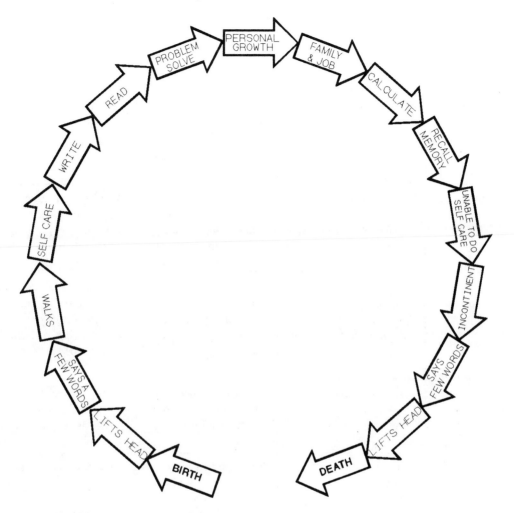

Figure 9–3 Circle of life: dependent, independent, dependent

ers. He does not remember the direction to his room or the dining room.

An important part of nursing care is providing support to the family. They are uncertain about their own behavior toward a loved one who no longer recognizes them. Some may desperately attempt to reorient the resident; others display their discomfort by avoiding visits altogether.

Alzheimer's Disease

The dementia called Alzheimer's is being labeled the disease of the century for the elderly population. It is not a new type of dementia; the pathology was described by a physician nearly two hundred years ago. In 1907 a German neurologist, Alois Alzheimer, studied and described the dementia in more detail. A

	STAGE I	FAMILY TEACHING	STAGE II
Memory	Forgetful with mild memory lapse. Long-term memory undisturbed.	Keep all items in familiar, specific places. Write messages, names, and phone numbers. Supervise and check frequently.	Recent memory is totally lost. Long-term memory deficits begin to show. Acquired routines are forgotten.
Behavior	Subtle personality changes. Forgets social courtesies. Withdrawal. Difficulty focusing attention.	Remind gently and tactfully when social courtesies are forgotten. Plan short activities with familiar content.	Confused to time, person, place, and event. Suspicious, argues, untidy, agitated. May strike out.
Ability to learn	Becomes very imaginative in covering memory loss. Reasoning is intact.	Reorient often and repeatedly. Encourage to keep performing skills.	Logic and judgement impaired. Loss of reasoning and ability to read.
Communication	Spoken sentences become shorter. Words may be missing.	Listen for missing words and help fill in the gaps. Use simple, short sentences.	Loss of sensory processing. Speech is garbled. Repetition of words or phrases is common.
Nutritional Status	Taste becomes flat. Food choices decrease.	Serve food in plain dishes. Offer hi-cal snacks, remind to eat at meal time, suggest favorite foods.	Appetite may increase, though may not be aware more food is being eaten. Mouth is always moving.
Physical status	Unsteady gait, trips easily, and drops things.	Pick up rugs, remove low tables and stools. Install rails, bars in hall and bathroom.	Loss of coordinated movement. Unable to walk, feed, or dress self.
Sensory status	Seems to tune out the world. Touch sense is intact.	Touch. Use name. Encourage old familiar friends and family to visit.	Unable to process what is seen and heard. Cannot initiate hugs, but can respond.

TABLE 9–3   An Overview of Alzheimer's Disease

FAMILY TEACHING NURSING APPROACHES	STAGE III	NURSING APPROACHES
Clocks and calendars in easy view. Picture or label contents of cupboards and drawers. Do not alter routine. Assist with hygiene and clothes	Impairment in all areas is evident.	Caregiver must perform all cares. Is no longer to perform routine functions. Is not safe to leave alone at any time.
Do not force to be involved in activities. Avoid stressful situations, crowds, travel, or changes in environment. Structure routine as much as possible.	Unresponsive verbally and physically except for reflexes.	Provide quiet soothing environment. Administer, with caution, medications as ordered by physician. Restrain only for safety, and as a last resort.
Do not expect the individual to draw conclusions or have opinions. Use name frequently. Remind of events, read mail.	Loss of ability to absorb or process new information.	Read to or play soothing music that is familiar. Identify yourself. Use resident's name often. Do not change routines.
Use low tones. Expect one word responses. Use eye contact. Never approach from behind.	Gutteral sounds or mute. Unresponsive to simple commands.	Use touch, smiles, and calm approach. Do cares with gentleness. Talk slowly and with reassurance as you work.
Cut food in bite-sized pieces. Offer finger foods. Monitor weight and activity level. Do not feed. Encourage to feed self.	Decreased appetite. Difficulty chewing and swallowing. Weight loss may be significant.	Spoon feed. Foods must be ground or blended. May progress to tube feeding.
Walk with cane, walker, or assistance. May be in a wheelchair. Caregiver may need assistance.	Spastic, rigid muscles. Immobile. May develop seizure activity.	Warm baths to relax muscles and limbs. Range of motion to decrease atrophy and contracture. Seizure meds.
Use short spoken phrases and smiles. Expect responses. Keep familiar smells, sounds, tastes, and pictures in home or room.	Unresponsive to sensory input. Responds only to painful stimuli.	Touch gently when doing cares. Use name and speak softly. Assess facial expression for signs of pain. Medicate carefully by physician order.

TABLE 9–3 (Continued)

woman had died in her 50s following several years of severe dementia. The autopsy revealed degenerating brain cells and neurofibrillary tangles in the area of the brain associated with memory. Little research was continued on this dementia until the 1960s. Changing demographics initiated new research on the growing aging population. The media picked up the message when entertainment personalities were diagnosed with the condition. Unfortunately, Alzheimer's became a "buzzword" that the public frequently attached to forgetfulness at any age.

Today, Alzheimer's still can only be diagnosed positively by autopsy. Physicans rule out organic problems, review the person's history and symptoms, and diagnose "Dementia–Alzheimer's Type." It is estimated that over 2.5 million Americans, mostly elderly citizens, are affected by this disease. Death is often the result of an infection or other complication. The life expectancy of Alzheimer's victims is much shorter than that of other elderly persons.

In addition to the neurofibrillary tangles found in the brain's nerve cells, neuritic plaques seem to develop around the neurons. There also seems to be decreased acetylcholine, the neurotransmitter that is involved in sending information between cells in the brain. Research continues to look for underlying causes of these changes and the symptoms demonstrated by the victims of the disease. Some findings include the belief that there is some familial tendencies; there seems to be an inherited predisposition. Other research has identified a defective chromosome associated with the neurofibrillary tangles and neuritic plaques. Older theories linked the disease to viruses with very long incubation periods, or aluminum. The traces of aluminum found in the brain are now thought to be more of a result, rather than a cause, of the dementia.

A thorough examination is required to determine a probable diagnosis of Alzheimer's dementia. The focus of the examination is to rule out other possibilites and establish the characteristic behaviors of the disease. The physical includes a thorough neurologic examination. A medication history and functional assessment is important. Differentiating Alzheimer's from other dementias includes confirming cognitive deficits, progressive impairment in memory, and difficulty in managing usual activities of daily living. Identifying behavior problems also include: *anomia*, the inability to name things; *agnosia*, the inability to recognize things; *apraxia*, the difficulty in accomplishing activities; and *aphasia*, the difficulty in speaking.

There is no treatment for Alzheimer's disease at this time. Experimental drug therapy is directed toward preventing the breakdown of acetylcholine in the brain. Supportive care for the patient and family is the therapy until research discovers the cause and an effective treatment.

The symptoms of Alzheimer's are described by characteristic behaviors demonstrated in three stages, table 9–3. Prior to Stage I, casual memory loss or other deviations from the person's "normal" behavior are often attributed to illness, stress, or old age. Family members tend to gloss over the changes, with comments such as, "Grandma is sure getting irritable in her old age!"

Stage I demonstrates more pronounced changes in areas such as memory, behavior, ability to learn, communication, and nutrition, and physical and sensory status. The older adult manages at home with a supportive family. Teaching the family about the disease and methods to cope can be very helpful to them and the elderly member with Alzheimer's. However, in this stage, many families may still be in denial and refuse to seek help.

Assistance is needed with activities of daily living in Stage II. The person is dependent. Recent memory is lost, confusion is increased, and the individual may become either agitated and aggressive, or extremely docile. Social behaviors demonstrated are opposite of those observed in younger adult years. For example, a woman during younger years was described as a kind and gentle supportive wife and mother. She now is abusive in language and strikes out at her husband when he visits. Her daughter, in confidence, recalls her childhood and episodes when her father would hit her mother.

During Stage II, some elderly victims of Alzheimer's can remain at home. This requires a number of supportive family members and community services to assist with respite care and other needs. At some time during this stage, many elderly are admitted to a long term care facility because the caregiver burns out. This is usually an elderly spouse with intermittent or no family help. The confused person does not know night from day, wanders, and does not allow the caregiver adequate emotional or physical rest.

Stage III demonstrates continued progressive impairment in physical abilities. Cognitive ability is gone and the individual requires total care. Safety concerns related to ambulation, such as wandering, or ingesting inedible items, are no longer risks. The effort of caregiving is physical in providing total care with the prevention of complications of bedrest. Maintaining a sense of dignity is ongoing. Because of the decreased cough reflex and immune response in aging, pneumonia is often the cause of death.

Family members may exhibit expressions of relief rather than sadness at the time of death. Often the grieving process began when the parent or grandparent could no longer recognize family members.

Caregiving to Alzheimer's victims will continue to be a challenge and an issue of health care in the next century. Today, there are limited funds for what is identified as "custodial care." Family caregivers become physically, emotionally, and financially exhausted. This is also true of caregivers and the payment systems in long-term care.

Nursing Intervention with Dementia Victims

Nurses have an expanding role in the care and management of elderly dementia victims. Since there is little treatment, the resident's physician does not have the active involvement with this condition as with other chronic disorders. Nursing collaborates with occupational therapy, physical therapy, and recreational or activity departments to attempt to keep the resident ambulatory and provide a quality of life.

The resident care plan related to dementia focuses on behaviors. The behaviors need to be evaluated carefully to determine the nature and possible causes; then intervention will be more appropriate and successful. Two basic approaches to behavior management are psychosocial measures and medications. Reality orientation is an example of therapies used with confused residents. Finally, the care plan must include the resident's family. They have a great need to know what is happening to their confused parent or other relative. Nurses provide support and reassurance in decisions regarding choices for care.

In establishing a data base for care plans focusing on mental impairment, the nurse can begin by determining the resident's mental status. Figure 9-4 illustrates a short mental status exam that you can complete during a brief interview. In the example, the 75-year-old resident was admitted ambulatory, accompanied by his wife and daughter. Mr. Brownington appeared alert, and his conversation seemed appropriate. His daughter had come from out-of-state to assist her mother with this event. She stated her mother was exhausted from her father's nocturnal wandering. After assisting him to place personal items in the room, the nurse sat beside Mr. Brownington to visit and complete the short mental status exam, figure 9-5.

Recall that it is best to plan an elderly interview early in the day when the person is more

SHORT MENTAL STATUS EXAM

Test Items	Maximum Score	Resident Score	Weight
1. What year is it now?	(1)	_1_	x 4 = _4_
2. What month is is now?	(1)	_O_	x 3 = _O_
3. Memory Phrase: Repeat after me: John Brown, 42 Market Street, Chicago			
4. About what time is it? (within one hour)	(1)	_O_	x 3 = _O_
5. Count backwards from 20 to 1.	(2)	_2_	x 2 = _4_
6. Say the months in reverse order.	(2)	_2_	x 2 = _4_
7. Repeat the memory phrase.	(5)	_3_	x 2 = _6_
8. Where are you now?	(1)	_O_	x 4 = _O_
9. What is your name.	(1)	_O_	x 4 = _O_
10. Who is the President of the U.S.?	(2)	_1_	x 2 = _2_

Total = _20_

Circle level of impairment:
Minimal = 0 - 8,   Moderate = 9 - 22,   Severe = 23 and above

Comments: _Became agitated when asked to_
repeat phrase. Got up out of chair
and walked to doorway x 2. Attempted
to cover-up inability to complete numerical
exercise; laughed, stated never good
c̄ numbers. Answer for President
incorrect, corrected self c̄ cue.

Figure 9–4   Sample of a short mental status examination

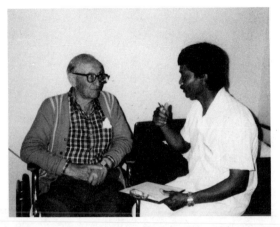

Figure 9–5 Visiting with a new resident will assist in completing a short mental status examination.

likely to be refreshed and alert. The elderly may demonstrate sundown syndrome if interviewed extensively late in the day. *Sundown syndrome* may be described as symptoms of agitation, restlessness, or disruptive behavior that are demonstrated in the late afternoon or early evening hours in persons who are usually alert, calm, and cooperative during morning hours.

Examining Behaviors

The resident's conduct, manners, and response to stimuli is not often addressed until it becomes a "problem." Problems are usually perceived to be disruptive actions or events that irritate or interfere with other resident's or caregiver's activities, or are unsafe to the resident and others. Examples are verbal or physical abuse, continual verbal bantering, or wandering into other resident's rooms. Table 9–4 presents disruptive behaviors that confused elderly may exhibit. How to cope with these behaviors in nursing intervention and prevention may assist you in providing care for confused elderly persons.

"Appears agitated," may be written in the chart. What is meant by agitated is not always clear. It is often a general term meaning in-

creased activity. Depending on the usual activity of a resident, it could be increased rocking motion in a chair, or an increased pace or amount of time spent in walking. Examples of other increased activity could be frequent attempts to get out of bed or climb over side rails, continual pulling on a catheter or other tube, or searching for items believed to be lost. Although most caregivers describe agitation in disruptive behaviors, a resident can demonstrate more quiet, but still agitated, behaviors. This is when agitation is manifested in less disruptive behaviors such as sleeplessness or poor appetite.

Agitation is described as aggressive when the resident could cause injury to self, other residents, or caregivers. The confused resident could attempt to strike or bump other residents with fists, canes, or wheelchairs. Sometimes a very confused agitated resident will refuse to cooperate with caregivers who are providing personal care. There may be an attempt to bite or scratch.

Another way agitation is demonstrated is in a change in speech pattern. Verbalization may be exaggerated normal speech, or very different speech patterns such as repeated speech or questions, such as, "When am I going home?" Resident's speech can also be louder, faster, less clear, or they may use profane language that has not traditionally been in their conversation.

Determining the cause — if possible — of the agitation, is helpful in calming the resident both physically and emotionally. If the confused resident cannot relate her fears or needs, the caregiver needs to be resourceful and discover the irritant. Caregivers assigned the same group of residents for a period of time learn the unique characteristics of each person. They can often see a pattern of events or situations that tend to promote agitation.

The feeling of tension or irritability may be precipitated by pain, fever, or other body response to acute illness, adverse reactions to medications, and other physical discomforts.

BEHAVIOR	DEFINITION	SYMPTOMS	INTERVENTIONS	PREVENTION
Violent reactions	An emotionally violent response to a seemingly insignificant incident.	Crying Verbal abuse Angry outbursts Frenzied restlessness and physical violence	Protect yourself. Do not try to reason with the individual. Ignore if behavior is attention seeking. Remain silent, be calm. Reassure and be tender. Do not use threatening body language. If physically violent, gently back into a corner using a shield such as a large sofa cushion. Restrain only as a last resort.	Be aware of what causes or triggers outbursts. Attempt to eliminate or minimize those sources. Correlate the time of day when incidents occur. Establish a trusting relationship with the individual by using a consistent touch communication type of approach. Very careful use of medication in low doses.
Delusions and hallucinations	A delusion is a fixed idea with no basis in reality but is stubbornly maintained.	The individual believes they or loved ones have another identify or have performed impossible feats. They see things that are not really there.	Do not try to talk the individual out of the idea. Do not agree or go along with the idea. Attempt to distract. Be gentle and supportive. Focus on real objects in the area.	Look for hidden meanings in the delusions. Rule out drug toxicity, infections, pain, or other physical stresses. Remove objects that may be involved in the hallucinations.
Paranoia	Unreasonable distrust, suspicion, or an exaggerated sense of one's own importance.	Suspicious and hostile. Blame others for what they forget or cannot find. Protect ego.	Do not argue or defend self if accused. Do not embarrass the individual. Be matter of fact. Look for missing objects. Rearrange schedules, make new appointments. Handle things for them.	Keep away from crowds. Become a confidant. Empathize. Never surprise. Write out all activities and do not deviate from the plan. Always be honest. Maintain eye contact.

TABLE 9–4 How to Cope With Disruptive Behavior in the Confused Elderly

BEHAVIOR	DEFINITION	SYMPTOMS	INTERVENTIONS	PREVENTION
Restlessness and wandering	Purposeless and repetitive movements or aimless walking with no direction or apparent purpose.	Sundowning. High agitation levels. Constant physical motion. Endless repetition of spoken phrases.	Attempt to lower stress level by taking care of needs such as exercise, food, toileting, pain relief, prevention of fatigue, and decreasing disturbing sights and sounds.	Identify the individual's agenda. Identify the things that motivate the activity. Carefully note time, behavior, and intervention. Develop care plan to prevent the behavior.
Self mutilation	The act of damaging the body by one's own self.	Finger or nail biting are common. Pick at one spot of the body. Hit head against the wall or other object. Pull out hair. Skin rubbing.	Keep hands busy with crafts or other activities that require the use of the hands. Increase daily exercise. Keep sharp objects out of reach.	Reduce stress level. Carefully note behavior and attempt to find a cause for anxiety. Divert or change the activity by substituting a safe activity.
Hiding or hoarding objects	To accumulate or gather objects by saving and/or hiding.	Objects in the household or living area are picked up and hidden.	Understand and have patience. Do not accuse. Find hiding places. The same ones are often used many times.	Lock up valuables. Lock doors to private areas such as offices and medication rooms.
Inappropriate sexual behavior	Behavior involving the genitals that is not appropriate in public.	Exposing the genitals. Masturbation or undressing in public.	Remove from public setting and take to room where behavior may continue. Establish a behavior modification program for each individual.	Supply touching and stroking that is appropriate. Check medication profile for possible new medications with side effects. Check for possible urinary tract infections or other infections in the genital area.

TABLE 9–4   (Continued)

Some predisposing factors related to psycho-social problems and agitation could be sensory deprivation, social isolation, increased environmental stimulation, and different caregivers.

Approaches to Behavior Management

A team approach is helpful in gathering data about the confused resident and his behaviors. Nurses, nursing assistants, therapists, and family members work together in planning the most successful approach. A calm approach in talking and moving is a good start in managing agitation. A gentle voice and touch is soothing to the internal tension. This may take a conscious effort since most long term care facilities are very active places. Other approaches include maintaining a routine, a schedule, structuring activities, and redirecting the resident to more purposeful actions. Keeping the environment quiet or moving the resident to a less stimulating place is also helpful. For example, it will be more calming to have a resident listen to soothing music in her room than to join a group having a sing-a-long with piano music.

Restraining a resident with physical devices or medication control should be a last resort. Using wrist, vest, or other physical restraints may increase agitation. Even when a caregiver attempts to hold a resident to protect both persons, the action may initiate further aggressive behavior. When it becomes necessary to use physical restraints, caregivers must follow facility protocol and use reasonable care. This includes obtaining a physician order and family approval. Nursing measures implement use of safety measures such as checking circulation, fastening straps in appropriate places, and staying with the resident if the situation still appears hazardous.

Restraint or control of behavior with the use of medications should also be implemented with extreme caution. Physicians may order psychotropic drugs such as Diazepam, Flurazepan, or Triazolam on a PRN basis. It becomes nursing judgement whether the medication is administered. Nurses must take time to evaluate the disruptive behavior and determine if psychosocial measures would be as effective as a medication.

One difficulty in administering medications as a treatment for behaviors related to confusion is the potential risk of undesirable side effects. Recall that the normal aging process affects the metabolism of medications. Some psychotropics have a very long half-life which may be extended longer in the elderly. Combinations and interactions of a few or several medications may exaggerate or change a behavior.

Careful observation and documentation of behaviors before and after administration of psychotropics is very important. This helps in determining the effects of the medication. The lowest therapeutic dose is always the most desirable. Nurses in long term care facilities collaborate with physicians to plan the medication for treatment of behaviors related to confusion in the elderly.

Reality orientation includes activities completed by nurses and other caregivers to increase awareness of time, place, and person in people with confusion or other memory impairments. This means of assisting the confused elderly in maintaining a quality of life has been used by nurses for over 25 years. The technique can be implemented during routine interactions with residents. For example, when awakening a resident, you may say, "Good morning Mr. Lyon, this is Sue Smith, I'll be your nurse today. It's Tuesday, 8 a.m. and time for breakfast." This is in contrast to, "Wake up Mr. Lyon, it's time to eat." The first statement provides the resident with his name, your name, the day, time, and activity. All caregivers can participate in this type of reality orientation. It is not a structured group activity like other therapies.

Long term care facilities promote reality orientation for all residents in a variety of ways. Calendars with facility activities are usually placed in each room. The date, in large numbers, is displayed near the nurse's desk or elevator, at eye level for residents in wheel chairs.

In facilities with public address systems, a morning greeting may include the date, time, and weather forecast, in addition to activity announcements.

A feeling of well-being is perhaps the goal of all therapies that focus on feelings and behaviors of the confused elderly. Any therapy should be revised or discontinued if it appears to agitate or irritate the resident. You must report changes; a team approach will again be used to revise the care plan.

Social Implications/Providing Family Support

Beginning confusion often starts during active aging years and the family attempts to cope. As the elderly family member demonstrates increased confusion in routine tasks, there is also an increase in problems with social interactions. Later, social isolation occurs; sometimes separating an elderly couple from social activities in the community.

Problems with social interaction as a result of increasing confusion may occur because the elderly person has difficulty in conversation. He may no longer be able to participate in an activity such as playing cards. The family continues to include the confused member; but friends and neighbors become uncomfortable in the social situation, and visits become more infrequent.

Family members of residents who have mental impairment need continued support by nurses and other staff members. The confusion may have surfaced after the resident was admitted. You need to establish a rapport with the resident's family and other visitors to provide support during this difficult time for them. Perhaps they need an explanation regarding the disease or condition. Explaining the disease process and expected behaviors may assist them in preparing for the days ahead.

Support groups are often helpful to family members. One example is the Alzheimer's Disease and Related Disorders Association. Hopefully, the family will have had an inter-action with home health nurses or other community resource persons while the confused family member was at home. Part of establishing rapport with the family will be to determine their support system. Nurses in long term care facilities become a part of that support system. They also can put the family in touch with organized support groups. Objectives of support groups include providing information as well as an emotional outlet to express feelings and frustrations.

Social implications for the resident in the long term care facility relates to maintaining interactions with other residents and staff for as long as possible. Meaningful relationships can provide cognitive stimulation, maintain communication skills, and promote self-esteem. There will come a time in late stages of dementia when social isolation occurs because of the loss of cognitive ability. As the resident's abilities deteriorate, the family still requires support and guidance from nurses.

Summary

The gradual loss of intellectual abilities means loss of decision-making control over personal activities. For the aging population this means eventual dependency and possible placement in a long term care facility for the remainder of life.

This psychosocial dependency in aging relates to changes in brain cells that are a result of chronic organic disease or in normal aging changes in cells and tissues. Like other conditions discussed in earlier units, some elderly are more prone to these symptoms of aging than are others in their cohort. Symptoms of intellectual dysfunctioning in the elderly are not to be interpreted the same as personality disorders of younger adults.

Confusion or disorientation is the major symptom demonstrated by older adults who have become dependent because of mental impairment. Confusion can be acute or chronic. Like other symptoms in the aging population, a sudden change in behavior is probably related to an acute illness. Delirium or acute brain disorder can usually be attributed to a toxic condition. These are usually short-term episodes and patients will return to previous levels of alertness. During the time they are confused, patients are unable to cooperate and follow directions.

Chronic brain syndromes demonstrate gradual progressive loss of intellectual abilities. These dementias are characterized by losses in intellect, memory, orientation, and judgement. Early signs of confusion are demonstrated in loss of recent memory and difficulty in concentration. There can be many causes of these chronic brain disorders, but it is estimated that perhaps half of the elderly demonstrating the symptoms have the Alzheimer type.

Nursing care for residents with progressive dementias focuses on maintaining independence for as long as possible. There is no cure and medical treatment addresses managing behaviors and acute conditions, such as infections. A majority of the care involves nursing intervention to manage the activities of daily living. Care plans also focus on other chronic disorders. The Nursing Process is a challenge for nurses, especially when residents are unable to verbalize their feelings and symptoms.

Two basic approaches to behavior management are psychosocial measures and medications. Psychosocial measures stress environmental control and therapeutic behaviors of caregivers. Treatment that is more constraining includes the use of physical restraints and psychotropic medications. This type of control should be used as a last resort after careful evaluation of behaviors and psychosocial methods implemented.

Reality orientation is a method of assisting the confused elderly to maintain a quality of life. Techniques of orienting the resident to time, place, and person can be implemented by all caregivers during usual interactions with the person.

A feeling of well-being by the resident is the goal of all care plans when addressing the problem of confusion and related behaviors. Some elderly are more comfortable emotionally when they continue to live in the past.

Social implications of aging and confusion often begin when the elderly are still at home. The isolation of confusion may begin when there is difficulty in communicating and interacting with friends and neighbors. Family members need the guidance and support of nurses and other caregivers when the elderly family member is confused. Support groups also assist in providing education as well as a place to share feelings and frustrations. In their support and guidance, nurses and others encourage family members to stay involved, and continue caregiving and visiting.

Giving of your time, your caring, and your touch can make a difference in the lives of all residents, including the confused elderly. A special moment, a tender touch, and individualized caring can be the environmental stimulation needed to promote self-worth and positive feelings in the confused elderly.

For Discussion

- In a small group: Identify words or short phrases that describe your feelings when caring for patients who are experiencing confusion. Discuss possible reasons for these feelings.
- In a small group: Share approaches used in implementing reality orientation. Evaluate each situation, focusing on patient response and changes in nursing intervention.

- Invite someone who can share a family's views on experiencing confusion in an elderly family member.

Questions for Review

1. What is delirium? *State of mental confusion*
2. What is dementia? *Impairment of intellectual function*
3. What is multi-infarct dementia?
4. What is chronic organic brain syndrome? *gradual progressive loss of intell abilities*
5. What is Alzheimer's type dementia?
6. What are two psychosocial interventions for confusion? *OT PT*
7. Why should restraints and medications be used as a last resort with confused elderly?

Psycho social
1. environmental control
2. Therapeutic Behavior

Unit 10
Experiencing Loss
in Dependent Aging

Objectives

After reading this unit you should be able to:

- Recall the stages of grieving or loss.
- Identify multiple losses of the aging population.
- Discuss loneliness related to losses in aging.
- Discuss depression and related situations in the elderly.
- Discuss elderly responses to dying and death.
- Describe implications for nursing care of elderly persons experiencing multiple losses.

"He's gone." "She's gone." "It's gone." Most of us have experienced loss in our lives. Perhaps it was a pet or favorite toy. Maybe a move to a new community resulted in a period of grieving for a special place in your home, your friends, school, or neighborhood. Many of us, whatever age, have experienced the death and loss of a grandparent, parent, or friend.

The aging population experiences multiple and compounding losses that involve their identity, life style, independence, and companionship, figure 10-1. Experiencing these losses may begin as early as middle age, when children become independent and aging parents begin to die. For most aging individuals, multiple losses begin at the time of retirement, and are compounded rapidly during the old old years.

This unit will focus on the multiple losses experienced by the aging population, their responses or reactions to the losses, and appropriate nursing intervention. A review of the stages of grieving will be presented. Perhaps you have studied them in other courses.

A discussion of losses will identify those experienced by the active aging as well as the compounded losses of dependent aging. Nurses in all areas of practice must be alert to the kinds of losses elderly patients experience. Patient interviews and nursing histories need this data when analyzing patient problems. Part of the nursing diagnosis will include the affect of loss on physical problems and behavior changes.

Loneliness can be experienced during all stages of life. The multiple losses with aging can intensify and extend the feelings associated with loneliness. This unit will identify some expressions of loneliness in aging.

Depression in the elderly is underestimated in this country. It is often masked by other complaints and ailments. It can result from deep extended loneliness, a reaction to medications, or other causes. Alcoholism and other abusive behaviors may be a result of depression or compound the symptoms. Suicide in the elderly is at an alarming rate for this population group.

The process of dying and the event of death is managed by the elderly as individually

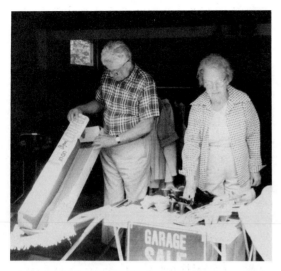

Figure 10–1 The elderly experience multiple losses with aging.

as it is with younger persons. Our society too often responds to these events in aging as if they are to "be expected" and "taken for granted." The elderly are not supported adequately. Most have a greater fear of dying alone than of death itself.

This unit will close with a discussion focusing on nursing intervention for elderly patients and residents experiencing multiple losses. Mental health is important in the nursing care for all age groups. Some studies demonstrate that nearly one quarter of the elderly population have significant mental health problems. This may be an underestimation as today's elderly grew up before effective treatment existed and they are from an era that believed mental health problems were a sign of "weakness of character"; few sought available treatment. Gerontology specialties and research are relatively new. There are few health professionals with education and experience in geriatric mental health. You will have the opportunity in your nursing practice to assist the elderly in maintaining meaningful life experiences.

Stages of Grieving or Loss

Elisabeth Kübler-Ross developed the stages of grieving, a coping mechanism, as a result of her experiences with dying patients. *Grieving* is an expression of sorrow or mourning in response to death or a significant personal loss. Most nurses are familiar with these stages because many nursing courses utilize them. Although the focus of study is usually the responses of a dying person, the same coping mechanisms can be observed in people experiencing a variety of losses throughout life. Examples can be loss of a job, loss of health in a chronic disease, or losses experienced as a result of a divorce. In this discussion the focus will be on the grieving of multiple losses associated with aging.

Denial

When an event occurs that is perceived as a major or catastrophic loss by a person, the immediate response is, "That can't be true!" It may involve only self, or perhaps someone with close emotional ties, such as a parent or friend. Comments regarding "mistakes" of identity, of tests, or other information are common. Instant reactions are that "It can't be that bad," or "It can be fixed."

This time of denial can be a "buffer" to allow the person to "work through" the information and his feelings. It is not a time for nurses or others to provide any more information than is necessary, or to attempt patient teaching. The person is often in a state of "emotional numbness" and could not process the information. You may have to repeat previous statements as the person is attempting to clarify and internalize the initial information.

Anger

The next stage may demonstrate quiet anger or active rage and resentment. The "not me" response is replaced with a "why me" reaction. Often the person is angry with God but lashes out at family members, the physician, caregivers, or whoever is present at the moment. Whatever the activity, nothing is right. A response may be, "Haven't I been through enough already?"

When you are confronted by a person who is grieving and angry, you must remember he is not angry with you; do not take it personally. Also do not try to stop his anger, but allow him to ventilate his feelings. Show respect by accepting him and listening to him.

Bargaining

This is often a time of negotiating. The individual has moved from the "why me" to the "yes, but" reaction to loss. Usually the bargaining is with God in events of severe or terminal health situations. The elderly, however, often want to bargain with children or others to maintain the life style that has been comfortable to them. Examples could be situations where they may have to give up driving cars or living in their homes.

Depression

This is a quieter, more nonverbal stage as the individual works through the process and realizes, "yes, it's me." Often the person wants to be alone as he works through memories and begins to "let go" of his job, his car, his home, his wife, or whatever loss he is experiencing.

Perhaps your patient is hospitalized because of a recent stroke. He is grieving the loss of previous good health and probably his home and life style as he faces admission to a long term care facility. During this stage you may complete procedures or care in silence, demonstrating an understanding of his needs at this time. It is not a time to be "cheerful," or to attempt to cheer a patient.

Acceptance

This is a time to sigh; it is a relief to reach this stage. It is not necessarily the outcome desired, but "I'm o.k." It may be a resignation,

"This is the way it'll have to be." There may be some feeling of victory if a compromise was possible.

Perhaps this is the time for patient teaching to assist the elderly in a change of life style and to meet new challenges. You may need to clarify information given earlier which the patient could not process. He may want to take control of his new situation. This is another opportunity for communicating by touch and listening.

Hope

Throughout life, and the stages of grieving and loss, there is hope. It seems to be the nourishment that sustains a person from day to day and from one stage to the next. The feeling or expectation that something will "change for the better" persists in all of us.

A conflict in hope occurs when the person needs hope for daily survival, and those around him express hopelessness. Another conflict may be when the person has accepted the outcome, such as death, and family or others are in denial and cling to unrealistic hope.

This process of grieving varies considerably with individuals; people do not always progress from one stage to the next as discussed. Some may remain in one stage, such as denial or anger, and be unable to move on to resolving the loss. Others may move back and forth between stages. The elderly may be in different stages of grieving for different events of loss.

As a nurse practicing in a clinic, hospital, long term care facility, or other setting, you will need to collect data related to the patient's life and experiences. Perhaps your clinic patient has an elevated blood pressure. He is still angry because after 30 years of employment he lost his job due to company reorganization. "Do you have any idea how much time and sweat I put into that place? This is the thanks I get!", he exclaims. In long term care a new resident is despondent as he is working through having to leave his home. He is not yet ready to accept and adjust to his new life in this facility. Figure 10–2 summarizes the stages of grieving.

Aging: A Time of Multiple Losses

As the elderly age, the number of losses are multiplied and compounded. They occur in areas of identity, life style, independence, and companionship. Some losses are sudden and unexpected, others are anticipated; neither is easily accepted or managed.

How the elderly react to the losses and manage grieving of losses is influenced by lifelong coping mechanisms and resources available to assist with coping. This includes family members and other support persons. Those who have had positive adjustments in life and to aging, and who are able to put events into proper perspective, may be more positive in outcomes to loss. Healthy aging involves a process of adaptation to changes. Maintaining positive self-esteem is the major factor in promoting mental health in aging.

Losses Related to Identity

Our identity is tied to activities and material goods, as well as our personality. There are parts of our identity that we develop and control such as educational achievements, the life style we choose, or perhaps the home we purchase. Other people in our environment place identity labels on us by the neighborhood we live in, the type of work we do, or our behavior in interpersonal communication. The elderly maintain the identities that are related to their personality such as "always smiling," or "agreeable," or "grumpy and irritable." It is the identity related to activities and material goods that they begin to lose.

Retirement and the loss of identity related to the type of work done, the responsibilites, and perhaps even the job title are the major identity losses in active aging. Men who devoted all, or nearly all, of their time to work are often at a greater loss because they do not have hob-

STAGES OF GRIEVING OR LOSS

GRIEVING — Expression of sorrow when responding to death or significant personal loss.

- Denial — "It can't be true!" — "Not me!"
  - disbelief of event or information
  - time needed for processing information and feelings
- Anger — "Why me?"
  - quiet anger or active rage directed at God, family, or anyone nearby
  - need to ventilate feelings
- Bargaining — "Yes but..."
  - negotiating with God or someone perceived able to grant requests
  - need time to work through stage
- Depression — "Yes, it's me."
  - quiet, more nonverbal response
  - need time to recall memories and let go
- Acceptance — "I'm o.k."
  - relief and resignation to outcome
  - time to readjust and make new plans
- Hope — "Things will change for the better!"
  - sustains people during stages and from day to day

Figure 10–2   The stages of grieving and loss

bies or other interests for the redirection of their identity and time.

For women remaining at home, there are identity losses related to children's activites or volunteer work in the school and community. Fewer elderly women today were in the work force when they were younger. Their work identity was attached to housekeeping expertise, cooking, and organizational abilities in the community. Making the best lemon meringue pie in the county, was an identity initiating as much pride and competition in today's elderly women as having the top real estate sales is in today's younger women.

Loss of income that is associated with work reflects on the identity of many elderly. This occurs when there are not adequate funds to maintain the life style previously enjoyed, and it is witnessed by friends, neighbors, and others.

Where we live is a part of our identity. This is as broad as the state we live in, and as specific as the street address or apartment building. Owning a home initiates great pride in all people, including today's elderly. Many never had a mortgage, or they "paid off" the house in a few years. When the elderly must give up their homes, for whatever reason, it is a great identity loss, figure 10–3.

The need to reduce the amount of personal possessions because of a move into a smaller home or into a long term care facility also reflects an identity loss. Relocation losses impact an individual's association of possessions with its identity and contribution to family and society. For example, a man with an extensive woodworking shop in his basement sold his tools when moving to an elderly high-rise apartment. He was well known for the projects he contributed to the community and the toys he made for his grandchildren. It was appropriate for him to feel the loss of his tools and the associated identity.

Women may have possession loss grieving related to items of furniture that are related to

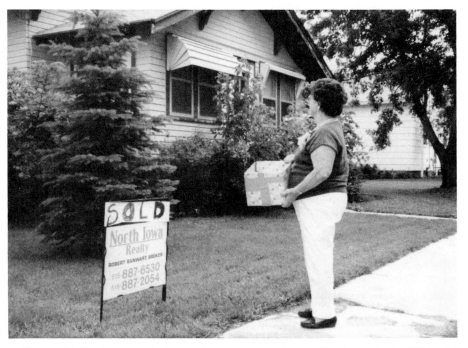

Figure 10–3   Leaving the home is a great identity loss for the aging individual.

long-time roles. For example, the need to give up a large table that seated all family members at holidays may indicate the loss of identity of "holiday cook" or the event of "Christmas at Mom's." The identity of hostess may be lost when moving to a one bedroom apartment and giving up the "spare" or guest bedroom. The homemaker identity loss is multiplied and compounded when a catastrophic illness requires admission to a long term care facility.

Caregivers in long term care facilities must be alert to the family and social histories of residents. Care must be taken to avoid stereotyping residents as frail, helpless, and with no redeeming past. It is important to maintain their dignity and self-esteem by focusing on abilities and previous roles.

Losses Related to Lifestyle

Life-style changes are impacted by losses in physical health and income. Physical limitations that occur due to gradual aging changes and reduced endurance are managed more easily than sudden acute events that initiate immediate drastic changes.

Mobility problems and sensory deprivation are two major influences in losses related to life style. Degenerative joint disease may rule out participation in recreational activities that were enjoyed for many years. Visual deficits may precipitate the need to give up needlework, playing cards, or other activites of individual enjoyment or social interaction.

Limited income and the need to reduce personal possessions may also impact losses related to comfortable life styles. Extensive travel or providing generous gifts to every grandchild may need to be exchanged for local travel and small gifts for special occasions. Entertainment may have to be curtailed. A widow traditionally invited over 100 family members for a holiday buffet in her home. When she moved to an apartment she could no longer continue with this event and felt the loss of this activity and her role.

The loss of life style is quite dramatic when the elderly person is admitted to a long term care facility. Activities are planned and coordinated primarily by the staff. An individual can maintain some related interests in hobbies, reading, dining out, or sports activities as they are offered, and the individual is able to participate. It can be expected that some residents will grieve the loss of a life style.

Losses Related to Independence

Limited activity related to a chronic disease or a deficit related to an acute illness can promote a level of dependency at any age. For the active aging, decreasing vision may precipitate the first loss related to independence: driving a car. This is an agonizing loss for the elderly, and often a frustrating and "nerve-racking" experience for their children. The elderly parent felt he managed his familiar environment without difficulty. His vision loss was so gradual he did not notice the potential hazards. Adult children see the increasing "near misses" of accidents, but cannot bring themselves to remove this major association with independence.

Advancing age or the exacerbation of chronic disease and aging begin to initiate some dependency in activities of daily living. This loss of independence can be in eating, bathing, or walking in the home. It means not being able to do what you want when you want.

Loss of independence continues when the elderly become residents of long term care facilities. They have lost some identity, lifestyle, and self-care abilities. The losses are now intensified as the individual must give up more personal possessions, perhaps her home, and now her privacy. Although caregivers use privacy curtains and other measures to protect the resident, seclusion is difficult to establish in a long term care facility. Most elderly must share a room with a stranger, have difficulties with eating witnessed by others in a dining room, and be bathed by a variety of caregivers.

Losses Related to Companionship

The most significant of the multiple losses is the loss of people and special relationships. For the elderly today, the loss of a spouse after decades of companionship is expected but devastating when it occurs. Often each person believes he or she will "go first" and be spared the grief and loneliness. Grieving the loss of a spouse may have started weeks or months earlier if the spouse was a victim of Alzheimer's disease or a debilitating stroke.

Professionals who advise widows or widowers in health, legal, or other concerns usually suggest that no major changes be initiated until a year after the loss of a spouse. The decision to sell a home and move to another community is often regretted after a period of time. Making as few changes as possible is the suggestion if health and finances permit. Many losses and changes in a short period of time can result in "bereavement overload," and the person is overwhelmed with the grief associated with multiple losses.

As the elderly become aged, they experience ongoing losses of friends and family. The social circle becomes smaller from debilitating disease, aging, and death. The lengthening life expectancy demonstrates that some old elderly are experiencing the death of their own aging children, as well as brothers, sisters, and other family members.

Residents of long term care facilities become separated from their traditional environment and the nature of the relationships important to them. Friends and relatives can come to visit, but they do not feel it is the same as before. It is helpful if they are still able to leave the facility and join the family for holiday dinners or other special occasions. For the elderly who no longer have family members to visit, nurses and other caregivers begin to take on the role of special relationships. The multiple losses associated with aging are summarized in figure 10–4.

Loneliness: A Response to Multiple Losses in Aging

We are social creatures. In the 1980s the group activity game Trival Pursuit gained rapid popularity as the excitment of video games waned. Some said this could be expected as humankind tolerates one-person entertainment for a period of time and then searches for interaction with others.

Loneliness or being lonely is a subjective feeling. It is unhappiness at being alone and longing for family, friends, or a former life style. Loss predisposes us to loneliness; this feeling is experienced by nearly half of the aging population at any given time. The incidence of loneliness increases in widowed or single men living alone and restricted in mobility. Many elderly fear the loneliness of old age more than death.

Complaints of loneliness tend to be occasional unless perceived isolation is present. The elderly can feel isolated socially as they lose the relationships of friends. Emotional isolation can occur after the death of a spouse. Limited activity or mobility can precipitate feelings of isolation.

Loneliness is painful. It can initiate feelings of anxiety, emptiness, and abandonment. It decreases self-esteem. The elderly present physical complaints and a perception of poor health more often than feelings related to loneliness. They do not identify the physical complaints with loneliness. Complaints of fatigue, sleeplessness, or aches and pains may be related to the stress and anxiety of loss. Responses indicating boredom, having "time on my hands," or self-pity may be observed.

Residents in long term care facilities where there is an abundance of people and activity can feel as lonely as the elderly living alone in the community. They have experienced many losses; the need for continued meaningful relationships in a strange new environment results in feelings of loneliness. There is fear of this

MULTIPLE LOSSES EXPERIENCED BY THE AGING

IDENTITY — Tied to activities and goods
- Job: profession, trade, or type of work, title and responsibilities.
- Income: funds that maintain life style and identity with those activities.
- Address: neighborhood and dwelling, and the identity perceived by others.
- Possessions: items that identify roles, such as host/hostess.

LIFE STYLE — Impacted by physical health and income
- Mobility: participation in recreational activities, such as fishing or golf.
- Vision/Hearing: activities of individual interest or social interaction, such as sewing or playing cards.
- Income: participation in interests, such as travel or purchasing gifts.
- Housing: home, because of physical health or income, such as a move to children's home, small apartment, or long term care facility.

INDEPENDENCE — Related to increasing physical or mental limitations
- Vision: visual acuity to drive a car, read price tags, identify numbers on paper money.
- Mobility or endurance: completing self-care and activities of daily living.
- Cognition: decision-making abilities to manage independently.
- Autonomy: planning daily schedules and activities when admitted to a long term care facility.

COMPANIONSHIP — Parting with special relationships because of a move or death
- Spouse: decades of sharing, assisting, and intimate companionship.
- Family: outlive siblings and even own children.
- Friends: shrinking social circle.

Figure 10–4   Multiple losses associated with aging

unknown territory and the resident needs someone in whom he can trust and confide.

In the multiple losses of aging and the resulting loneliness, perhaps one of the deepest losses of human need is that of touch. In our relationships with friends we seek continued communication by responding, "keep in touch." We turn the pages of a photo album or squeeze an old teddy bear to keep in touch with our memories. Friends and family are greeted with hugs or handshakes. The intimate touch of a spouse or companion lingers in quiet memories. The elderly often hunger for touch.

Nursing care implements touch in all interactions with with residents. Holding a hand while listening to a resident or giving an extra pat on the arm or shoulder in passing contributes to the need for human touch, figure 10-5.

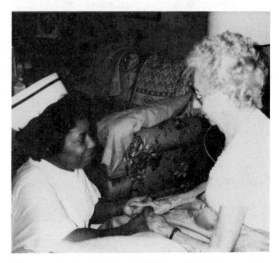

Figure 10–5   Nurses fulfill the elderly's need for touch.

Depression and Suicide in Aging: A Response to Hopelessness

Estimates of significant mental health problems in the aging population range from 15 to 25 percent. Discussions indicate that the number is probably underestimated and that these disorders in the elderly are underdiagnosed and undertreated. One problem is that diagnostic measurements have not been developed and validated for this age group as they have been for younger population groups.

People of all ages experience stress; the elderly are not excluded. Younger adults experience stress related to employment goals and other achievements. In aging, stress is related more to losses. During middle age years workshops on coping with stress are designed to assist people during job changes and other stressful events. Society has not yet met the challenge of teaching the aging to cope with their stresses associated with loss.

Depression

Depression may be described as feelings and expressions of sadness, helplessness, hopelessness, dejection, gloominess, or low spirits. A decrease in functional ability and activity is observed. It is the most common mental disorder in the aging population. It may not be recognized as it is masked by other disorders of aging. Elderly depression is considered to be reactive or situational rather than an affective disorder of major depression seen in younger age groups. This is because it is a response to the stresses and multiple losses of aging.

Assessing for signs of depression in the elderly must include a comparison with usual or previous behavior patterns. Some changes or characteristics include: (1) social withdrawl, (2) loss of motivation or energy, (3) envy or criticism of others, (4) increased demands on others, (5) feelings of unworthiness and helplessness, (6) changes in appetite, (7) changes in sleep patterns (sleeplessness or an unnecessary amount of sleep) (8) indecisiveness and inability to act on decisions, or (9) poor outlook about the future. The elderly may deny feelings of sadness or worry, but continue to focus on physical ailments.

In long term care facilities, the resident requiring some assistance with activities of daily living may demonstrate more signs of depression than the totally dependent resident. The independent resident is able to interact with staff, with others in group activities, and with family members. The totally dependent resident is also less depressed because he has more frequent contact with caregivers.

A perceived loss of control in elderly depression can contribute to learned helplessness. This is dependent and passive behavior that results in increased time with caregivers. It is uncertain whether caregivers (1) promote the helplessness by doing more for the individual and thereby increase the dependency; or if (2) the elderly promote the helplessness in a search for control of activities and the attention and acceptance of caregivers.

Depression in the elderly is a complex problem. When first suspected, a physical and mental examination is completed, drug therapies are reviewed, and other avenues to potential problems are persued. This is to rule out other possibilities for physical and behavioral changes and complaints. Nurses and other caregivers should not confuse depression with dementias. There is no cognitive loss with depression and it is treatable with drug therapy and psychosocial interventions.

Alcobolism in Depressed Elderly It is estimated that 10 to 15 percent of persons over 60 years of age have problems related to drinking. Studies suggest that drinking among the elderly population is a continuation of a lifetime responses to social and emotional events. However, the onset of alcoholism in older adults seems to be associated with stress and losses, including loss of a support system, figure 10-6.

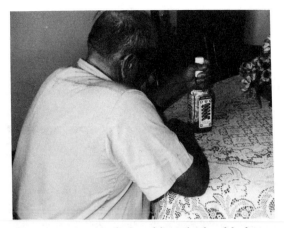

Figure 10-6 Alcohol problems in the elderly are often associated with the stresses and losses of aging.

The disease is being recognized as an increasingly serious problem with the elderly. There is an increased risk of suicide in older alcoholics.

Alcohol dependency in all ages interferes with personal health, interpersonal relationships, and financial stability. The disease in the elderly may be accepted or ignored because there are other physical and social situations that contribute to declining health, social isolation, and reduced income.

Tolerence for alcohol seems to decrease in the elderly. This combined with aging sensory and mobility limitations increases the probability of accidents and injury. Additional risks include the masking of cardiovascular and other system disorders, and serious interactions with the numerous medications taken by this population group.

Health professionals need to include questions regarding the the use of alcohol in patient interviews and assessments. Patient teaching with elderly must include information about interactions of alcohol and medications and the affect of alcohol on chronic health conditions. Referral for inpatient or outpatient treatment options are as pertinent for the elderly as for younger persons.

Suicide

The suicide rate among the elderly in this country steadily increased during the last decade. For the population over age 65, the percentage of suicides is greater than for any other age group. This number may be underestimated since it is based on death certificate statistics; suicide in old age may be underreported. Elderly white widowed males have the highest suicide rate.

Suicide in the elderly is considered to be a response to a quality of life they do not want, or cannot accept. They believe medical technology has prolonged death, not life. The choice is sometimes referred to as "rational suicide" when the individual calmly examines his life to determine whether it is worth living. Current circumstances are evaluated and their future projections may indicate helplessness and a burden to others. They feel there is no other alternative.

The feelings prior to suicide relate to losses, depression, and a sense of hopelessness. Unlike younger persons who may wish to be "found" or "stopped" in a cry for help, the elderly DO want to carry out the event. This may be one reason for the higher incidence of suicide in this age group.

Nurses and other caregivers need to be alert to signs of potential suicide such as meticulous planning, giving away treasured possessions, sudden happiness, or statements of death wishes. Assisting to promote self-esteem and meaningful activities may resolve or obstruct the intent of suicide. For the elderly who feel suicide is the only solution to their situation, they will eventually carry through with a suicide act. Caregivers and family members need support and perhaps counseling to resolve their grief and avoid associated guilt.

Some studies have focused on the impact of severe emotional trauma in younger years to increased aging depression, suicide, spouse abuse, and other mental health concerns in specific population groups. For example, elderly Jews who are Holocaust survivors are compared with ethnic cohorts living in the United States during World War II. Similar mental health aging concerns in the twenty-first century will focus on southeast Asian refugess of the 1970s. These are examples of population groups having no control over their destiny, that are subsequently thrust into a new culture and life style with limited time for grieving and emotional healing. Emotional conflicts may then resurface during aging. Figure 10-7 summarizes aging depression and other concerns.

Dying and Death and the Elderly

The final stage of living is dying. Although we all know that death is certain at some time, the elderly are faced with their mortality on a more impending basis. *Thanatology* is the study of dying and death. College courses and community education classes are available for this specialized study.

Dying is a process that can occur over hours, days, or weeks. As biological processes slow and begin to shut down, there are psychological and sociological responses made by the elderly and their families. Nurses and the elderly are involved together in dying and death as over 70 percent of deaths occur in health care facilities.

Unlike younger people who are expected to "fight it" and demonstrate a will to live, society expects the elderly to face dying in a passive accepting manner. The elderly present two common responses to death: a positive acceptance or a premature giving up. In positive acceptance, the person has accepted a terminal

DEPRESSION IN AGING

DEPRESSION
- Significant mental health problem in the elderly.
- Considered underdiagnosed and undertreated.
- Related to stresses associated with aging.
- May be masked by other aging problems.
- Expressed in feelings of sadness and hopelessness.
- Seen in long term care facilities: residents having less contact with caregivers, peers, and family.

ALCOHOLISM
- Estimates of 10 to 15 percent of adults age 60 and older have problems related to alcohol consumption.
- Continuation of lifetime habit.
- Elderly onset related to stresses in aging.
- Tolerance of alcohol decreases in aging.
- Increased potential for accidents and medication interactions.
- Referral for treatment options important for elderly.

SUICIDE
- Percentage of suicides greater than in any other age group.
- Old age suicide may be underreported.
- Response to undesired quality of life; feel there is no other alternative.
- Desire to carry out suicide event; no wish for rescue.
- Unresolved emotional trauma of younger years may increase risk in aging years.

Figure 10–7   Depression and associated concerns of aging

diagnosis and continues to enjoy life on a day-to-day basis. Those who demonstrate a premature giving up express a futility in life and can be in a chronic state of bereavement for their own life.

Nurses and other caregivers assisting the elderly facing death can support the resident by helping to put the past into perspective. This maintains self-esteem even in times of total dependency. Promoting involvement in the present helps find meaning in each day's activities. The focus is to motivate the resident to look forward to the next day's events. Nurses also support the dying elderly by assisting the resident and family to prepare for the event of death. The nurse is often the liaison who arranges for clergy visits, private meeting areas, and other requests of the resident and family. During the final minutes of life, it is often the nurse who holds the slender frail hand and comforts the old.

Long term care facilities usually have memorial services on a monthly or periodic basis for the residents to remember and mourn those who have recently died. When residents have few or no family members, the facility staff may be the majority in attendance at a funeral. Nurses in long term care facilities must be in touch with their own feelings about dying and death to effectively manage the psychosocial aspects of care for the elderly.

Nursing Care: Assisting the Elderly Experiencing Loss

Recovery from loneliness and depression does not occur overnight. It is a long process; for some it is an ongoing effort to manage an acceptable quality of life. For nurses, it is a special challenge to integrate psychosocial nursing and meet elderly mental health needs in an increasingly busy, task-oriented workplace.

Nursing care that assists the elderly who are experiencing multiple losses occurs in all practice settings. Some approaches are informal

while others such as life review and pet therapy can be more structured.

Life Review and Reminiscence

Gerontologist Robert Butler originated the term *life review* when describing reminiscence as a positive measure in giving significance and meaning to life for the elderly who are questioning their self-worth. Activating long-term memories explores and assesses one's life. Today nurses, social workers, and others implement this technique with individuals or small groups of elderly. A formal approach includes specified meeting times and topics of discussion.

The process of life review assists the depressed elderly in realizing their life accomplishments. It also assists those with recent memory loss and others having unresolved conflicts. It can be a pleasant time to relive and share memories and plan for the time that is left. For some elderly, the process may be painful. Life review should be terminated when it is not therapeutic.

All caregivers can implement reminiscence when assisting residents with personal care and other activities. It provides the caregiver with an opportunity to get to know the person and realize how his past is a part of his personality today. Reminiscence improves communication, helps establish rapport, and individualize care. Self-esteem improves with the resident who realizes that he is valued as a person.

This informal style of reminiscence is implemented spontaneously. For example, Mr. Holloway is watching television when you enter the room to give him his medications. A new car advertisement flashes on the screen and he comments about all the "new-fangled gadgets." You respond, "Tell me about your first car, Mr. Holloway."

Pet Therapy

Some long term care facilities have pets as a part of their "staff." Activities departments in other facilities bring in a dog or other animal for a visit on a routine basis. Elderly who live alone and are capable of caring for a pet may receive one as a gift from family members.

Studies demonstrate that pets are very therapeutic because they satisfy the need to touch and they give unconditional love. For those living at home alone, they provide a sense of security and companionship, and fulfill the need to nurture or care. Cats and dogs are the most popular pets and seem to help alleviate the anxiety and loneliness of loss and aging. It is thought that contact with animals can lower blood pressure and relieve tension, figure 10-8.

When the use of live animals or pets is not practical, stuffed plush animals are given to residents. Throughout life we respond to stuffed animals and they generate a feeling of well-being. Residents in long term care facilities can meaningfully relate to the plush animals by touching and perhaps attaching a name from a pet they owned in the past. Pets and plush animals become topics of converstaion and a means of communication between residents and staff.

Spirituality and the Elderly

Spirituality and the need for maintaining belief systems is vitally important to the elderly in a time of aging and experiencing multiple losses. It becomes especially difficult when deficits in mobility or other limitations prohibit the elderly from attending services or participating in their traditional religious activities. Spiritual need may be the most important need for the elderly, but the most hidden.

During nursing interviews it is important to learn about the elderly's spiritual needs and religious beliefs and practices. Learning just the basic information will help determine if the resident wants visits from clergy or other persons. Helping a resident in spiritual distress can include listening or sitting beside him in silence. It is important to support the elderly with their spirituality needs by providing them the time, people, and prayer books or other items necessary for meaningful rituals.

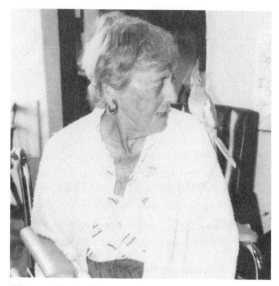

Figure 10–8   Pets are therapeutic for the elderly.

Supportive Care for Multiple Losses in Aging

Supportive nursing care for active and dependent elderly experiencing loss includes encouragement to take one day at a time. These older adults should be assisted to set small goals for each day that reflect meaningful activity. Suggested activities are those that promote self-care, involvement with people, and a positive outlook. Loneliness is nonproductive. Some elderly can be encouraged to help others, make new friends or join a group. In any situation of active or dependent aging, measures should be taken to avoid isolation and self-pity.

One of the most challenging and rewarding aspects of nursing practice is to provide psychosocial nursing care to the elderly experiencing the multiple losses of aging and finally dying and death. It is also emotionally taxing to the nurse; you must have a support system to be successful. Figure 10-9 summarizes nursing interventions to assist the elderly who are experiencing nultiple losses.

ASSISTING THE ELDERLY EXPERIENCING LOSS

Implemented informally and formally in all practice settings:

- Life Review
  — activate long-term memories to explore and assess meaning of own life
  — acknowledges life accomplishments
  — assists managing unresolved conflicts

- Reminiscence
  — improves communication
  — assists in establishing caregiver/resident rapport
  — improves self-esteem

- Pet Therapy
  — satisfies need to touch
  — provides unconditional love
  — provides companionship and security
  — assists in alleviating anxiety and loneliness
  — plush stuffed animals may also generate a feeling of well-being

- Spirituality
  — maintaining belief system important at a time of multiple losses
  — support traditional beliefs and practices
  — listening, sitting in silence, and touch support spiritual needs

- Supportive Care
  — encourage managing one day at a time
  — set small goals
  — plan meaningful activity
  — encourage self-care
  — promote positive outlook

Figure 10–9 Nursing interventions to assist the elderly person who experiences multiple losses

Summary

The elderly population experiences multiple and compounding losses in aging. These losses include parts of their identity, independence, lifestyle, and long-time companions.

Grieving losses can be ongoing and the elderly can be in different stages of grieving for recent as well as past losses. Kübler-Ross identified these stages of grieving as denial, anger, bargaining, depression, and acceptance. Throughout all stages there is hope.

A common response to the multiple losses in aging is loneliness. This is unhappiness about being alone and a longing for family, friends, possessions, or other losses. Usual complaints are related to physical ailments such as fatigue and aches and pains. Other complaints may focus on boredom or self-pity. Comments about loneliness are seldom expressed.

Nearly half of the elderly population experience loneliness at a given time and almost half of those have significant mental health problems. Situational or reactive depression is the most common problem and is related to multiple losses. Characteristics of elderly depression include feelings of sadness and hopelessness, loss of motivation or energy, enviousness, and changes in appetite and sleep.

Other concerns with mental health and aging, and potentially dysfunctional lives, are alcoholism and suicide. There is an increased incidence in this population group and symptoms are often masked by other aging conditions. Mental health problems are treatable, but are considered underestimated, underdiagnosed, and undertreated in the elderly.

As the elderly age and become more dependent, they face their own mortality daily. Society expects the elderly to accept dying and death in a passive role. It is not that easy; they are fearful of dying alone. Two common responses to death are positive acceptance and premature giving up.

Nursing care to assist the elderly who are experiencing loss includes encouragement to take one day at a time and set small goals to make each day meaningful. Life review is a technique that helps the elderly put the past in perspective by reminiscing and realizing their life accomplishments. It promotes self-esteem, manages depresssion, and assists in resolving earlier life conflicts. Pet therapy is known to be helpful in dispelling anxiety and loneliness; animals satisfy the need for touch and to nurture.

At the close of life, maintaining spiritual and religious traditions is vital to the emotional health of the elderly. Nurses support these needs by implementing patience, listening, and arranging for clergy, prayer times, and other specific individual needs. Supporting the elderly through aging and loss can be one of your most rewarding nursing experiences.

For Discussion

- In small group discussions, share some personal loss and how you managed the grieving process.
- Invite one or more of the following as guest speakers:
  - A nurse or social worker to share experiences in implementing life review or reminiscense therapy.
  - A widow or widower to share experiences of loss in aging as well as positive outcomes.
  - A mental health counselor to give a profile of aging clients and their problems.

Questions for Review

1. What are the stages of grieving?
2. What are four general losses associated with aging?
3. What is lonelines?
4. What are four symptoms of loneliness demonstrated by the elderly?
5. What is situational depression?
6. What are four symptoms of elderly depression?
7. What are two common responses to death presented by the elderly?
8. What is life review?
9. What are two nursing interventions used to assist the elderly in managing the stress of multiple losses?

Unit 11
Dilemmas Confronting Dependent Aging and Caregivers

Objectives

After reading this unit you should be able to:

- Define ethics and dilemmas.
- Identify issues concerning the right to live or die.
- Discuss issues related to quality of care.
- Identify family caregiver dilemmas.
- Discuss professional caregiver concerns.

Choices! The freedom to make choices is what health care dilemmas are all about. First, there is the opportunity to make choices or decisions that will influence outcomes of health or illness situations. Second, choices have to be evaluated and decisions made to manage the outcomes of the earlier choices. For example, an active 70-year-old has an unexpected stroke. His physician and family decide to admit him to intensive care and all lifesaving measures, including a respirator, are implemented. The family believes he will "pull through" since he has been so healthy. He may not be his "old self," but certainly will not need all this equipment. The patient does recover to manage independent breathing, but he is not responsive and cannot eat. Now what? Should a feeding tube be inserted to manage nutrition and prolong life? Where will he receive his total care? Making choices may mean confronting additional issues or dilemmas.

The dilemmas, choices, and decisions pertaining to health care in the United States have mushroomed during the last decade, and will be with us for some time. The elderly population is in the forefront of discussions because of their growing numbers, the high cost of care, and their limited income.

This unit will identify some of the dilemmas facing the dependent aging and their caregivers. Ethics will be defined and discussed briefly as an influence in decision making. The dilemmas will be introduced under four broad categories: (1) right to live or die issues, such as resuscitation orders and living wills; (2) quality of care issues, such as access to care and elderly abuse; (3) family caregiver issues, such as burnout and guardianship; and (4) professional caregiver issues, such as use of restraints and inadequate staffing. The discussion will present factors on the issues, but will not provide answers or actions. They are still being wrestled with by individuals and society.

Nurses, as primary caregivers, are often confronted with the dilemmas that face the elderly. This is because they are the health professionals providing direct care in the hospital, clinic, home, or long term care facility when the dilemma arises. Choices are outlined by the physician; a decision must be made. Perhaps you are the hospital nurse caring for a stroke patient. A son says to you, "Dad can't live at home alone anymore. I don't know what we're going to do." As a clinic nurse, you hear an elderly woman who is the caregiver for her husband with Alzheimer's sigh, "I don't know how long I can last. He is up most of the night now."

Patients, residents, and family members do not expect you to provide the answers. You are the person who is just there at that moment. This is the reason for being aware of the dilemmas that surface when caring for the elderly. Your role is to be a good listener, provide information, and refer them to resources that will be helpful. It is also most likely that, at sometime in your lifetime, you will be confronted with these dilemmas for yourself or a family member.

What Are Ethics and Dilemmas?

Ethics can be broadly defined as standards of conduct, moral judgement, and philosophy. These are standards to evaluate principles of right and wrong. The standards reflect our value system. In this country, values are based on individual freedoms and the governing mechanisms or laws.

Dilemmas are events in which all choices seem to be equally unfavorable; any outcome will be unfavorable to someone. It is value conflicts between individuals, or groups in which memberships have the differing values, that result in dilemmas.

The value of individual rights sets up the conflict of choice between the greatest good for one or the good for the greatest numbers. Should thousands of health care dollars be spent on neonatal intensive care for one high-risk infant or for prenatal care or child immunizations for many people? Should legislation provide more dollars to support the care of the fewer elderly in long term care facilities, or for programs to assist the larger numbers of dependent elderly outside these facilities? The shrinking health care dollar has highlighted this issue.

Another issue is that right and wrong and good and bad are not the same thing. Something that seems good may not be right. A classmate is a good person; she panicked when failing a course and cheated on a test. That is wrong. A mother may say she always loves her children, but does not always like them. In both situations the people were held in high regard; it was their actions or behavior that caused the conflict. Actions, and what can be changed, should be the focus of ethics. Unfortunate events do occur; that is not failure.

Is health care a right or a privilege? The United States was founded on beliefs of individual's rights. Some people are saying that health care has become a privilege for those who can afford it; a national health care policy should be developed. This creates the dilemma of establishing something for the good of all which is contrary to the individual rights philosophy of the framer's of our Constitution.

Many of the ethical dilemmas arising in health care today are the result of high technology. In decades or centuries in the past, humankind survived on individual stamina. Perhaps what we call comfort measures were implemented; water was offered or cool cloths applied to the body. Some cultures held vigils over the ill while others abandoned the sick. Today, the use of machinery and drugs to prolong life has introduced many people and "things" into the picture. Who makes the decision to use the equipment? Who makes the decision to take it away? Individual rights has not clarified the answer. We will hear more about these dilemmas as this country struggles with its health care delivery system, figure 11-1.

Nursing, like other professions, has a code of ethics. This value system, as developed by the American Nurses Association, is based on duties of nurses. Conflicts arise for nurses when patient care choices have to be made. For example, a dying resident needs extra time for care and comfort, but 25 other residents need their medications. Often, the duty of tasks and pro-

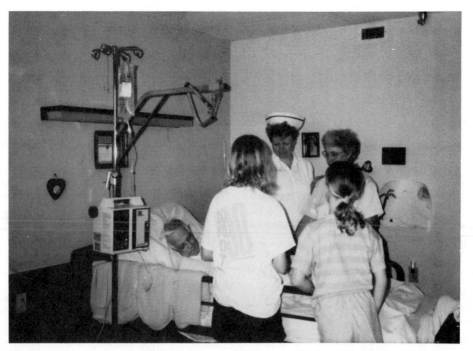

Figure 11–1 Struggles with health care dilemmas will be with us for a long time.

cedures wins as nurses are held accountable for these duties. They are not held accountable for the time involved in meeting the psychosocial needs of people.

Right to Live or Die Issues

Measures to prolong life, at the very least the continuation of vital signs and brain activity, or measures to stop these activities are a part of right to live or die issues. Another part is who makes the decisions. The conflict is primarily between the individual's right to bodily integrity and autonomy, and professional duty to preserve life. In legal situations and court proceedings, the reference is to the state's duty to preserve life.

Actions for outcomes are more clear when

the person is able to give informed consent regarding directions for activities that influence bodily integrity. The dilemma, and legal action, often occurs when the person is unable to provide informed consent and make choices for treatment. Who then should be authorized to make those decisions? One problem with legal decisions in right to live or die issues is that these ethical dilemmas are entwined in moral values. They are not the same for everyone.

Some of the right to live or die issues confronting the elderly are "do not resuscitate/do not intubate" (DNR/DNI) directives, withholding food and/or fluids, providing nutrition via feeding tubes, living wills, and euthanasia. These are not easy choices to make, and when made may not be implemented because of the unclear liability of health care professionals. Also, many elderly are uninformed about their rights and the specific nature of lifesaving procedures.

Organ Transplantation

Organ transplantation in elderly persons is not a major issue today. The elderly are usually not good candidates because of multiple system disorders, plus many are poor surgical risks. The transplantation of organs or tissues may be an aging issue in the future because of today's research. One example is the use of fetal tissue for the treatment of Parkinsonism.

Resuscitation/Intubation Directives

Resuscitation as an emergency intervention to restore vital signs includes a range of procedures from rescuer cardiopulmonary resuscitation (CPR) to advanced life support with mechanical devices at a trauma center. Intubation interventions include the use of endotracheal tubes for mechanical ventilation in resuscitation efforts, as well as the insertion of other tubes, such as intravenous feedings. DNR and DNI directives do not mean the same thing. A person with a chronic respiratory disorder may wish to be intubated, but not to have CPR. Another person may wish to have CPR, but with no advanced life support systems including intubation and use of a respirator.

The individual's consent for DNR or DNI is documented on his medical record and chart as a physician's order. They are referred to as "no-code" orders and the DNR/DNI is noted on the care plan. One of the dilemmas with the elderly is that the outcome of successful resuscitation efforts is often poor. Other dilemmas occur when family members cannot agree on treatment directives when the elderly person did not make prior decisions for care.

Withholding Artificial Nutrition/Fluids

Withholding or withdrawing artificial nutrition and fluids is a controversy in rights of life and death. Is the artificial nutrition a medical treatment or is it meeting a basic need? Elderly patients and residents most often receive artificial nutrition by nasogastric or gastrostomy tube feedings. They may not be able to swallow because of a stroke, be too weak to eat enough food for adequate nutrition, or may have refused to eat.

The right to refuse treatment of any nature is a decision made by the patient or resident with informed consent. Information about a treatment's risks or benefits is provided by the physician. Again, the dilemma with the elderly is often that they are in a weakened physical state, confused, or have other limitations that interfere with making or directing a decision.

Living Wills

Living wills, also known as advance directives, are written instructions about treatment. They are in the laws of 40 states. The living will may also name a proxy or surrogate decision maker. States may differ in the definition of terms and in various restrictions. Some states recognize only prescribed formats while others accept a specific personalized document. Figure 11-2 is a sample living will document.

Conflicts with living wills include the fact that they need to be specific to be implemented accurately and therefore do not reflect the person's general feelings about treatment. The elderly and their families should be encouraged to discuss wishes regarding medical treatment and the withholding of life-preserving measures when in a terminal condition. Family physicians, lawyers, agencies on aging, or other elderly advocates are good resources regarding states' living will laws.

Euthanasia

Euthanasia means easy and painless death to end suffering. It is sometimes called "mercy killing." It has received a considerable amount of attention in recent years because elderly people have been tried in courts and jailed for killing a spouse, often one suffering from Alzheimer's disease. Books have been written by people who have assisted a parent or other loved one to achieve their goal of death. Some express their guilt for not assisting. Others express guilt for helping in what today is considered illegal measures. People and the courts will have much to contemplate in the future to determine policies for the termination of treatment decisions.

Quality of Care Issues

Concerns directed at quality of care are those of access in getting into the system as well as those issues directed toward the actual care. Factors influencing access are related to geographic location, insurance, available finances, receiving information about available services, and seeking care. Issues about the actual care received include the setting where care is provided and elderly abuse.

Access to Care Issues

All issues related to access to health care can be traced to allocation of health care dollars. In this country we are losing the ability to pay for the health care we want. Choices have to be made whether to place limited dollars on health care, education, or other social needs. Total health expenditures in the United States averaged just over $1000 per person in 1980. They are projected to average over $5000 per person in 2000. Today, there are over 37 million people who have no health insurance.

Other factors that influence rising costs include the aging population. By 2030, when the youngest Baby Boomers become 65, it is projected that the 65 and older group will be over 20 percent of the population. Today, that group is just over 12 percent and accounts for one-third of the health care expenditures in this country (most spent in the last year of life). These are dilemmas for the country as a whole.

For the elderly individual, where he lives may determine the care he receives. Many elderly live in rural areas where hospitals are

closing; they are no longer affordable to operate. Physicians leave rural areas because the patient loads are overwhelming and the income uncertain. Public transportation is not available to take the elderly to communities where health care is available.

Medicare is available to adults 65 and older, but many elderly do not have the finances to pay the deductible or purchase supplemental insurance. They may qualify for Medicaid but are not aware of the process or are too proud to accept what they call "welfare." Illnesses are managed or ignored until a crisis occurs which costs the elderly and the health care system considerably more for curative treatment or long-term care. Affording health care is a dilemma facing urban as well as rural elderly. The elderly often have to make choices whether to put their Social Security check in shelter, food, or health care.

Receiving knowledge about available health care services is part of access to care issues. The health care system is very complex; many elderly do not understand it. They also do not realize they are now more responsible for managing their own health. Even when information has been presented, some elderly choose not to seek medical attention. They may be fearful about the outcome.

Where health care is received, or physical limitations are managed, is also a dilemma. Decisions relating to moving and disposing of possessions is always difficult. There is a considerable amount of decision making and planning, and sometimes there are few choices when deciding whether to provide care for a dependent elderly person in the home or in a long term care facility. Appropriate services, caregivers, and support persons are evaluated.

Access to care is an emerging dilemma of the veterans of this country. They have been guaranteed health care as partial payment for military service. To cut costs, the federal government is looking at covering only service-related health problems. This is a financial, political, and philosophical dilemma.

MINNESOTA

Health Care Declaration

NOTICE:

This is an important legal document. Before signing this document, you should know these important facts:

(a) This document gives your health care providers or your designated proxy the power and guidance to make health care decisions according to your wishes when you are in a terminal condition and cannot do so. This document may include what kind of treatment you want or do not want and under what circumstances you want these decisions to be made. You may state where you want or do not want to receive any treatment.

(b) If you name a proxy in this document and that person agrees to serve as your proxy, that person has a duty to act consistently with your wishes. If the proxy does not know your wishes, the proxy has the duty to act in your best interests. If you do not name a proxy, your health care providers have a duty to act consistently with your instructions or tell you that they are unwilling to do so.

(c) This document will remain valid and in effect until and unless you amend or revoke it. Review this document periodically to make sure it continues to reflect your preferences. You may amend or revoke the declaration at any time by notifying your health care providers.

(d) Your named proxy has the same right as you have to examine your medical records and to consent to their disclosure for purposes related to your health care or insurance unless you limit this right in this document.

(e) If there is anything in this document that you do not understand, you should ask for professional help to have it explained to you.

TO MY FAMILY, DOCTORS, AND ALL THOSE CONCERNED WITH MY CARE:

I, _____, being an adult of sound mind, willfully and voluntarily make this statement as a directive to be followed if I am in a terminal condition and become unable to participate in decisions regarding my health care. I understand that my health care providers are legally bound to act consistently with my wishes, within the limits of reasonable medical practice and other applicable law. I also understand that I have the right to make medical and health care decisions for myself as long as I am able to do so and to revoke this declaration at any time.

(1) The following are my feelings and wishes regarding my health care (you may state the circumstances under which this declaration applies):

Figure 11–2   Sample living will declaration (Courtesy Minnesota Board on Aging)

(2) I particularly want to have all appropriate health care that will help in the following ways (you may give instructions for care you do want):

(3) I particularly do not want the following (you may list specific treatment you do not want in certain circumstances):

(4) I particularly want to have the following kinds of life-sustaining treatment if I am diagnosed to have a terminal condition (you may list the specific types of life-sustaining treatment that you do want if you have a terminal condition):

(5) I particularly do not want the following kinds of life-sustaining treatment if I am diagnosed to have a terminal condition (you may list the specific types of life-sustaining treatment that you do not want if you have a terminal condition):

(over)

Courtsey of Society for the Right to Die, 250 West 57th Street, New York, NY   10107

Figure 11–2   (Continued)

(6) I recognize that if I reject artificially administered sustenance, then I may die of dehydration or malnutrition rather than from my illness or injury. The following are my feelings and wishes regarding artificially administered sustenance should I have a terminal condition (you may indicate whether you wish to receive food and fluids given to you in some other way than by mouth if you have a terminal condition):

(7) Thoughts I feel are relevant to my instructions. (You may, but need not, give your religious beliefs, philosphy, or other personal values that you feel are important. You may also state preferences concerning the location of your care.)

(8) PROXY DESIGNATION (If you wish, you may name someone to see that your wishes are carried out, but you do not have to do this. You may also name a proxy without including specific instructions regarding your care. If you name a proxy, you should discuss your wishes with that person).

If I become unable to communicate my instructions, I designate the following person(s) to act on my behalf consistently with my instructions, if any, as stated in this document. Unless I write instructions that limit my proxy's authority, my proxy has full power and authority to make health care decisions for me. If a guardian or conservator of the person is to be appointed for me, I nominate my proxy named in this document to act as guardian or conservator of my person.

Name: _____

Address: _____

Phone Number: _____

Relationship: (If any) _____

If the person I have named above refuses or is unable or unavailable to act on my behalf, or if I revoke that person's authority to act as my proxy, I authorize the following person to do so:

Figure 11–2   (Continued)

Name: _____

Address: _____

Phone Number: _____

Relationship: (If any) _____

I understand that I have the right to revoke the appointment of the person named above to act on my behalf at any time by communicating that decision to the proxy or my health care provider.

DATE: _____

SIGNED: _____

STATE OF _____

COUNTY OF _____

Subscribed, sworn to, and acknowledged before me by

_____ on this _____ day of _____ 19 _____

_____

NOTARY PUBLIC

OR
(Sign and date here in the presence of two adult witnesses, neither of whom is entitled to any part of your estate under a will or by op eration of law, and neither of whom is your proxy).

I certify that the declarant voluntarily signed this declaration in my presence and that the declarant is personally known to me. I am not named as a proxy by the declaration, and to the best of my knowledge, I am not entitled to any part of the estate of the declarant under a will or by operation of law.

Witness _____ Address _____

Witness _____ Address _____

Reminder: Keep the signed original with your personal papers. Give signed copies to your doctors, family, and proxy.

Figure 11–2   (Continued)

Quality of Care Issues

In any setting, one dilemma related to quality of care is elderly abuse. It is estimated that every year over 1.5 million elderly are victims of physical or mental abuse. The abuse may be a commission or omission that causes harm to the elderly by physical, verbal, or psychological means. Most abusers are family members. Examples of abuse include leaving a dependent person in the same position for hours or days, not providing hygiene or treatments, leaving them unattended for long periods of time, or exploiting them by spending their money.

The statistics for elderly abuse are based on reported cases. Many go unreported because the elderly are fearful and feel they have no control over the situation. Much of the abuse is attributed to caregiver stress. The stresses may be related to the caregiving, or other personal or family concerns. In family caregiving, family dynamics play a role. The family may have been dysfunctional for years or violence may be part of the normal family functioning.

Elderly abuse is also reported in long term care facilities. This is often also traced to caregiver stress. In any health care setting, nurses and other professionals are obligated to report the facts of the abuse. Many states have vulnerable adult laws and methods for reporting elder abuse. The coverage varies regarding age, type of abuses covered, reporting rules, and penalties for failure to report. All long term care facility residents are considered vulnerable adults. Nurses in any setting must evaluate the areas of vulnerability for their patients, and assess for potential problems as well as visable signs of abuse.

Resident's Bill of Rights

Quality of care is assured to residents of long term care facilities through state laws often referred to as "Nursing Home Resident's Bill of Rights." The document is given to residents at the time of admission, and addresses rights related to several issues such as medical treatment, personal possessions and traditions, and the opportunity to file grievances. Despite these assurances, many elderly residents find that privacy is a dilemma. Because of costs, there are few private rooms and few can afford them. The elderly must live in a small room with few remaining personal possessions and a roommate who is a stranger. The elderly usually do not have a choice of roommate and may be paired with someone who is confused. This dilemma also infringes on our value system of individual rights and autonomy.

Family Caregiver Dilemmas

At the end of the twentieth century we are focusing on providing care for the elderly in the home as we did nearly 100 years ago. More than six million elderly require some assistance with basic personal needs; two million are residents of long term care facilities. Two-thirds of the group needing help live at home and receive free care given by family and friends. Most of the caregivers are women; many are elderly spouses with their own aging problems, or daughters with jobs and other family responsibilities.

Dilemmas may occur because the caregiver has not received adequate information about the disease or condition and how to take care of the family member. Another problem is inadequate assistance from other family members, home health team members, or respite caregivers. An accompanying problem is that assistance tends to "dry up" after a period of time; often by the time a spouse has been a caregiver for three years. Friends and even family find it "gets old" to be running to help and they find there are other demands on their time. Government and private insurance payers cover only a limited number of visits; soon the home health care visits are infrequent or terminated. The caregiver is too busy with caregiving to seek alternative assistance.

Caregiver Stress/Burnout

The result of the dilemmas of caregiving in the home is stress and burnout of the family caregiver. It is the reason for many long-term care admissions. In elderly couples, the caregiver may be the first to die.

Stress in the spouse or other family caregiver may be manifested in hypertension, gastrointestinal disturbances, and sleeplessness. Musculoskeletal complaints appear as lifting becomes a more difficult task. Incontinence in the dependent person increases the work load and fatigue occurs with increasing caregiving time and laundry and other housekeeping tasks. At a time when more emotional support is needed, the caregiver feels a lack of socialization and increased isolation. There are support groups and community services, but studies have shown that only a small percentage of the caregivers seek these avenues.

Guilt surfaces and is expressed in many ways. Children living miles away feel guilty because they are unable to help. Other children living nearby express guilt if they feel they are not helping enough. The caregiver spouse feels guilty if the needs of the dependent spouse are not met because of his/her own limitations or advancing fatigue and stress. The major guilt for all occurs when placing a dependent family member in a long term care facility. Sometimes there are feelings of personal failure or guilt because of promises made earlier.

Guardianship

Guardianship becomes a dilemma when gradual confusion is occuring and the elderly begin to have difficulty in problem solving. It is somewhat like taking the car keys or car away from an elderly parent. Potential hazards are witnessed, but taking action is always difficult. It is usually a crisis that initiates a guardianship or management of some personal or financial affairs. Examples are bills that do not get paid because mail is tucked inside magazines, or there are insufficient funds because Social Security checks were not cashed. Fraud also plays a role. Unscrupulous persons often prey on the elderly. For example, a newspaper carrier

made daily collections from an elderly confused woman who lived alone.

Limited guardianship and powers of attorney can be arranged with lawyers when the person is still competent. There are many reasons that a person may need assistance with financial or legal matters in the future. Planned alternatives can help alleviate inappropriate guardianship and the total loss of personal rights.

Professional Caregiver Concerns

Nurses experience dilemmas and also have choices to make. The problems are related to direct resident care as well as the working conditions and continual changes in the responsibilities of nurses and other caregivers. Issues are entwined as they ultimately affect the care of the elderly.

One recent issue related to resident care is the use of physical restraints. The dilemma for nurses is that restraints are usually "prn orders" and are to be applied only when necessary, but nurses are also responsible for the safety of the resident. Since the nurse cannot watch the resident every moment, any clue of potential hazard such as confusion, weakness, or past history of falls often initiates the use of a restraint.

Studies demonstrate that applying restraints may lead to earlier increased dependency. For example, a confused resident may be restrained because he fell attempting to get out of bed by himself. Because he is restrained a majority of the time, he will probably be bedbound sooner. Mental status will also probably deteriorate.

Another problem that arises with restraint issues is conflicts within families about the use of restraints. One member may want safety at all costs and another feels the elderly's freedom is more important. Additional caregiver dilemmas reflect that once a caregiver applies a restraint, others do not question the continued need by reevaluating the situation.

The question with restraints as with other dilemmas is who makes the decision. Should individual rights dictate that the patient can take the risk of freedom or autonomy over safety? We all take risks, but nurses feel a tremendous pressure with the liability involved in this issue.

Nurses feel the dilemma of understaffing and heavier patient or resident assignment loads in the issue of quality of care. Staffing is usually tied to DRGs or other measurements of patient care requirements, and nursing salaries are budgeted out of monies collected from resident room rates. Nurses want competitive salaries for their expertise. The conflict arises in a health care delivery system that is attempting to cut costs which includes careful management in scheduling, and often increased workloads.

Work related stress and burnout occur in nurses too. Some of the predisposing causes include the increased amount of time and care residents need, the increasing amount of documentation and paperwork, and the shortage of nurses. Some say the shortage is due to the fact there are more opportunities for nurse employment. Also, there are fewer nursing students as today more career opportunities are available to women, while nursing remains primarily a women's profession.

Dilemmas on the job include expectations of the resident's family. The media has focused more on health care issues which makes the family more informed. Part of their guilt is expressed in making sure the long term care facility "does everything." The expectations may be unrealistic. The dependent elderly dilemmas become shared between the nurse and the family.

One result of health care cost containment is the increase in lower paying, less skilled caregivers. Nurses find themselves responsible for the care given by these workers. However, these workers are increasingly responsible for more technical skills. Expanded roles over time are demonstrated in the fact that decades ago only physicians were considered qualified to measure blood pressure. Over the years nurses and other professionals became qualified to complete this task. The current federal nursing assistant curriculum guidelines include teaching trainees the procedure for taking blood pressures.

Because nurses provide direct patient care to residents facing many life preserving dilemmas, they are also directly involved in the research and studies on bio-medical ethics. Many facilities are beginning to have ethics committees and nurses are members. They represent nursing views and also express their patients' and residents' feelings.

Summary

"It was the best of times, it was the worst of times," wrote Dickens in the *Tale of Two Cities*. It is often that way for the elderly of today. Technology has improved the quality of life in so many ways and moved the life expectancy from 47 years to 74 years in this century. However, technology has also created dilemmas that some believe prolongs death rather than life.

The ethical questions arise with a conflict between individual rights which are prized in this country and the duty to preserve life. Where once humankind had to survive independently, today there are many people and much machinery that is involved. Who makes the decision?

Elderly individuals are confronted with growing issues related to preserving life as well as a quality of life. Some of those issues include: resuscitation and intubation orders, artificial nutrition and fluids, and living wills. Before these are even considered, some elderly do not have the access to health care because of where they live, financial limitations, and inadequate health information.

A majority of dependent elderly are cared for in their homes by family members, most often an elderly spouse. The caregiver suffers guilt, and becomes a victim of caregiver stress and burnout. Meanwhile nurses also share these dilemmas with the elderly because they work directly with the resident and family. They also experience resident care dilemmas such as use of physical restraints and professional concerns such as overwhelming work loads.

What does the future hold? We cannot project solving these bio-medical ethics, but just managing them will be a challenge in the next century.

For Discussion

- Read several references on one or more topics presented:
  a. Two or more students present opposing issues on the topic.
  b . Discuss the role of the nurse and possible actions in each situation.
- Obtain a copy of your state's living will. Discuss items covered and decisions that must be made by the person making the advanced directive.
- Obtain a copy of your state's elderly abuse law. Discuss the nurse's responsibility related to the directives.
- Invite a guest that is willing to share his/her family's decision making in a health care dilemma.

Questions for Review

1. What is ethics?
2. What are dilemmas?
3. Why are ethical dilemmas so difficult to manage?
4. What are DNR/DNI directives?
5. What are living wills?
6. What are two family caregiver dilemmas?
7. What are two professional caregiver concerns?
8. Why is it important for nurses to understand some of the health dilemmas the elderly face?

Unit 12
Care Plans for the Dependent Aging

Objectives

After reading this unit you should be able to:
- Identify nursing diagnoses common to dependent elderly.
- Discuss family and socioeconomic influences in developing resident care plans.
- Discuss the comprehensive nature of resident care plans in long term care facilities.
- Describe adaptations in the nursing process that are required to meet the needs of dependent elderly in long term care facilities.

Quality of life! Quality of care! These are two issues facing all generations today. Previous discussions have focused on technology and costs and the dilemmas they present. Quality of life and quality of care are also important considerations in developing and implementing care plans for residents in long term care facilities. The resident care plan is the framework for all activities of daily living and monitoring of health needs. It is an outline of the delivery of care and reflects standards of care set by health professionals and other providers of care.

The Nursing Process is not new to you. You have implemented the five step process of assessment, nursing diagnosis, planning, implementation, and evaluation in other course work and patient care assignments. This book has used steps of the nursing process as parts of many presentations. In this unit, the more specific use of care plans in long term care facilities will be discussed.

In acute care settings, care plans utilizing the Nursing Process address short-term needs of an acute illness event. They may also focus on a crisis or exacerbation of a chronic condition. Time alone does not usually allow for extensive research into patient, family, and social history

to include information and events that would improve a patient care plan.

Holistic nursing care is a goal all nurses want to implement for their patients. It reflects the idea of *holistic health* which focuses on the whole person; all interactions with his/her environment. The nature of the health care system today makes this goal even more of a challenge in acute care nursing.

In long-term care, a holistic approach in a comprehensive care plan is required to meet the needs of residents. Some residents have a short-term placement of several weeks to a few months. This is designed as a rehabilitative period between the hospital and return to home. It is a direct result of the cost containment efforts and short hospital stays of the past decade. However, for most residents, the comprehensive care plan must reflect all their needs, as the facility is their home for many years; often the remainder of their lives, figure 12-1.

Care plans for residents also tend to reflect the nursing model. The *nursing model* focuses on needs related to accomplishing tasks of daily living and mainataining a level of health. Nursing intervention focuses on nursing measures that will assist residents in accomplishing those

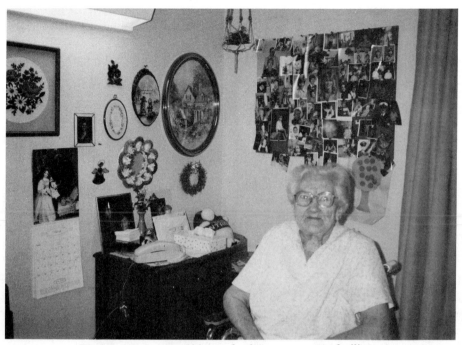

Figure 12-1   A resident of a long term care facility

tasks and maintaining the highest possible level of functioning. For example, encouraging a resident to walk to the dining room for meals, and walking with him to evaluate his abilities and needs, promotes joint mobility and a level of independence.

Medical treatment for diseases related to joint mobility might include anti-inflammatory drugs and physical therapy, or possibly surgical intervention. When patient or resident care plans reflect nursing actions that are directly related to physician orders, they are said to reflect a medical model. The focus is more on curing or improving a disease process.

The payment system for health care is also reflected in resident care plans. The system tends to respond to charges for medical treatment. Some facility resident care plans may reflect the medical model because of state and/or federal reimbursement guidelines. Federal medicare guidelines require the review of resident care plans every 30 days by a nurse, and every three months by a multidisciplinary team. Many regulations influence each resident's care plan.

Most elderly residents are dependent because of problems with mobility or memory. This unit will introduce you to the data collection initiated by a broad network of people who make assessments for placements in long-term care and then the development of an individualized comprehensive care plan.

Nursing diagnoses will include those that demonstrate difficulties in functional abilities. *Impaired Physical Mobility* and *Altered Thought Processes* are two diagnoses that reflect the dependency problems with mobility and memory.

Planning begins before a resident is admitted to the long term care facility. It continues during the approximately ten-day admission period. After that time, an initial care conference is arranged. Needs are identified and formalized into a plan of care. The resident, family, nurses, social worker, dietitian, housekeeper, and others participate in developing the plan to manage all aspects of the resident's care.

Implementing a resident care plan requires comprehensive nursing skills. In long-term care today and in the future, nurses will utilize a broad range of medical and surgical nursing skills in addition to adaptations related to the aging process.

Evaluating the outcomes of a resident care plan is an ongoing process. The major goal is always to promote the highest level of functional ability possible for each resident. Keen observation monitors the potential of an acute illness as well as changes in chronic conditions. A measure of practicality needs to be used in evaulating changes and outcomes. Are goals realistic? A resident usually recovers from an acute event, but often it exacerbates dependency by adding another degree of unrecoverable weakness.

As developers and implementers of resident care plans, nurses wear many hats. They may become an extension of the family as they develop a special bond with or between the resident and family. Nurses are the front line defense for observing health needs and alerting physicians to a change in the resident's status, figure 12-2.

There are many personal and professional rewards in providing care and assisting the dependent elderly in a long term care facility. You have the opportunity to learn from their rich life experiences, promote continued dignity and self-esteem in their aging, and most of all provide a quality of life.

Assessment: Expanding Baseline Data

The assessment step in developing a resident's care plan involves two phases of data collection. Government regulations influence the framework for both phases. The admission, or

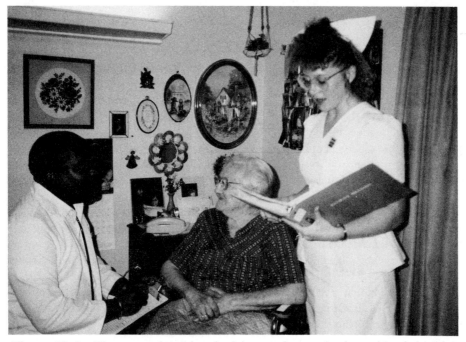

Figure 12-2   The nurse alerts the physician to changes in the resident's health status.

"placement," of an elderly person to a long term care facility requires pre-admission screening of the individual for government funding of costs. The second phase of data collection occurs during the 10 days following admission to the long term care facility. Again, government policies are involved, requiring a resident care conference and formalized care plan to be in place after ten days.

Data Collection Before Admission

Before the staff nurse begins the admission interview and data collection, many people have collected lots of data to determine if the long term care facility is the best place for the individual to live and receive care. Many people could have raised the question, "Isn't it time for Mary to get help or move to a nursing home?" A spouse, other family members, clergy, friends, neighbors, physicians, and many others could be the concerned person that initiates a pre-screening process. Even Mary herself may realize that she and her husband can no longer manage as she becomes weaker.

The public health nurse and a social worker are often the professionals designated by the county or community to collect data and evaluate if alternative services would meet continued care needs, or if long-term care is required. If placement in a long term care facility is the best choice, the individual and family are usually asked if they have a preference for a particular facility. Most often a family's knowledge of a facility is acquired by "word-of-mouth." Families, especially spouses, are concerned about the location of the facility in relation to transportation and being able to visit.

When the family has no information about choosing a long term care facility, the pre-admission screening nurse can provide names of facilities in the community. Additional information can be given that assists in selecting a long term care facility. These may include: (1) location and ownership of the facility, (2) types of services provided (physical therapy, speech therapy or other needed services), (3) ability to

have own furniture or other possessions in the room, (4) availability of the individual's physician, (5) approval by Medicare or other reimbursement system, and (6) activities planned for residents. The State Board on Aging, Ombudsmen services, community senior citizen groups, and others usually can also offer guidelines for selecting a long term care facility.

In the hospital, discharge planning nurses will evaluate the patient's physical condition and functional abilities to determine if continued care needs can be met at home, in a convalescent facility, or a long term care facility. There are interviews with the patient and family. The discharge planner collaborates with the physician, social worker, and others to establish the method and setting of continued care. This often is a difficult process because the patient may have been a very active aging person and a recent catastrophic event is changing her life style.

Admission to a long term care facility is no longer "immediate" or unplanned. There is a lot of groundwork planning before the elderly person actually enters the facility. Once the pre-admission screening process indicates that placement is appropriate, the facility social worker begins to make admission plans with the family, figure 12–3. The elderly person, although consulted, may not be directly involved

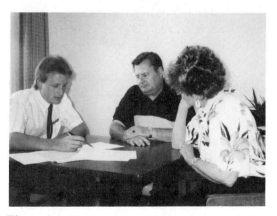

Figure 12–3 Admission plans are initiated by the facility social worker and the family.

with the meetings and other activities. The individual is often ill or weak with the health crisis that is initiating this move.

At the beginning of this phase, basic information is gathered about the elderly person's health and living needs. This is to determine if the facility has the appropriate resources to meet the identified needs. For example, does the facility have the equipment and staff to meet the needs of a respirator patient? The director of nursing, social worker, and other administrative staff make these decisions.

The facility social worker is usually the liaison between the facility and the family. In small facilities where there may not be a social worker, the director of nursing assists the family during the admission process. Facilities may provide packets of information and meet with the family to plan the move and explain policies and procedures.

Information and planning at this stage include financial arrangements. The family may or may not have an understanding of government funding for elderly health care, or the status of the parent's personal insurance and other assets. Explanations include payments to the facility as well as managing additional costs that are not reimbursed by insurance. Unfortunately, many still believe that Medicare pays all or most of longterm care costs. Family members, and later the resident, also receive a copy of the Resident's Bill of Rights and information about vulnerable adult laws. All long term care facility residents are considered vulnerable adults, although states vary somewhat in the implementation of laws. At this time, or during the admission process, the "code" or DNR/DNI choices need to be made by the elderly and/or family.

Groundwork planning with the family includes decisions on personal belongings that can be a part of the resident's living area in the facility. A favorite chair, a television, and pictures to hang on the wall are examples. The amount and type of clothing and how it will be marked and laundered is another discussion. Families are given tours, activities and schedules are explained, and procedures discussed. Often, residents and families do not have a choice of rooms, because they are limited. Many long term care facilities have waiting lists. When possible, residents are matched according to physical and mental abilities. More facilities are beginning to allow married couples to share the same room.

Data Collection on Admission

This is the stage of resident admission where you, as a staff nurse, may become involved. During the groundwork planning with the family, the admission date is arranged. The time is often planned around resident unit schedules, such as during the afternoon when the nurse may have more time. You may receive the information several hours or the day before to help in organizing your time.

Housekeeping, nursing assistants, and others prepare the resident's room for her arrival. It is your job to check that everything is ready and any special equipment is available. Although you will not have many details at this time, you will have basic knowledge of the resident's needs.

It is wise planning to be alert to your communication skills and body language, which will be observed by the new resident and her family. Hospitality skills such as friendliness are important at a time that is difficult for the resident and her family. A majority of the elderly, even when they agree this is the best place for care, do not want to move into a longterm care facility. For many of today's elderly, this may be their first move for decades, perhaps since they were married or young adults. In the future, because of today's more mobile society, the elderly will have experienced a variety of homes and communities. For the family the time is difficult, perhaps because of the stress of the elderly's acute illness, dealing with the sale of a home or moving personal belongings, and guilt related to the inability to care for the person at home.

Welcoming the new resident includes introducing yourself and explaining the events of the first few hours. Usually this includes an orientation to her room, an introduction to her roommate if it is not a private room, and placing her personal belongings in the room, figure 12-4. During this time you are informally collecting data about the resident's physical and mental abilities and limitations as well as the family interactions with the resident. Basic information, such as the hours meals are served, should be provided. Be careful not to "overload" the new resident with schedules and activities. Each day can include new information for her to absorb. The admission day should include items she feels are important, such as how to call the nurse or how she will receive telephone calls from her family.

Sometime before you leave your workday, the initial nursing interview for the resident's chart will need to be completed, figure 12-5, as well as a short mental status examination if indicated. During your informal data collection you will make a nursing judgement regarding the appropriate time for the interview. She may appear to be more secure if you stay in her room and complete it now, or perhaps she needs a nap first.

A systematic approach to data collection is implemented in this initial physical and functional assessment. It will be used as baseline data during the following days while additional data is collected for the first care conference.

Your data collection may include a hospital discharge summary and information received from the social worker's family interview.

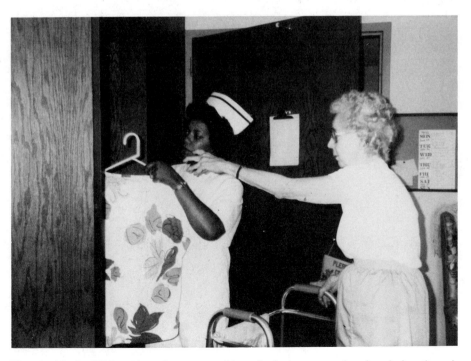

Figure 12-4 Welcoming the new resident includes arranging her belongings in the room.

SAMARITAN BETHANY, INC.
NURSING ADMISSION/READMISSION DATA

NAME_____ ADM./READM. DATE_____ TIME_____

MR #_____ CLINIC # _____ DOB _____ AGE _____

SEX:___M___F

ADMITTED VIA: AMBULANCE _____ CAR_____ W/C ___SELF____

ADMITTED FROM: HOSPITAL _____ NURSING HOME_____ HOME____

ORIENTATION TO SAMARITAN: TOUR_____ ROOMMATE_____CALL LIGHTS_____

      BEDSIDE STAND_____ DRAWERS_____ CLOSET_____BATHROOMS_____

      MEALTIMES_____ ACTIVITIES_____ FLOOR_____NURSES_____

PHYSICIAN_____ PHARMACIST_____

CODE STATUS_____ ALLERGY_____

REASON FOR ADMISSION: _____

DIAGNOSIS: _____
_____
_____

MEDICATIONS: _____
_____

MENTAL STATUS
____Alert
____Oriented
____Disoriented
____Forgetful
____Lethargic
____Semi/comatose

COMMUNICATION
____Normal Speech
____Speech Impairment
____Language Barrier/
    uses gestures
____Inappropriate Cont.
____Unable to Speak

HEARING
____Good ___R___L
____Poor ___R___L
____Deaf ___R___L
____Aid ___R___L

VISION
____Good ___R___L
____Poor ___R___L
____Blind ___R___L
____Glasses

TEETH
____Natural
____Dentures ___U___L
____Partial ___U___L
____No teeth

DRESSING
____Independent
____Upper Torso
____Lower Torso
____Ties shoes
____Fasteners
____TEDS

GROOMING
____Independent
____Oral care
____Scalp care
____Peri care
____Shave
____Hair(assist.)
____Beauty Shop

BATHING
____Shower
____Century Tub
____Bed bath
____Spec. foot care
Day _____
____Assist. c Bath
____Assist. in/out tub

EATING
____Independent
____Tray Set Up
____Assist. c Eating
____Total Feed
____Gastrostomy Tube
____Spec. Utensils
____Dining Room
____Floor Lounge

BOWEL & BLADDER
____Continent
____Incont. of Bladder
____Incont. of Bowel
____Ostomy
____Bathroom
____Commode
____Bedpan
____Undergarments
____Catheter
____Constipation
____Last bowel movement

MOBILITY
____Independent
____Cane or walker
____Crutches
____Wheel chair
____Geri chair
____Bedfast

TRANSFERRING
____Independent
____1 or 2 Assist.
____Hoyer Lift
____3 man lift

ROM
____Limited upper ext.
____Limited lower ext.
____Unable to turn self
____Prosthesis
____Trapeze

Figure 12–5 Sample nursing interview (Courtesy of Samaritan Bethany, Inc., Rochester, MN)

SAFETY
_____ Wanderer
_____ Gait Belt
_____ Grey Belt
_____ Posey
_____ Siderails
_____ Water mattress
_____ Air mattress
_____ Egg crate mattress
_____ Sheepskin mattress
_____ Foam w/c cushion

THERAPY
_____ Physical
_____ Occupational
_____ Activity
_____ Remotivation
_____ Reality Orientation
_____ Psychiatric

BEHAVIOR
_____ No problem
_____ Minor problem
_____ Moderate problem
_____ Disturbs others
_____ Verbally abusive
_____ Physically abusive

PHYSICAL ASSESSMENT

Condition of skin: _____

_____

Indicate on diagram below: All body marks, such as, scars, bruises,
     lacerations, decubiti, contractures, or other body abnormalities.

ADMISSION VITALS: _____ B/P ____ Pulse ____ Temp. ____ Resp. ____ Wt. ____ Ht.
                      24 HOUR-EVERY FOUR HOUR VITAL SIGNS

DATE	TIME	BLOOD PRESSURE	TEMP.	PULSE	RESP.	SIGNATURE

ASSESSMENT SUMMARY: _____

_____

_____

NURSE'S SIGNATURE: _____   DATE: _____   TIME: _____

                                                      SBH
                                                      R N7 11/85

Figure 12-5 (Continued)

Although this information is important and helpful, nurses should always document objective and subjective data collected at the time of the interview. The resident's health could have changed, or other events occurred that makes your data different from what others have collected. Figure 12–6 summarizes baseline data collected for an expanded assessment when the elderly are admitted to a long term care facility.

Nursing Diagnosis: Mobility and Memory Problems

The facility staff, especially the nurses and nursing assistants who work most closely with the resident, continue to collect data and make assessments for the care plan that will be developed at the initial care conference, 10 days following admission. While continually gathering data, the caregivers also validate it to be sure it is accurate. It is organized within basic needs,

times of day, and other measurements to look for patterns that point to specific needs. Ongoing assessments assist in determining the resident's needs for all his activities of daily living as well identifying major health problems.

Recall that a *nursing diagnosis* focuses on actual or potential health problems that a nurse can identify and treat independently. For example, dyspnea can be identified and treated with nursing measures such as raising the head of the bed and pacing the person's activities. In contrast, a medical diagnosis focuses on diagnostic tests to determine the cause of the dyspnea, such as asthma, and the appropriate medical treatment. These activities require a licensed physician. When nurses implement the medical treatment, such as administering a bronchodilator, it is called "delegated medical treatment." These activities require a physician's order; they are not nursing measures. Many nursing education programs and health care facilities use the North American Nursing

---

EXPANDING ASSESSMENT FOR LONG-TERM CARE PLACEMENT

Data Collection Before Admission
- Obtained through pre-screening process implemented by discharge planner, public health nurse, and social worker.
- Evaluates physical condition and functional abilities to determine alternative services or long-term care placement.
- Assists family in the process of selecting a facility.
- Determines health and living needs to assure facility has appropriate resources.
- Assists family in planning financial arrangements, and understanding government and facility regulations, policies, and schedules.
- Includes decisions on personal belongings that will be a part of the resident's living area.

Data Collection on Admission
- Includes informal observation of physical and mental abilities and limitations.
- Includes subjective and objective information on chart nursing interview.
- Includes a short mental status exam, if indicated.
- Determines all physical and functional abilities related to activities of daily living.
- Compares data obtained with hospital discharge summary, pre-screening assessment, or social worker's family interview.
- Provides information for interim care plan.

Figure 12–6 Baseline data for resident admission

Diagnosis Association (NANDA) nursing diagnostic categories.

The problems experienced by the elderly that initiate dependent living and admission to a long term care facility are usually related to mobility and memory. Figure 12–7 lists the major nursing diagnoses that relate to these problems as well as the more common diagnoses long-term care nurses implement when developing resident care plans.

During the assessment, potential problems are frequently validated with a variety of flow sheets. Nurses in long term care facilities have become creative in organizing data into specialized flow sheets. Figure 12–8 is a sample flow sheet for collecting data related to potential

MAJOR NURSING DIAGNOSES

- Impaired Physical Mobility
- Activity Intolerance
- Altered Thought Process

CONTRIBUTING NURSING DIAGNOSES

- Potential for Injury
- Potential for Infection
- Self-Care Deficit
  (One or more personal care needs)
- Altered Nutrition: Less than Body Requirements
- Potential Fluid Volume Deficit
- Functional Urinary Incontinence
- Constipation
- Chronic Pain
- Impaired Skin Integrity
- Anxiety
- Social Isolation
- Impaired Communication
- Knowledge Deficit
- Ineffective Coping
  (Individual and/or Family)

Figure 12–7 Common nursing diagnoses in dependent long-term care residents

elimination problems. Caregivers throughout the 24-hour day collect and document data that will assist in determining needs for all hours of patient care, figure 12–9.

Actual or potential problems also need to be validated with the resident's family. Residents who have been admitted after a period of home care probably have a functional assessment that was completed by the home health nurse. Those admitted from the hospital, having had an acute illness episode, may not have discharge information related to a total functional assessment. For example, a resident admitted following surgery for a hip fracture will have information about his ambulation and physical therapy. He would be expected to be independent in eating. However, if he was not able to cut meat or peel a banana at home because of arthritic fingers and generalized weakness, he will not be able to complete those tasks now.

Family caregivers can explain the elderly's abilities prior to hospitalization or how they managed at home before the long-term care admission. If they were in a weakened debilitated state because of an acute illness, you can expect some areas of independence and self-care to improve. Remember, the medical diagnosis with expected symptoms and responses may not correspond with the resident's functional ability. Assume nothing!

Planning: A Multidisciplinary Approach

Approximately 10 days after the resident enters the long term care facility, a multidisciplinary team meets for input into the care plan. The members include all those active and interested in the resident's quality of care and quality of life. The resident and family are the most important members. Nurses, nursing assistants, social worker, dietitian or dietary supervisor, physical therapist, activities director, and housekeeper are other members. Additional persons, such as a speech or occupational therapist, may

Samaritan Bethany Nursing Home
Rochester, Minnesota

Bowel and Bladder Assessment

NAME: _____ DR. _____

MR#_____AGE_____RM#_____

1. Diagnosis relating to incontinence problem.

   _____

   _____

   _____

2. Previous pattern of elimination prior to onset of problem.

   _____

   _____

   _____

3. Is the resident ambulatory?_____

4. Is the resident able to communicate needs?_____

5. Diet_____

6. Appetite_____

7. Dentures_____

8. Medications relating to bowel or bladder problems.

   _____

   _____

   _____

9. Urinary Catheter?_____

10. After data collection is complete, determine: Is this resident a candidate
    for Bowel/Bladder Retraining?

    Yes_____   No_____

11. Proceed to Care Plan.

Figure 12-8 Sample flow sheet for collecting specialized data (Courtesy of Samaritan Bethany, Inc, Rochester, MN)

DATA COLLECTION

Date:	N	D	E	N	D	E	N	D	E	N	D	E	N	D	E
1. Time of incontinence.															
2. Amount (S-M-Lg)															
3. Was bed wet?															
4. Fluid Intake															
5. Was urge present?															
6. Type of incontinent product used?															
7. Orientation (Confused or alert)															
8. Was resident awake when incontinent?															
9. Was resident incontinent during activity or mealtime?															

Figure 12–8   (Continued)

SAMARITAN BETHANY HOME
CARE CONFERENCE – NURSING ASSISTANT INPUT SHEET

NIGHT SHIFT   THE FOLLOWING RESIDENTS HAVE CARE CONFERENCES SCHEDULED FOR _____

BED MOBILITY (Turn self?)				
PROTECTIVE UNDERGARMENTS?				
BEDPAN/COMMODE/BATHROOM				
BOWEL/BLADDER CONTROL				
MAKE NEEDS KNOWN AND USE CALL LIGHT?				
ORIENTATION				
BEHAVIOR PROBLEMS? (Describe)				
SKIN CONDITION/SKIN CARES				
PAIN (Describe)				
RESTRAINTS? (type)				
OTHER COMMENTS?				

Figure 12–9 Sample data collection tool for determining new resident needs (Courtesy of Samaritan Bethany, Inc., Rochester, MN)

be involved depending on the needs of the resident. This group begins the planning for a comprehensive care plan, figure 12–10.

Major influences on the framework of the care plan include the resident's and family's requests and preferences, the medical treatment reflected in the doctor's orders, and insurance and other funding for care. If the family has not been available to assist in validating assessments, the observations can be clarified at this time.

The resident's preferences are noted in all areas of biological, sociological, and psychological needs. At the time of admission the social worker's assessment will include some social and family history. Information that will assist the facility in maintaining the resident's lifestyle includes noting family, cultural, and religious traditions. For example, one resident wanted to be left alone for an hour every morn-

ing after breakfast for personal prayers and meditation. Birthdays and other family holidays are important traditions to maintain.

The family will be encouraged to be involved in the care. Some prefer to take care of the personal laundry, and arrange to take the resident out for lunch. One gentleman, his wife a victim of multiple deficits from a stroke, drove to the facility every morning to visit and feed her lunch. There are countless ways that family members continue being involved in the quality of life of their elderly member. Others cannot or will not be involved.

Medical treatment is included in the plan of care; the physician's orders arrive with the resident at the time of admission. The multiple chronic conditions of dependent elderly indicate that most residents will have several prescription medications. Most facilities also have "standing order" forms for physicians to com-

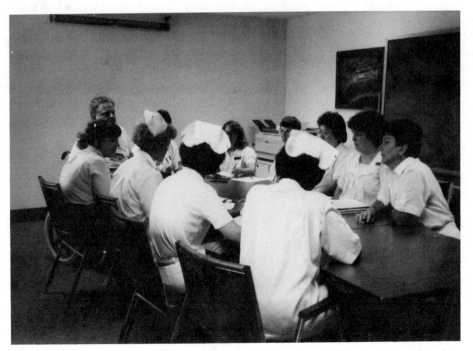

Figure 12–10   The multidisciplinary team meets for the care planning conference.

plete. Examples could include acetaminophen for complaints of mild discomfort or fever and bisacodyl suppositories for intermittent constipation. These orders address general complaints, such as a headache, that people usually treat themselves. The facility is now the resident's home, and the nurse, after usual data collection for reasonable care, can administer "standing order" medications and treatments.

Nurses observe the results of medical therapies and keep physicians informed. Government regulations require physicians to visit residents, on a routine basis, in the long term care facility. Acute care illness situations will require the resident to be transported to the physician's office by a medical van, or the family may take the resident.

Funding of care influences the resident's care in a number of ways. Medicare pays only for a limited number of initial days in the facility. If the resident is financially indigent, Medicaid continues the payments. Private insurers pay a limited amount, leaving most of the costs to be paid out-of-pocket by the elderly or their families. Supplies and equipment are not uniformly reimbursed by all funding sources. This is important for nurses to know. Before you can arrange for a resident to have her dentures relined, send her to a podiatrist, or make an appointment at the beauty shop, you have to know who is going to pay the bill! Some funding sources will not pay for multiple vitamins or laxatives.

Funding also influences the number of caregivers and other services available to assist the resident. The government is in the process of designing a prospective payment system for long-term care as it did for acute care. Recall that in acute care the Medicare program pays according to the patient's diagnosis; it is called the Diagnostic Related Groups (DRGs).

Case Mix is being implemented in some states for reimbursing costs in long-term care. *Case Mix* is a type of payment system that reimburses operating costs based on the condition and needs of residents. The classifications focus on the amount of assistance the elderly need with activities of daily living rather than their medical diagnoses. In Minnesota, an A through K method of classification identifies levels of dependency. A resident identified as "A" requires minimal assistance in bathing, eating, toileting, and other daily personal activities. A resident who is in the "K" category may be totally dependent and require special nursing skills. The payment system reimburses on a daily rate, and may be less that $50 for an "A" and almost $100 for a "K." Total reimbursement to a facility will be reflected in budgets, staffing, and supplies.

Nurses are directly involved in the costs and funding of long-term care. They assist in being "thrifty" with the limited dollars of the residents. They may suggest friends or family give a gift coupon for a haircut or permanant. Nurses document the abilities and limitations of residents, which utimately reflects on reimbursement for the care. This discussion may not seem pertinent to planning in the nursing process, and the development of resident care plans. It is!

The plan also includes goals. The goals focus on the resident's physical and emotional strengths. Utilizing the strengths will increase self-esteem followed by increased motivation, abilities, and cooperation. There will be less time on task for the resident and the caregiver. Figure 12–11 summarizes factors influencing planning in the development of dependent elderly care plans.

Implementation: Adaptations for Dependent Care

Care plans for dependent elderly are implemented primarily by nurses and nursing assistants with intermittent direct or indirect care provided by other members of the multidisciplinary team. Nursing assistants provide or assist with much of the personal care while nurses administer medications, implement special treatments or procedures, and make continual assessments.

The difference in implementing care for active and dependent elderly is in patient teaching and monitoring health. The active aging are given more responsibility for their own health which requires increased patient teaching by nurses. The dependent aging continue to live longer and become even more dependent, which increases the responsibility of nurses in areas of monitoring residents' health and basic needs. For example, a resident having dysphagia as a result of a stroke may receive nothing by mouth and all nutrition and fluids via a gastrostomy tube. Nurses and other caregivers are totally responsible for the assessment and administration of this resident's nutrition and fluids. Observations will be made regarding weight changes, skin turgor, condition of mucous membranes, and characteristics of urine. They will evaluate the number of calories received in the tube feeding and the amount of water instilled.

Observations and nursing interventions that are implemented by nurses in long-term care can be discussed in three general categories. They are (1) the tasks that are involved in continuing acute care needs, (2) administering and monitoring medications, and (3) ongoing or long-term nursing observations.

Continuing Acute Care Needs

Until recently, the term "acute" did not even surface in long term care facilities. Many of the then "nursing homes" would not accept residents needing an indwelling catheter or perhaps supplemental oxygen. Today, people have a variety of tubes and specialized equipment, and receive "high tech" care in their homes and in long term care facilities.

MAJOR INFLUENCES ON THE PLANNING PHASE

Resident's and Family's Requests and Preferences
- Reflects biological, sociological, and psychological needs.
- Focus is on maintaining resident's previous life style: family, cultural, and religious traditions.
- Determine's family's ability and willingness to participate in care.

Medical Treatment
- Reflected in physician's orders.
- Focus is on multiple chronic conditions.
- "Standing orders" require nursing judgement.
- Influenced by government regulations.

Funding for Care
- Source of funding influences payment for treatments, supplies, and equipment; reflected in treatment approach and number of times implemented.
- Resident or family must cover many uninsured costs; may influence decisions for plan of care.
- Government funding based on condition and needs of resident; regulates care strictly by reimbursement.
- Reimbursement influences budgets; budgets influence number of caregivers to implement plan.

Goals: Maintain highest level of functional ability utilizing the resident's existing strengths.

Figure 12–11   Factors that influence the planning phase of care plans

Nurses manage continuing acute care needs of residents dismissed from hospitals after an acute medical or surgical event, or monitor ongoing tube feedings, oxygen therapy (including ventilators), intravenous therapy, and other equipment currently considered "high tech" for long-term care.

Residents returning from an acute episode in the hospital or a new resident admitted from the hospital require ongoing assessments similar to acute care nursing. Examples include more frequent monitoring of vital signs, inspection of surgical wounds with dressing changes, and evaluation of each body system to assure return to the resident's previous "normal" functioning. You will be removing sutures and staples when ordered by the physician. The resident would not be transported to the office for this procedure.

The resident's recovery and progress is documented in the chart and reported to the physician through telephone consultation. In the future more acute illness episodes will be treated in the long term care facility. For example, pneumonia and dehydration will be treated with supplemental oxygen and intravenous fluids and antibiotics, and the resident will remain in his room. Some sources say the resident will have an easier time recovering without the disruption of a different environment; they may avoid the episodes of confusion that often occur.

Residents may receive continuous oxygen therapies with chronic respiratory problems or nasogastric or gastrostomy tube feedings when unresponsive or unable to swallow. These are two examples of procedures that require frequent skilled assessments and knowledge of equipment, figure 12–12. In long-term care, there are no respiratory therapy departments to "run up" and take care of equipment problems or assess the resident. You will need to become knowledgeable of therapies and equipment for procedures where you are employed. A sample of special procedures and key assessment points are listed in table 12–1. Always consult a nursing skills reference to review a procedure you have not implemented for a period of time.

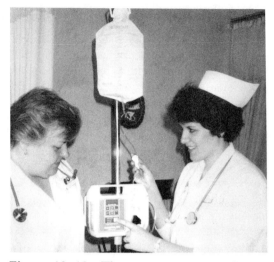

Figure 12–12   The nurse assesses equipment as part of a tube feeding procedure.

Administering and Monitoring Medications

Administering medications to dependent elderly residents, monitoring the results, and observing for potential side-effects involves a considerable amount of the nurses' time in long-term care. First, these elderly have several chronic conditions that are managed with medications. Nurses are responsible for as many as 30 residents; it is not unusual for a major medication pass to take two hours. Second, due to normal aging changes or disease problems, a resident may have difficulty swallowing or other problems when taking medications. Third, this is a time when busy nurses take time to make assessments. Residents also know this is a time they can "catch" the nurse to share a concern.

Additional time is involved in monitoring the medications. Recall that normal physical changes in aging affect the absorption, metabolizing, and excretion of drugs. Residents may have taken a medication for years and still have an adverse reaction. Many residents are not alert, are confused or dysphasic, or for some other reason cannot verbalize symptoms that could be related to medication reactions. You have to be a keen observer and good detective,

KEY ASSESSMENTS	RATIONALE

Oxygen Needs
• Nasal cannula for supplemental oxygen
  — check cannula frequently: placement of cannula prongs in nares, adjustment of elastic band
  — check oxygen equipment, including flow rate
	— elderly at higher risk for skin breakdown in nares and on ears
	— resident may dislodge cannula
	— resident's or facility's portable containers may need filling; therapeutic flow rate and resident response is monitored

• Inhalation devices: Atomizers and nebulizers for metered dose medications
  — check package instructions for correct assembly and operation of device
 	
  — observe resident's ability to manage device independently
 	
  — verify sequence of multiple inhalation medications
  — assess effectiveness of procedure and medication; include chest auscultation
	— assure that medication is administered correctly, resident receives full dose ordered
	— fatigue, weakness, or hand tremors may indicate the nurse must manipulate device
	— meet objectives of opening airway and reaching deeper airways
	— fatigue may prevent resident from complying with directions for inspiration and expiration
	— residents with prn orders may over-medicate and may demonstrate side effects
	— physician may change device or medication because of resident response or nurse assessment

• Suctioning: oropharyngeal, nasopharyngeal, tracheal
  — assess positioning: semi-Fowler's if conscious, lateral if unconscious
 	
  — maintain clean and sterile techniques with equipment and procedure
  — select correct suction pressure
 	
  — suction only during withdrawal of catheter, no more than 15 seconds
	— semi-Fowler's promotes lung expansion, lateral promotes secretion drainage and prevents aspiration
	— reduces transmission of microorganisms; elderly are higher risks for infections
	— elderly may need lower pressure to reduce risk of injury to mucosa
	— elderly are at greater risk for hypoxia, may tolerate only 10-second period of suctioning

TABLE 12–1 Special Procedures for Dependent Elderly

KEY ASSESSMENTS	RATIONALE
Oxygen Needs (continued) • Pacemaker Monitoring — check if pulse is slower than preset rate (Preset rate is usually noted on the front of the resident's chart.) — implement telephone monitoring by following equipment directions, (resident has small transmitting device for a monitoring service) — assess for signs of unusual dyspnea, chest pain, pulse irregularities, or dizziness	— slower pulse may indicate pacemaker malfunction — single-lead ECG monitors for abnormalities, resident and physician are notified regarding results — may indicate other cardiac or pacemaker complications

Nutritional and Fluid Needs
• Tube Feedings: Gastrostomy and Nasogastric
— check position of resident
 	
— check placement of tubing
 	
  1. Attach syringe to tube and aspirate contents with asepto syringe.
    — return contents to stomach
  2. Inject 10–20 cc air into tube after placing stethoscope on abdomen.
— check and maintain patency by introducing 30–60 cc water before and after feedings and medications
— clamp tubing when instillations are completed or disrupted
— check feeding pump or other equipment
(Bolus feedings are introduced by gravity with an asepto syringe. The intermittent feedings are not usually given to the elderly as they tend to induce diarrhea.)
— monitor intake of feeding and water, skin turgor, urine characteristics, weight changes
	— elevating the resident's head to 30 degrees prevents aspiration of feeding
	— may become dislodged, reduces risk of aspiration
	— results indicates tube is in stomach
	
	— avoid electrolyte losses
	— air entering stomach produces a whooshing sound
	— verifies patency of tubing, flushes tubing to prevent residue, clogging, and bacterial growth
	— prevents air from being introduced into the stomach
	— meters amount of feeding prescribed by physician,
	— slow, regular rate reduces gastrointestinal distress
	
	— evaluate nutritional and hydration status; most commercial tube feedings are approximately 1 calorie/1cc

TABLE 12–1 (Continued)

KEY ASSESSMENTS	RATIONALE

Nutritional and Fluid Needs (continued)
• Monitoring Intravenous Fluids
  — regulate flow rate
  (must know physician order and drop factor of infusion set)
  $$\frac{\text{volume per hour} \times \text{drop factor}}{60 \text{ minutes}}$$
	— prevents fluid volume excess or deficit
	
	Example:
	Physician Order:
	1000 cc D5W @ 75 cc/hour
	Drop factor: 15 drops/cc
	$$\frac{75 \times 15}{60} = 1075 \text{ gtt/hour or 18 gtt/minute}$$
	or 4–5 gtt/15 seconds

Safety (Infection Control) Needs
• Dry Dressing Changes
  — verify acute care physician's orders; observe resident's surgical dressings
 	
  — implement sterile and aseptic techniques and facility's protocol for gloving and disposal of contaminated dressings and supplies
  — document observations: drainage on dressing removed, condition of incision, sutures, and area, and type of dressing applied
• Incision Suture Removal
  — verify physician order
 	
  — identify each suture
    1. Hold two ends or knot with forceps.
    2. Slip point of sterile scissors under suture.
    3. Cut suture.
 	
    4. Gently pull suture in direction it was inserted.
	— post operative dressings may be occlusive or nonocclusive; incision may require cleansing, or application of specific medications.
	— prevents nosocomial infections and post operative complications in the high risk elderly
	
	— promotes continuity of care, and notes progression of healing and recovery
	
	— need physician order to implement procedure
	
	— identifies and separates one suture from another
	— clearly identifies where suture will be cut
	
	— cutting cleanly one time avoids leaving any suture fragments in wound to initiate infection
	— reduces discomfort resident may experience

TABLE 12–1   (Continued)

KEY ASSESSMENTS	RATIONALE
Safety (Infection Control) Needs (continued) — document type of sutures removed and condition of incision and wound area Skin Staples: (Some surgeons use surgical staples to close an incision. This requires a special staple remover instrument; it may need to be obtained from the hospital or physician's office.) — slip point of instrument under center of staple, squeeze handle, rotate wrist, and lift staple	— promotes continuity of care; notes progression of healing process — most surgical staples have a small projection that secures it in the skin; the action flattens and releases the staple, and reduces resident discomfort
• Wet-To-Dry Dressing Changes — implement clean and sterile techniques; follow facility protocol for gloving and disposal of contaminated dressings and supplies — carefully remove dressing; DO NOT moisten if dressing adheres to tissue — inspect wound carefully; note areas with good blood supply (red), purulent drainage (yellow), and necrosis (black) — apply one gauze moistened with normal saline or prescribed solution; cover all exposed tissue — apply dry gauze	— prevent nosocomial infections; promote healing in high risk elderly population — the reason for this dressing is to debride a wound; the moist dressing absorbs exudate and tissue debris — evaluates the status of wound healing; documentation may require actual measurements of areas — saturated gauze will not permit the debriding of the wound; tissue cells need moisture — becomes absorbent layer to pull moisture from surface of wound
• Pressure (Decubiti) Ulcer Treatment — consult resources to verify action and correct application of prescribed topical medication or dressing 1. Ulcers requiring cleansing: may be treated with detergent or oxidizing solutions; may be harmful to healthy tissue.	— physician choice of treatment may depend on depth and extent of ulcer — solutions such as half strength hydrogen peroxide cleanse ulcer and increase oxygen supply to tissues

TABLE 12–1 (Continued)

KEY ASSESSMENTS	RATIONALE
Safety (Infection Control) Needs (continued)	
2. Infected ulcers may be treated with antiseptic or antimicrobial solutions such as providone iodine.	— reduces bacterial growth, some solutions may be harmful to healthy tissue or may be toxic if undiluted — cover area with solution; may leave open to air

3. Ulcers that are deep and require debriding may be treated with enzymes such as collagenase.
  — secreting ulcers may be treated with agents such as dextranomer
  — ulcer may need to be irrigated to remove agent
	— agents debride dead tissue; apply thin layer of ointment avoiding healthy tissue; cover with dry dressing
	— agents absorb exudate; pack wound with granules, cover with dressing

4. Ulcers that require skin protection may be treated with emollients or protectants such as aluminum paste or benzoin tincture. — implementation includes careful assessment, detailed documentation, and frequent repositioning to facilitate circulation and resident comfort	— areas surrounding ulcer may be irritated by tape or agents treating the ulcer; apply sparingly and carefully as they may inactivate other topical treatments — promote healing in elderly skin which is fragile and requires meticulous ongoing care

TABLE 12–1   (Continued)

always watching for changes in behavior or any clue to a potential problem. Table 12–2 identifies some of the more common medications the dependent elderly receive and the side effects to monitor.

Administration of medications to residents begins, as in any other setting, with the five rights: right resident, right drug, right dose, right route, and right time. Also check for drug allergies and carefully document in the medication record. If you have any questions, consult the physician's order, a drug reference, the resident's chart, or other resources. The physician may order a laboratory test to evaluate the serum level of a drug.

Special considerations in the administration of medications to the dependent elderly include the need to crush medications for easier swallowing, or other alterations of the form in which the medication was manufactured and intended to be consumed. The pharmacist is your best resource when determining if you can crush the medication without altering its action. When the resident begins to have difficulty in swallowing, consult his physician to see if a liquid form can be ordered. Table 12–3 presents guidelines for special considerations when administering medications to the dependent elderly.

Long-term Nursing Observations

Nurses need to be continually alert to monitor the basic needs and activities of daily living of all the residents. There are challenges to maintain a functional level of activity and func-

---

REMEMBER

- to check resources to know drug actions, interactions, and side effects.
- a drug's concentration and solubility is affected by aging changes of proportion of fat, lean tissue, and water.
- decreased gastric motility may slow gastric absorption of medications.
- drugs are cleared by the kidney and liver.
- the smallest dose may still be toxic to the elderly.
- the key to safe drug therapy is good assessment.

MEDICATION _____	SIDE EFFECT/ AGING CONSIDERATION _____
A. Cardiac Glycosides	— Observe for confusion, restlessness, anorexia or blurred vision that are new symptoms or changes in behavior. — A narrow therapeutic range results in toxic serum levels due to decreased renal and hepatic functioning; monitor apical pulse. — Toxic symptoms may occur because of nutritional or diuretic dehydration.
B. Antihypertensives	— Observe for signs of lightheadedness or fainting, postural hypotension, lethargy, dizziness, or confusion. — Monitor vital signs. — Elderly require a higher blood pressure for adequate cerebral perfusion; higher measurements are more acceptable in the elderly. — Elderly hypertension is related more to vascular changes and dosages are carefully individualized.
C. Diuretics	— Observe carefully for signs of dehydration: weakness, hypotension, poor skin turgor, weight loss, or confusion. — Elderly have decrease of total body water content and may have poor fluid intake placing them at high risk for severe dehydration. — Dehydration and accompanying electrolyte imbalances may complicate preexisting gout and diabetes.

TABLE 12–2 Common Medications Administered to the Dependent Elderly

MEDICATION	SIDE EFFECT/ AGING CONSIDERATION
D. Sedatives/ Antianxiety Agents	— Observe for excessive sedation or residual drowsiness even with small dosages. — Elderly are sensitive to central nervous system effects; may demonstrate sedation or confusion in the daytime. — Many agents have a long half-life and accumulation of drug in circulation may result in stupor or confusion.
E. Bronchodilators/ Spasmolytics	— Observe for adverse effects of restlessness, dizziness, insomnia, palpitations, or tachycardia. — Interactions may occur with beta-adrenergic blockers. — Monitor dosages; anxious elderly residents want extra medication.
F. Anti-inflammatory Agents	— Observe for signs of gastrointestinal distress and occult blood loss. — Increased capillary fragility in elderly predisposes to serious bleeding being more common. — Long term corticosteroid use in chronic respiratory conditions may result in incidental fractures and infections; the need for more careful monitoring of diabetes in elderly receiving this treatment.

TABLE 12-2 (Continued)

tioning body systems. Because of increasing dependency and decreasing activity, all residents have the potential for difficulties with skin integrity, joint mobility, food and fluids, and bowel elimination. The potential for injury is always present. Falls, often in the resident's room, are the most common cause of injury to the elderly. Prevention is the best treatment for all these problems.

The elderly's skin is very fragile and needs continual attention. Nursing measures to main-

tain skin integrity include assisting the resident with adequate intake of nutrients and fluids, and using moisturizers on the skin. This helps keep the skin healthy. Frequent repositioning also relieves pressure areas and promotes circulation to bring nutrients to the cells. Signs of potential skin problems should receive immediate nursing intervention to prevent additional problems that may require medical treatment. Once there is a break in the skin it takes a long time for healing to be complete.

REMEMBER

- to consult the resident's physician when you have a question or problem regarding the medication order or resident's reaction to a specific medication.
- to consult the package inserts or facility or resident's pharmacist when you have a question or problem regarding altering the nature of a prescribed medication.

SITUATION	CONCERNS
• Resident has difficult swallowing or can not swallow. Tablets or capsules need to be crushed or opened to mix with water or food for easier swallowing. They may need to be administered via a nasogastric or gastrostomy feeding tube.	• Altering the nature of the medication may not provide the intended action of the drug. 　a. sustained-release capsules: when crushed alters covering that dissolves; resident receives more drug over a shorter period of time which may have adverse reactions; some "beads" may be mixed with food if they are not chewed. 　b. liquid-filled capsules: may irritate the mucous membranes of the oral cavity. 　c. enteric-coated tablets: if crushed the drug will be released in the stomach instead of the small intestine; will not be absorbed correctly or may be inactivated. **ALERT!** Some drugs such as Theo-Dur Sprinkle are intended to be activated in food. **ALERT!** Medications to be administered via feeding tube should *never* be mixed with a feeding preparation.
• Resident does not have finger dexterity to manage picking up tablet and placing in his mouth.	• Tablets may get lost in bed linens or placed under the tongue. Use spoon to scoop tablet out of medicine cup and place correctly in resident's mouth.
• Resident is to receive medication by injection and appears to have very little subcutaneous or muscle tissue.	• Medication may not be injected into correct tissue or cause undue discomfort to resident. Select needle gauge appropriate for medication and needle length appropriate to administer in desired layer of tissue; needle length may be shorter than usually used for younger adults.
• Resident receiving periodic injections has very limited activity, is unable to use lower extremities, or has poor tissue integrity.	• Medication may be poorly absorbed because of inadequate circulation; injection sites may become sites of lesions. Upper extremities may be more appropriate sites because even limited activity in eating or other self care increases circulation.

TABLE 12–3   Guidelines for Administering Medications to the Dependent Elderly

Skin wounds are categorized according to color, figure 12–13. The tissue in red wounds is traumatized but still has a good blood supply and potential for healing. A yellow wound is infected and has purulent drainage. The physician will probably order some method of cleaning and a wet-to-dry or other type of dressing. A topical and/or systemic antibiotic may be ordered. A black wound has at least some margins of necrotic tissue. Debridement, perhaps surgically, will remove this dead tissue to promote granulation and healing of viable tissue. Healing of any of these wounds is a long process in the elderly because of the compromised immune system and other aging changes in the body systems.

A variety of treatments that include pharmaceutical products and "in-house-remedies" developed by nurses and physicians are implemented to heal and protect damaged and infected skin.

A plastic-like permeable film is sometimes used to protect the skin. Other agents such as povidone-iodine are used to prevent bacterial growth on the skin. Nursing measures to keep the skin dry are also implemented.

The resident may have had joint mobility problems for years, related to joint stiffness and osteoarthritis. Residents can maintain a degree of joint mobility for independence by walking to the dining room for meals and completing self-care. Problems occur when a resident has experienced a stroke or other event that resulted in paralysis, or becomes weakened to the point that self-care is not possible. Stiff joints and contractures can occur in a very short time.

Nursing measures to promote continued joint mobility include encouraging and assisting the resident to complete as much self-care as possible. Perhaps she can wash her upper body, feed herself with the assistance of adaptive uten-

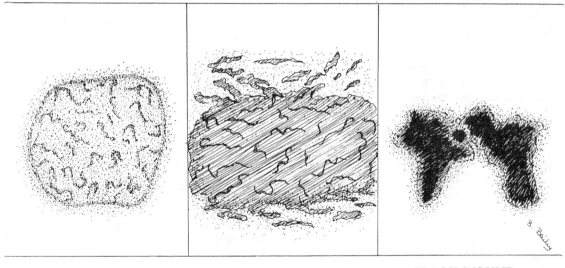

RED WOUND   YELLOW WOUND   BLACK WOUND

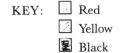

KEY: ☐ Red
      ☑ Yellow
      ◪ Black

Figure 12–13 Categorizing wounds according to color (Adapted for use by Brian Bailey)

sils, and complete grooming tasks, figure 12–14. It takes nursing time to allow residents to compete self-care. Some caregivers feel frustrated with time constraints and believe it is more efficient to do the care themselves. That will not promote joint mobility and eventually results in the resident requiring total care.

Passive range-of-motion (PROM) exercises assist in keeping the joints mobile in all residents. It is more commonly implemented with those who are confined to a bed or a wheelchair, figure 12–15. The procedure needs to be completed several times a day and on a daily basis to be effective in maintaining joint mobility.

Adequate intake of food and fluids becomes more of a concern as the elderly become more dependent. The caregivers become increasingly responsible for offering and assisting residents with their nutritional needs. Every system in the body requires water for adequate functioning; the importance of providing water cannot be underestimated. The usual seasonal respiratory and gastrointestinal viruses can dehydrate the elderly in a very short time.

Most elderly persons cannot drink a glass of water in several gulps like younger people. You need to offer and encourage them to take several sips frequently. Be sure to offer extra liquids between meals such as when medications are administered, when implementing a foot soak, or just by taking a moment to stop when you walk by the room.

The resident that needs to be fed should be included in the event, if possible, to maintain his self-esteem and a desire to eat. Prepare "finger foods," such as bread or crackers, that the resident can handle while you assist with foods that are more difficult to manage. If the resident cannot feed himself at all, allow him the choice of what he wants to eat first.

The potential for chronic constipation is apparant in all dependent elderly because of physical aging changes and limited activity. Some weak elderly do not have the energy to expel stool.

Caregivers must encourage an adequate fluid intake and higher fiber foods to promote a stool consistency that is easier for the elderly to pass. Most long term care facilities have bulk-producing, or evacuation-stimulating, preparations that are not medications in their bowel management programs. These may include unprocessed bran that can be added to cereal, prunes or prune juice, or other combinations, administered to those having chronic constipation problems.

Nurses also implement nursing measures to

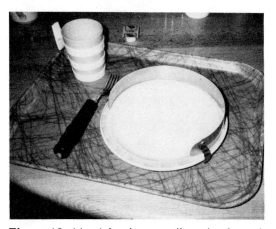

Figure 12–14 Adaptive utensils assist the resident to maintain some independence.

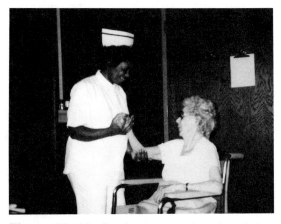

Figure 12–15 Passive range-of-motion helps maintain joint mobility.

promote bowel elimination such as providing privacy, allowing adequate time, and padding a toilet seat to decrease the discomfort of bony prominences. Remember, elimination has been a very personal and private event for the elderly. Caregivers must protect the resident's privacy and dignity.

Physicians may order stool softeners or laxatives such as docusate calcium or docusate sodium, psyllium, or milk of magnesia. PRN suppositories and enemas may also be included in a resident's standing orders. The focus today is to avoid medication preparations as much as possible and to promote improved nutrition and fluids and normal bowel evacuation.

Evaluation: Meeting the Highest Functional Level

Evaluation is an ongoing cycle of the Nursing Process in assessing, goal setting, and implementing. The single goal is quality of life.

Part of the evaluation is in documentation. Clear concise facts indicate observations and care implemented; they point the way for future care. Documentation has always been important and part of nursing care. Government regulations now require extensive documentation for quality assurance in evaluating the type and standard of care, and the fact that the care was given, for reimbursement purposes. Practicing nurses will attest to the fact that they are spending more time in charting and other documentation, and more people are reading what they write!

Government regulations dictate that the care plan be reviewed by a registered nurse every 30 days, and by the multidisciplinary team every 3 months. The resident's caregivers are in a continual process of evaluation of every part of his activities of daily living to promote quality of life.

Evaluation determines if the resident has the appropriate caregivers assisting him. As his

acuity level changes he may require more skilled nursing. Rehabilitative therapies are also evaluated for long-term benefits. They are costly and families may have to decide if therapy should continue. Funding sources, unfortunately, justify reimbursement for improving a disease process more than to improve functional ability.

Families are a part of the multidisciplinary team, and also evaluate care and the elderly's abilities and progress on a daily or weekly basis. Conflicts sometimes surface because a family member has unrealistic goals set for the resident. It is often the nurse's responsibility to explain to the family the physical and mental changes that are occurring which result in increased dependency. Remaining strengths can be identified, and measures of quality of life discussed.

The resident's response is the most important when evaluating the care plan. She may not want aggressive care and therapy. When the nurse takes a few moments to sit and visit with the resident, she will probably share her views and goals and how she wants to live in the long term care facility, figure 12–16.

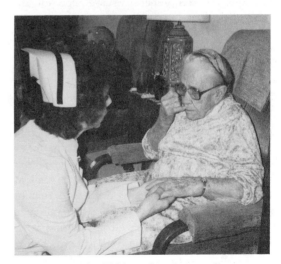

Figure 12–16 Taking the time to listen to a resident's views will help to meet her goals.

Summary

Providing a quality of care and quality of life to residents in a long term care facility is primarily the responsibility of nurses. This is a big responsibility because the end of a person's life is controlled and directed more by nurses than by the individual. Think about how you may influence the last years, months, or even days of a resident's life.

One method of assuring the resident's quality of care is in a comprehensive care plan. Nurses have always complied notes and some type of plan to meet their patient's needs; this was even before government regulations!

The Nursing Process is a problem-solving process to develop a comprehensive resident care plan. The assessment phase includes data collection before the elderly person is admitted to a long term care facility. A pre-admission screening team evaluates physical and functional limitations to determine the best setting for care. Social workers meet with families prior to admission to explain policies and procedures and determine the elderly's and family's concerns and requests.

A multidisciplinary team provides data and develops the comprehensive care plan for the resident in long-term care. This team includes the resident, his family, nurses, nursing assistants, dietitians, social workers, therapists, housekeepers, laundry personnel, and others who may be involved in the activities of daily living. Caregivers use a variety of specialized flow sheets to collect data and assess potential resident problems.

Nursing diagnoses in most residents relate to problems with mobility and memory. Other diagnoses reflect on these concerns as well as exacerbations of aging and disease. Actual or potential problems may have to be validated with the family. Nurses need to determine the resident's abilities when he lived at home before establishing realistic goals for the care plan.

A formalized care plan is developed after the resident has been in the facility for 10 days. The multidisciplinary team meets for a care conference. The resident's preferences are considered as well as physical and functional abilities and limitations. Family, cultural, and religious traditions are implemented in the plan; this is the resident's new home. The plan includes medical treatment and is also influenced by government and other funding sources.

Implementing the resident's care plan may mean a continuation of acute care nursing. Often, residents are admitted to the long term care facility from a hospital and are recovering from an acute medical or surgical event. The acuity of physical health of residents indicates that long term care nurses implement more sophisticated or "high tech" procedures.

The administration and monitoring of medications involves a considerable amount of the nurses' time. Many residents receive several drugs which treat a number of chronic conditions. Nurses must be alert to side-effects because many dependent, often confused elderly, cannot verbalize symptoms.

Implementation of the care plan includes long-term observations of potential problems in all dependent elderly. These include managing skin integrity, joint mobility, bowel function, and adequate nutrition and fluids. Preventing injury, especially falls, is continuous in a number of safety measures.

Evaluation includes all steps of the Nursing Process as it determines the need for additional data, a new focus on goals, or a different method of implementation. The entire multidisciplinary team is involved in ongoing evaluation. Documentation is a vital part of this step; caregivers and funding sources focus on documentation for quality of care.

The final judge of quality of life is the resident. How he feels about his care and life during his remaining years is the nurses' ultimate performance appraisal. What a challenge!

For Discussion

- Reflect on what is important in your life. Identify several personal, family, social, or religious traditions that you would want incorporated in a care plan.
- Visit with a resident in a long term care facility. Ask what traditions he/she is able to continue. What traditions would he/she like to continue that are not now a part of his/her shedule?
- Review a resident's chart. Identify nursing diagnoses related to his/her dependency.

Questions for Review

1. What are two nursing diagnoses common to dependent elderly?
2. Who are members of the multidisciplinary care plan team?
3. What are four socioeconomic factors that influence the resident's care plan?
4. What are three ongoing nursing observations in the elderly?

Section 4
Leadership Skills for Managing a Resident Unit

The aging population has been identified and a comparison made between active and dependent aging. The second group has special needs and problems that often cannot be managed at home. They also do not require acute care in a hospital. The long-term care setting is usually the alternative for the dependent elderly requiring skilled care. In Section 4 the role of the nurse in this setting will be defined and explored.

Nurses are involved with leadership and management tasks at every level and area of practice. The understanding of those functions is becoming more important in long-term care. Today there are ongoing changes of health care delivery in this setting. One of the changes is the increasing acuity of the residents' health. *Acuity* refers to unstable or severe health conditions. Other changes include sweeping rules and regulation changes in state and federal government policies. There is also a tightening of budgets at all levels. These changes necessitate the need for greater efficiency in the delivery of health care to the dependent elderly.

Leadership and management share some similarities. Both suggest that someone is in charge and helping workers. The difference is in how this is done. *Leadership* can be described as having the capacity to guide, and the ability to influence, lead, enable, and inspire. This is done by participating in or guiding the activity. *Management* is the act of controlling, handling, arranging, directing, or supervising an activity. This is accomplished by being responsible for the activity and controlling its movement. What was once reserved entirely for the director of nursing service is now included, in part, in job descriptions of every level of nursing in long-term care.

This section will focus on leadership and management skills implemented in resident care. These skills are applied to nursing care as well as the management of a resident unit in long term care facilities. Examples of patient care experiences in clinical assignments will be identified to assist you in adapting leadership skills to a resident unit. For purposes of this discussion, a resident unit in a long term care facility will be defined as a group of 30 residents, 3 nursing assistants, and 1 first-line manager nurse.

Unit 13 will describe levels of nursing management within a facility. The major responsibilities of each level and the interaction with other departments will be discussed. Leadership skills that are used in patient care will be adapted to managing resident care in Unit 14. These include managing own time, prioritizing tasks, and using effective communication techniques. Using leadership skills to manage a resident unit will be discussed in Unit 15. Characteristics of leadership that are abilities in patient care will be adapted to the role of the first-line manager nurse. New responsibilities of delegating tasks and appraising the performance of nursing assistants will be presented.

Unit 16 will discuss factors outside the resident unit that influence the functioning of the unit. These influences include the geographical setting and ownership of the facility, and behaviors of the first-line manager nurse expected by the facility and the public. Styles of management are discussed in Unit 17. This includes how giving directions, and including the caregivers in decision making influences the functioning of the resident unit. Unit 18 presents situations that require decision making by the first-line manager nurse. The flow of activity and decisions will assist you in understanding the process of problem solving on the resident unit.

After reading this section you should have basic ideas about the skills and activities required to direct the care on a resident unit. Putting the process in action successfully will take experience and practice.

Unit 13
Management Levels in
Long-term Care Nursing

Objectives

After reading this unit you should be able to:

- Define leadership and management.
- Describe three management levels in nursing practice.
- Describe differences between the management levels of long-term care nursing practice.
- Identify the role of the Licensed Practical/Vocational Nurse and the Registered Nurse in long-term care.

In long term care facilities, as in many other businesses, there are lines of authority. These lines illustrate where each position fits within the network of personnel. It also defines lines of responsibility, or who is responsible to whom. Most long term care facilities have a diagram which clearly demonstrates the relationship of all the departments from the administrator to the resident living in the facility. All department supervisors are usually directly responsible to the administrator, figure 13-1. This supervisor position may also be titled manager, director, or department head. Each department has its own levels of staff. There are also lines of responsibility at the department level as shown in figure 13-2. The lines of responsibility in this unit will focus on the nursing spoke of the management wheel.

The LP/VN practicing in long-term care in the position of first-line manager needs to have an understanding of the major responsibilities of the levels of nursing management. This is because the interactions between the first-line manager nurse and other management levels of nursing occur more frequently in the long-term care setting.

Who Are the Nurse Managers?

There are many ways to organize a nursing service in a health care facility. Figure 13-3 illustrates lines of nursing responsibility in three long term care facilities. Note that there are more nursing positions in Facility A than Facility C. This indicates changes in lines of authority and responsibility. The number of nursing positions depends almost entirely on the number of residents in the facility. The organizational structure of the facility and the acuity of the residents also influences the nursing positions and structure of nursing service. Obviously, a facility with many resident beds requires several nurses to accomplish the tasks completed by the director of nursing in a small facility.

All of the models in figure 13-3 place the director of nursing service at the top of the management tree. This position is identified as the *third-line manager.* A person in this position is responsibile for all nursing service personnel. All members of the department are ultimately responsible to this nurse. The nurse manager as director of nursing service is responsible to the administrator of the facility.

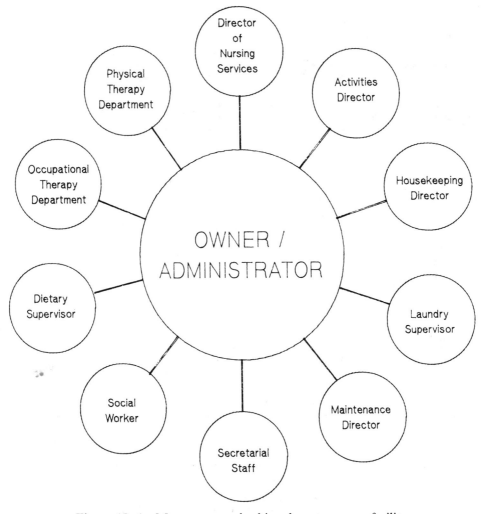

Figure 13–1   Management wheel in a long term care facility

The supervisor is a Registered Nurse and is primarily responsible for a specific area or section of a large facility. The staff and residents in this area are under direct supervision of this nurse. The responsibilities include 24 hour management of day-to-day activities. This supervisor is accountable to the director of nursing and in some facilities this nurse may hold the position of assistant director of nursing.

The *second-line manager* is a Registered Nurse or Licensed Practical/Vocational Nurse. This

nursing position is responsible for a facility floor, wing, or nursing station unit. Responsibilities include management of the staff and residents in this area; the position is accountable to the nursing supervisor or director of nursing service.

The staff nurse, as the *first-line manager,* is an LP/VN. This nurse is accountable to the second-line manager nurse. The scope of tasks ranges from direct resident care to responsibilities of management of the floor in the absence

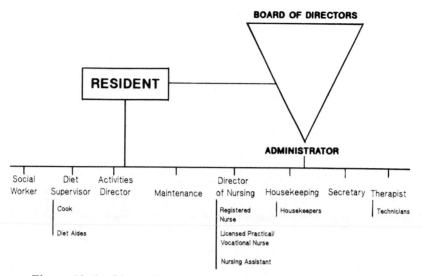

Figure 13–2   Lines of communication in a long term care facility

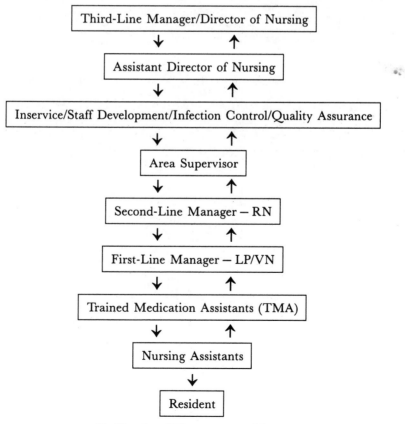

Facility A — 200 or more residents

Figure 13–3   Lines of responsibility in nursing service   (Continues)

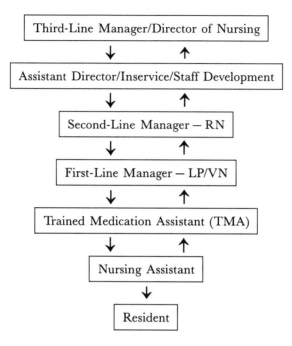

Facility B — Less than 200 residents

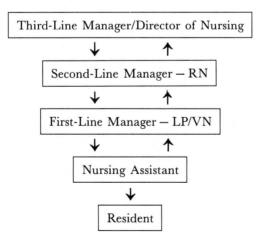

Facility C — Less than 60 residents

Figure 13-3 (Continued)

of the second-line manager. This nursing position is a bridge for residents to all departments and all services available in the facility.

Communications within the nursing department may be simple verbal instructions or more structured written memos, depending on the size of the facility. The communications between levels of nursing in a small facility may be informal, with direct routes between all levels. In larger facilities there may be more indirect routes of verbal and written communication. The resident always has the opportunity to have direct communication with all levels of nursing. Figure 13–4 illustrates an example of lines of communication in the nursing department.

The First-Line Manager: Licensed Practical/ Vocational Nurse

The Licensed Practical/Vocational Nurse is the licensed nurse having the most frequent interactions with the resident, figure 13–5. For this reason you are vital to the success of the nursing department. Your duties will vary from one facility to another, but you will always be expected to perform a wide range of tasks.

One important task in this position is the administration of medications, figure 13–6. Your knowledge base of drug therapy must be

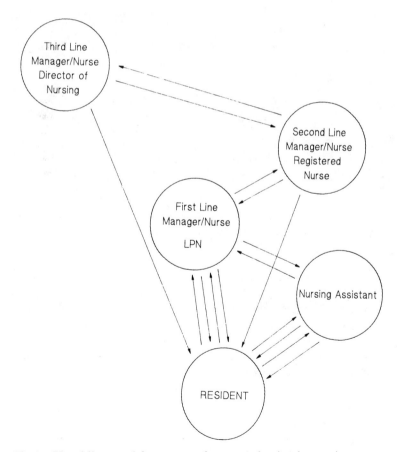

Figure 13–4   Usual lines and frequency of communication in nursing management

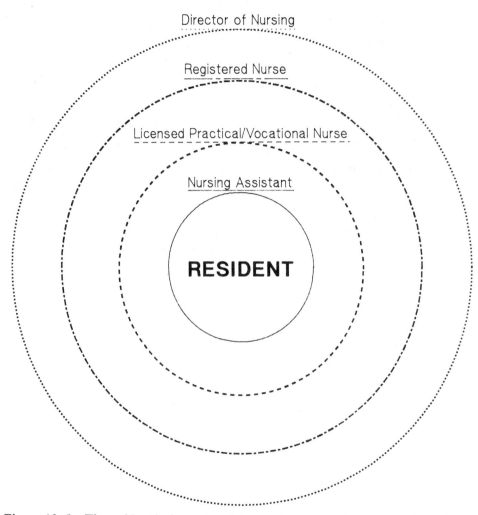

Figure 13–5 The resident is the center of the nursing service department circle of care.

current in order to keep pace with the rapid changes in the development of geriatric medicine. Any adverse reaction must be recognized and reported.

Another responsibility of the first-line manager is to administer medical treatments to the resident. These treatments may vary from applying a lotion or cream to dry but intact skin, to cleansing, treating, and redressing open, draining wounds. Recall caring for residents in long-term care also involves working with tracheos-

tomy tubes and suctioning, gastrostomy tubes and feedings, a variety of catheters, oxygen therapy, and other equipment. Although you may not always be directly responsible for these procedures, you are the caregiver responsible for the resident; therefore you must be alert for equipment that is not functioning properly, 13–7.

Your assessment skills will be implemented with every resident as you learn to note differences in behavior, responses to care, physical

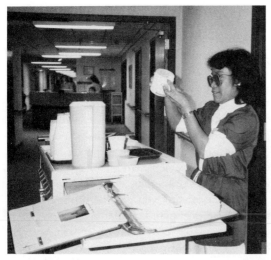

Figure 13–6 Administration of medications is an important task of the first-line manager nurse.

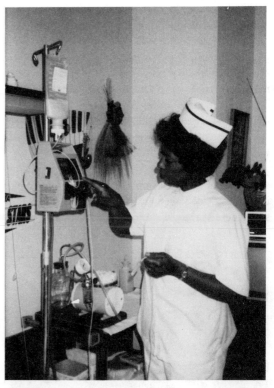

Figure 13–7 The nurse rechecks equipment to be certain it is functioning properly.

abilities, vital signs, and general appearance. With practice and experience, you will learn to put these observations together to make an assessment and nursing diagnosis of this resident's current status. Experience fine tunes these skills and you will document what you see, hear, feel, and smell with more ease and accuracy.

Functional ability can be more accurately assessed if the resident is not aware that an observation is being made. Pain can be evaluated and the source identified by watching facial expression and body movements during care. Mental status is easily monitored in the resident who is comfortable and relaxed in the presence of his caregiver. Skin condition is assessed by touch during care; you have made similar assessments when caring for patients in the hospital.

Documentation is one of the most important tasks of the first-line manager caregiver. It is probably one of the less desired tasks of nurses at any level. Perhaps one reason is the lack of standardized formats and methods in nursing practice and health care facilities. We

have all heard "if it wasn't documented, it wasn't done." This makes us realize the importance of documenting care, figure 13–8.

The importance of accuracy cannot be overemphasized. The resident's record is a legal document. What is written must be legible, concise, and informative. Narrative notes explain how the resident responded to care and his ability to participate in that care. Other documentation includes medications, treatments, and vital signs. Flow charts and resident status report forms are completed at the end of your workday. This information provides data for the resident care plans, the physician's treatment plan, the nurses on the next shift, facility support services, other departments in the facility, and the resident's family. This documentation is the link from the resident's bedside to the nursing service department and subsequently other departments.

Interaction with other members of the nursing staff should be comfortable and congenial. Be certain that nursing assistants understand medical terminology and medical jargon. *Medical jargon* means abbreviations and code words that signal expanded information.

Care must be taken when communicating with family members and staff from other disciplines. Be sure that your information is clear; avoid unfamiliar terminology. Courtesy and tact in all your contacts with others will make for smoother working relationships. A professional

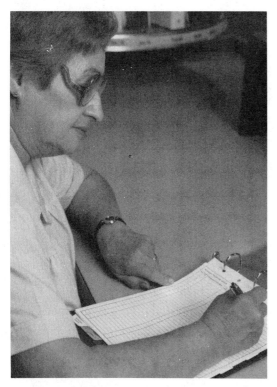

Figure 13–8 Documenting care is an important first-line manager task. (From Hegner and Caldwell/*Assisting in Long-Term Care,* copyright 1988 by Delmar Publishers Inc.)

attitude and appearance is also important in interactions with others.

Resident care plan conferences bring all health care disciplines, the resident, and the family together. Your documented information will be considered with the data presented from other caregivers. A plan of care will be developed from this data. This plan will include: (1) the identification of deficits or problems, (2) establishment of goals to decrease the deficit or solve the problem, and (3) approaches or ideas to achieve the goals.

The major link you provide in the development of the care plan is in data collection. Data collection is vital. Caregivers observe and record much of the information presented in the resident care planning conference. Your observations and assessments help to identify problems. In analyzing your data, you may suggest approaches to solutions. When implementing the care plan, your responsibilities include following the written care plan. As the resident progresses and goals are met, you will document successes in the narrative notes. If care plan approaches are not successful, this too must be documented. An alternative approach is discussed and care plans amended.

The first-line manager provides a leadership example when working beside the nursing assistant during the management of a group of residents, figure 13–9. You set the working pace, attitude, and example for the nursing assistants. If you do not follow the directions of the care plan, why should they follow it? If you perform procedures incorrectly, why do they need to do it perfectly? If you are less than courteous to your co-workers, do you have a right to insist that the nursing assistants always be pleasant to each other?

It will be challenging to work beside the nursing assistant directing resident care one day and then assume the responsibilites of a charge nurse the next day. The nursing assistant's responsibilities have not changed, but yours have. You may be tested and questioned by the

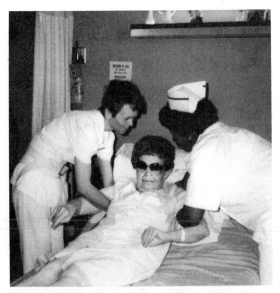

Figure 13–9 First-line manager nurses set examples when they work with nursing assistants at the resident's bedside.

nursing assistant who does not understand this role change. Your professional attitude and leadership ability will help you overcome any difficulties. Managing by making assignments and assuring that they are completed will result in a successful day for the resident and all team members.

Another task for the first-line manager may be to complete performance appraisals for the nursing assistants. Under the direction of the second-line manager you will complete this record for the nursing assistants on your resident unit. Appraisals are completed on a regular schedule regardless of the format chosen by the administration of the facility. Staff members at all levels need and deserve fair and objective evaluation of their work. This is done periodically to assist in personal growth as well as to give constructive comments on how to improve work performance. The appraisal should focus on strengths. It is a time to give a well earned "pat on the back." In some facilities the second-line manager nurse will complete the appraisals and you will be asked to provide objective observations of a nursing assistant's work performance.

Another important function of the first-line manager is evaluation of the tools of resident care. In addition to evaluating the resident's response to care, you will be evaluating procedures and equipment. During this evaluation process it may become apparant to you that facility procedures need to be written or current procedures revised. Situations when this may occur are when new or different equipment is used or when there are changes in regulations; the current procedures are no longer workable. Throughout your workday you will be involved in a continual problem-solving process.

Is it no longer feasible to follow the procedure due to equipment changes? Was the nursing assistant taught the correct method to complete the task? Were there "short-cuts" used that interfered with the objectives of the procedure? You will be expected to follow facility procedures and teach nursing assistants to use the same procedures. Continuity is important in completing procedures as well as in evaluating the need for change. The problem-solving process begins again.

As a first-line manager you may also be asked to be a member of one of the facility's networking committees. A safety committee is an example of a group that is concerned with the safety of all staff and residents. The infection control committee works to prevent infections before they need to be controlled. The pharmaceutical committee is concerned with the safe delivery of medications, including the safe storage of drugs as well the compliance with the five rights of administration. You are an ideal member for these committees as you are at the resident's bedside.

During your workday you will communicate with other staff members in your area in an informal sharing of information and observations. As data is collected and documented, information is formalized to be reported to the nurses following resident care during the next work shift. This formal report is the key to assuring the continuation of activity in the nursing service department. It provides continuity for the resident's care. Resident care reports may be written, given verbally, or taped.

In smaller facilities the third-line manager nurse reports to the entire oncoming nursing team. Other facilities tape the report for the staff, and only the charge nurses confer directly. Facilitating the report may be delegated to you if the charge nurse is occupied with an admission of a new resident, an emergency, or if you have been in charge of the unit for the entire work time. Figure 13-10 summarizes the responsibilities of the first-line-manager.

The Second-line Manager: The Registered Nurse

Registered nurses in long-term care function in a variety of positions. In facilities of 200 or more residents, a registered nurse may be staff development co-ordinator, quality assurance nurse, infection control nurse, wing supervisor, or the assistant director of nursing. These nurses may not be in daily direct contact with the residents, or have direct responsibility for the daily management of the resident unit. Their responsbilities are more specialized and administrative than those of the second-line manager registered nurse.

The second-line manager is in the middle of the nursing management tree. The scope of practice will be discussed in more detail here as this postition may be held by a registered nurse or a Licensed Practical/Vocational Nurse.

Responsibility for a facility wing or floor belongs to the second-line manager nurse. There may be 15 to 60 or more residents per wing. The staff assigned to the area may include LP/VNs, nursing assistants, and Trained Medication Assistants (TMA). *Trained Medication Assistants* are persons trained in state approved programs to specifically administer medications

- Administration of Medications
  - Knowledge of current drug therapy for elderly
  - alert to side-effects of medications in elderly
- Administration of Medical Treatments
  - Knowledge of equipment for advanced technical care
- Nursing Assessment of Elderly
  - Physical, emotional, behavioral observations
- Documentation
  - Resident records, insurance and government forms
  - Assist with writing care plans, procedures, and nursing assistant performance appraisals
- Communication
  - Interactions with resident, family, nursing staff
  - Resident care conferences, networking committees
- Leadership Example for Nursing Assistants
  - Follow nursing procedures and facility policies
  - Demonstrate nursing assistant tasks

Figure 13-10 Responsibilities of the first-line manager nurse

in long term care facilities. Some states identify this position as Qualified Medication Assistant or by some other title.

Large units of 60 residents will have one or two nurses who are responsible to the second-line manager nurse. This often depends on the acuity of the residents. Several nursing assistants assigned to assist in resident care as well as a TMA will complete the unit staff.

In a small unit of 15 residents, the second-line nurse may be the only licensed nurse assigned to the area. The same tasks must be completed on this small wing as on one of 60 residents. There will be fewer staff members having a wider range of tasks to accomplish. The duties of this nurse in charge will be expanded because many of the tasks require the abilities of a licensed nurse. Nursing assistants cannot administer medications, perform treatments, assess residents' conditions, or manage the unit. The challenge to this nurse may be greater.

Team and resident care assignments are made by this nurse. The key in making assignments is to blend and match the team members' abilities and resident care tasks. The end result is to be an efficient, organized team and unit. It is essential that the second-line manager nurse be familiar with all tasks required for the wing to function.

Key ingredients to a smoothly functioning nursing team are: (1) knowing the strengths of each staff member, (2) rotating assignments periodically, and (3) assuring that the staff members have working knowledge of procedures implemented on the unit. The success of working relationships and quality resident care is in the resident assignments and division of tasks that need to be accomplished.

The second-line manager is often responsible for teaching facility policies and nursing procedures to the staff, figure 13–11. This assures continuity and safe delivery of care to the residents. Use of equipment will be demonstrated, and staff members may complete return demonstrations to assure safe operation of the equipment and safety for the resident.

Supervision of the staff is another responsibility of this nurse. Each staff member is

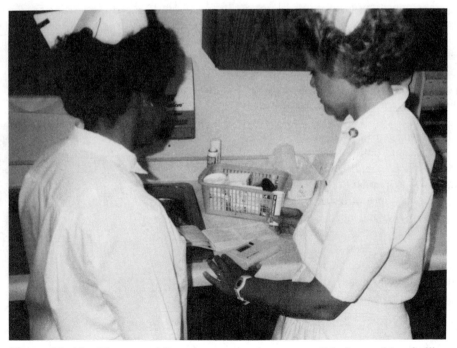

Figure 13–11   The second-line manager is often responsible for teaching facility policies and procedures.

observed and evaluated in the growth and development of work performance. Appraisals are completed as scheduled for some or all of the nursing staff. On a large wing this nurse may oversee those appraisals assigned to the first-line manager. Observations of work habits, use of procedures, and work relationships may be difficult to measure. The tasks will be made easier if the nurse makes a point to make daily observations, listen carefully to interactions, and identify clues to potential problems. Frequent documentation is again important.

When observing the performance of the staff, the second-line manager is also able to assess the resident. Since this nurse does not have the advantage of providing direct care, assessment must be based on observational skills and data from direct caregivers. Data collected in the assessment of the resident by the first-line manager will be utilized by this nurse in developing the resident's care plan. The second-line manager is part of the multidisciplinary team completing a functional assessment for the plan of care.

Documentation of a variety of data becomes a primary function of the second-line manager nurse. Medicare reimbursement forms, insurance company reports, and state payment systems require documentation and signatures of registered nurses. Most of the information required by these agencies is data documented in narrative notes and on flow sheets in the resident's record. When careful complete notes are documented on a regular basis, completing reports becomes a more efficient task for this nurse. The reports should not be left until the end of the workday. At that time they may be done in haste, omitting details that may lead to incomplete records. This could result in denial of reimbursement by a funding agency.

This nurse may accompany the attending physician during visits and examinations of the residents. These periodic visits inform the physician of the current health status of the resident. The nurse prepares the resident physically and emotionally for the visit and is present at the bedside during the examination. Residents may be confused and consequently uncooperative during the visit. The presence of the nurse will provide emotional comfort for the resident and assistance for the physician during the examination.

In some states *Gerontological Nurse Practitioners* may precede the physician visit. Gerontological Nurse Practitioners have received additional education and credentialing beyond their registered nurse licensure. Their scope of practice varies from state to state, and governing bodies are currently addressing changes in the law to clarify the practice of nurse practitioners. The nurse practitioner usually is employed by a clinic or a physician, and practices under the direction of a physician, figure 13–12.

Orders and progress notes written by the attending physician are interpreted by the second-line manager and incorporated into the care plan. Oral reports and written directions to other nurses are the usual methods of communication. If taped reports between work shifts are used, new orders are also included in this report. This nurse may also report these changes to the director of nursing in an oral report or written memo.

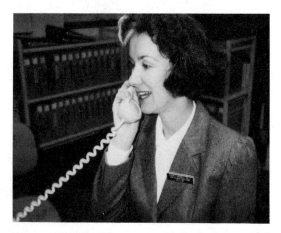

Figure 13–12 The gerontological nurse practitioner consults with a physician regarding a resident's treatments.

The second-line manager nurse may be a member of several networking committees within the facility. Often this nurse is a chairperson or leader of a group. Developing new procedures, and reviewing and revising existing procedures are important functions of networking committees.

Ongoing changes in local, state, and federal regulations usually involve the networking of several committees to assure compliance by the facility. Advancing technology changes the practice of medicine, nursing, and basic caregiving. Writing procedures and responding to new situations are part of the organized thinking of this nurse. Staff members from other disciplines look to nurses to help guide the way to change.

Residents in many skilled care facilties need specialized care which requires the attention of the second-line manager nurse. Specialized care includes feeding pumps, respirators, intravenous fluids, and catheters. This care has become commonplace outside of hospital walls. Nurses in long-term care have become comfortable working with a variety of machines and new methods of treatment. Resource persons from hospitals, medical equipment rentals, or other sources assist the long-term care staff to understand and operate the equipment. Through discharge planning, hospitals and long-term care facilities often work together to provide continuity of care for the resident. The second-line manager may be involved in teaching hospital staff during the exchange of information when they discuss approaches to geriatric nursing care.

The advances in technology and changes in the health care delivery system are addressed by the governing body of the facility. The policies established by this group clarify the limits and conditions of resident care that the staff will be prepared to implement. For example, to admit a resident requiring a respirator means assuring continual staffing of licensed nurses, policies and procedures for operating the respirator, and a community business to service the equipment. The facility's governing body evaluates if they can provide quality care to this potential resident. Nurses have direct input into this evaluation and the development of appropriate policies and procedures which must follow the guidelines and framework of established policy of the facility and standards of nursing practice. A chain of events follows with writing procedures, teaching staff, and implementing care.

The resident unit nursing staff communicates with the second-line manager primarily on an informal basis. Information concerning residents is exchanged verbally. As questions are asked, decisions are made on data collected and advice is offered. This nurse is expected to have the answers or be be knowledgeable of resources to find the answers.

The nurse in charge prepares the report for the oncoming nursing team and makes the decision regarding the type of delivery: oral, written, or taped. All facilities have a system or routine for reporting the activities of the workday to the oncoming staff. This overview of the tasks of the second-line manager nurse demonstrates that this nurse has tremendous communication responsibilities.

The Third-line Manager: The Director of Nursing

The director of nursing in a long term care facility is a registered nurse responsible for all aspects of nursing services. The management tree places this nurse directly responsible to the administrator. The following of all facility policies must be demonstrated in the directing of nursing services.

There is a wide variety of tasks and responsibilities for the director of nursing. Most of the responsbilities are managerial in nature. The scope of responsibility is usually reflected in (1) the number of residents in the facility, (2) the structure of the nursing service, and (3) the geographic location of the facility, and

(4) availability of qualified licensed staff. In small facilities in remote rural areas, the director of nursing may be one of only two or three licensed nurses on the entire staff. It is clear that this nurse will be responsible for resident care tasks as well as those of nursing service management. In large corporate facilities in metropolitan areas, this nurse will primarily oversee the operation of the nursing service. Some management tasks, such as scheduling or interviewing applicants, may be delegated to second-line manager nurses or the human resources department.

To assist you in understanding your interaction with the director of nursing, an overview of the role of this nurse will be discussed here. The director of nursing is viewed as a nursing consultant to the staff. Knowledge of nursing practice and agency policies are essential in assisting and guiding the staff in making decisions. This leadership is vital, demonstrates professionalism to the nursing staff, and is a role model for nurses in long-term care, figure 13–13.

A working knowledge of local, state, and federal regulations is not a usual nursing function. The director of nursing must acquire this knowledge as nearly every activity in a long term care facility is controlled, to some degree, by a regulatory agency. When nursing procedures are written or revised, the director reviews them to assure quality of nursing care and compliance with regulations. Your suggestions for a procedure change may seem ideal, but may not fit a current regulation.

Part of the regulatory process is the on-site visit by teams of reviewers from state and federal agencies. The director of nursing is accountable for verbal and written documentation during these visits. You may have a reviewer observe your medication administration as part of the evaluation process.

Medicare forms, insurance forms, and state reimbursement documents may be completed by the director of nursing. Portions of these documents may be delegated to you, but the

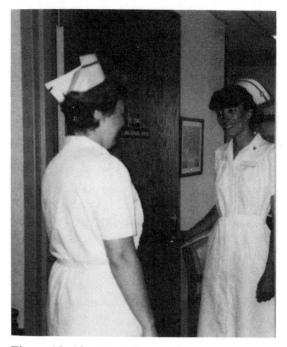

Figure 13–13 The director of nursing is the role model for nurses in long-term care.

director reviews the forms to maintain consistency and uniformity in documentation.

The director of nursing is a member of internal committees that function to keep the entire facility running smoothly. Health and safety concerns of the residents and the nursing staff, from a nursing perspective, are the director's primary responsibility in these committees. You may observe the need, and request lighting changes in resident or staff working areas. When channeled through the appropriate communication line, the director of nursing, requests will reach the committees.

Staff development to promote personal and professional growth is a responsibility of the director of nursing. In some facilities an in-service or staff development nurse is delegated to organize and implement specific programs or classes. Regulatory agencies often require annual updating of safety information and policies. The director of nursing is required to provide staff development through inservice education, and post other opportunities provided by schools, hospitals, or other resources. It is your responsibility to attend and be informed.

In most facilities the director of nursing interviews and employs staff for the nursing service department. The orientation process begins with this position. As a staff nurse you will be delegated a portion of the process that addresses first-line manager responsibilites. You are expected to be a role model representing nursing as practiced in the facility.

Accompanying the function of employing staff is the responsibility of disciplining, and terminating employment of members of the nursing staff. You are indirectly involved in this process. Your objective comments on performance appraisals may be included as data in the decision and action of the director of nursing.

In smaller facilities scheduling of staff is completed by the director of nursing. All schedules must be reviewed by this nurse as regulatory agencies require a specific number of nursing staff to comply with the number of residents and degree of skilled nursing care required. Requests for changes in working days should be in writing to the director or other person responsible for scheduling.

The director of nursing often serves on several advisory boards. They are usually programs preparing persons for employment in long term care facilities. Nursing programs, nursing assistant courses, and classes for assistants or technicans in dietary, activites, or physical and occupational therapies are examples. The director is a resource person addressing current practice in long-term care, who assists programs to meet desired competency levels. One of the members of the advisory committee of your school or program probably is a director of nursing from a long term care facility.

The director of nursing wears many hats. Families and residents with questions and problems often approach this nurse for assistance. The director is often a detective, advocate, diplomat, or minister as compliments and complaints often reach the office of the director of nursing.

Communications with the director of nursing are more formal in nature. An appointment should be made to allow time in the director's schedule to hear your concerns or requests. The appointment may be accomplished through a secretary, a telephone call, or a verbal request. The smaller the facility, the less formal the process. Requests for schedule changes, vacation time, or leave of absence should be in writing. It is wise for most interactions requiring the attention of the director of nursing to be requested in writing. Table 13–1 compares the levels of nursing management.

Summary

Leadership and management skills are people skills. Some natural ability to organize is essential to all nurses. Some natural ability to lead and manage is desirable to most nurses and especially those practicing in long term care facilities. Many nurses have learned their management skills by trial and error. This is a painful process. During your clinical experiences you have observed nurses successfully directing a nursing team and others struggling to manage similar tasks.

The first-line manager nurse is expected to be versatile and flexible. The responsibility may range from caregiver, to manager of a resident unit, to member of a networking committee. When seeking employment in a long term care facility, it will be important for you to have a basic understanding of the management tree and lines of authority in that facility. This information should be presented during your initial orientation. Policy manuals or handbooks should include the information and be available in the office of the director of nursing. In most facilities they are available on nursing stations.

Nurses at all levels of management are

involved in resident assessment, documentation, communication, and networking with family, visitors, staff, and other disciplines. Other responsibilities include assessing areas of safety, and evaluating the implementation of policies and

procedures. It will be your responsibility to learn what portion of each is delegated to you. Then it will be your responsibility to follow through to assure safe resident care and nursing practice.

TASK	FIRST-LINE MANAGER	SECOND-LINE MANAGER
Resident care	Implements	Supervises
Care plans	Input	Develops
Nursing procedures	Input	Develops
Performance appraisals	Completes for Nursing Assistant	Completes for LP/VN
Resident data	Collects documents, reports	Documents, assesses, plans
Medications for resident	Administers	Supervises, works with pharmacy
Medical treatments for resident	Administers, observes, reports	Supervises, revises Care Plans
Communication within nursing team	Informal	Informal or formal
Responsible to:	Second-line Manager	Third-line Manager

TABLE 13–1 Comparing First- and Second-line Nurse Manager Roles

For Discussion

- Request copies of facility and nursing management charts from facilities where you have clinical assignments. Compare the charts for similarities and differences in lines of authority.
- Visit with a nurse employed in a long term facility. Determine the type of caregivers and the acuity of residents on this nurse's unit.

Questions for Review

1. What is leadership? *guiding, influencing, a group or activity*
2. How is management defined in relation to nursing practice?
3. What is the difference between first-, second-, and third-line managers in long term care facilities?
4. What are three management tasks common to each management level?

1. assessment   4. safety   6 staff (network)
2. documentation 5 policies   family
3. communication

Unit 14
Using Nursing Skills in Nursing Management

Objectives

After reading this unit you should be able to:

- Identify skills to organize own time.
- Describe use of communication skills within the nursing team.
- Discuss time use in managing the care of a group of residents.
- Identify legal aspects in the role of the first-line manager.

You have had experience practicing basic concepts of leading and managing in caring for patients in other assignments. Recall that leadership means guiding, influencing, or inspiring a group or activity. Management is controlling, arranging, or directing the activity. When organizing patient care you followed the care plan to guide the patient to become more independent. You inspired the patient when teaching, coaching, and praising his ambulation efforts. The morning activity was arranged around scheduled activities of medications and treatments.

How have you managed the care of one or two patients assigned to you? What did you do first? Why was that activity your choice? Schedules and routines are parts of nursing management. If the morning vital signs are to be taken after the report is completed, your decision was easy. How did you decide when to assist the patient with his bath and walk in the hallway?

Perhaps an assignment looked overwhelming and you started at the top of your list of tasks copied from the kardex. Many inexperienced student nurses start with the bed bath and bedmaking. They perceive it as a lengthy task and feel they may not get it completed before lunch!

In preparing for the role of first-line manager in a long term care facility, the nurse must expand the organizational skills of patient care. Many long term care facilities expect the first-line manager nurse to direct the care of 30 residents and oversee the activities of at least three nursing assistant caregivers.

Organizing your time is a career skill; it does not happen overnight. If you had another career or other employment before your nursing education, you may have organizational skills to adapt to nursing practice. This unit will present skills for organizing time. The focus will be on adapting these skills to nursing practice in a long-term care setting. Communication skills will be reviewed with a discussion of adaptations to the nursing team. Legal aspects of the first-line manager nurse in long-term care will complete this unit.

Organizing Your Time

In any work or activity, organizing means taking the tasks to be accomplished and arranging them in an efficient manner. Organization leads to completing the activity "on time" or in a timely manner. The focus is on the product or end result of the activity. The process of completing the activity may involve an individual or group of people. If the work is well organized the person feels good about the results. This is probably because the person exercised control over the activity.

Organizing and control go hand in hand because there is planning. Planning does not add to the work time; it helps get more work done in less time. Again, recall your clinical assignment of one or two patients. You felt good when you thought through the patients' morning care and gathered all the linens and supplies before you started. Perhaps another time, when events did not unfold as you had hoped, you felt the situation was "out of control." Planning ahead helps keep the progression of activities in balance. Planning means setting goals of excellence, not perfection, and feeling good about a job well done, figure 14-1.

Establishing Goals

You are acquainted with goals as part of the patient's care plan. In utilizing the nursing process the patient's problems are identified and then goals or outcomes are established. Nursing interventions are identified to assist in achieving the goals.

Goals are results expected after a given period of time. Specific interventions or tasks are identified and planned to assist in meeting the goal. Goals may be short term or long term. Short-term goals in long-term care are usually those that can be accomplished in a day, a week, or a month. Long-term goals may take several weeks or months to accomplish. Sometimes goals and objectives are used interchangeably. Other times objectives are short-term activities designed to meet a long-term goal.

When setting goals to organize your time you should follow the same guidelines as resident care plan goals. First, goals should be realistic; they can be achieved with good organization. For example, if you are reassigned or "floated" to another unit, can you expect to administer medications to this group of residents as efficiently as on the unit where you are usually assigned? The answer is probably No! Your goals for the new assignment would include

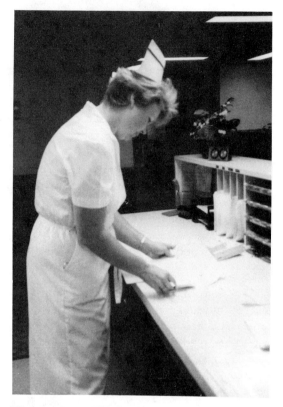

Figure 14–1   The first-line manager nurse plans ahead in organizing own time.

top priority items, such as medications and treatments. The goals would probably exclude tasks which are not "musts" for the day.

Second, goals should be acceptable to you. Are they satisfactory and worthwhile? Sometimes goals that are merely adequate have to be OK. If goals are not comfortable or acceptable, look again to see if they are realistic.

Goals need to be simple. That means they need to be clear and concise. If a goal seems to be too confusing and too complex, it probably needs to be restated.

Goals must be measurable. There must be a means of determining that the goal is met. Note that at the beginning of each unit in this book there are stated measurable objectives.

Objective statements and goal statements include action verbs:

> **Goal Statement:**
>> All nursing assistants will *demonstrate* the aseptic handwashing procedure by October 1.
>
> **Objective Statements:**
>> *Review* handwashing procedure with all nursing assistants.
>>
>> *Demonstrate* the handwashing procedure to all nursing assistants.
>>
>> *Observe* all nursing assistants complete the handwashing procedure.

Goals should motivate you! If they meet the criteria above, and have objectives identified to achieve the goal, you should be on your way! If you are thinking about when you should start, something is not right. The goal needs to be reevaluated. Samples of goals are shown in table 14–1.

Setting Priorities

Experts in time management present methods of setting priorities for tasks to determine what should be done first. Many factors are involved in prioritizing, including numbers of tasks, urgency, length of time to complete a task, and internal and external policies of the workplace.

Prioritizing is placing events or tasks in order of immediacy and importance along a time line. Taking the time to think this through saves time on tasks by being better prepared and completing tasks in the right sequence.

The "To Do" list is the recommended method of identifying tasks to be completed. If this exercise is not carried out, more time is spent on rethinking which tasks are done, which ones are left to do, and were any forgotten. A written list helps put tasks in order of importance.

Items on the "To Do" list can be ranked with an A, B, or C, depending on their importance. As are the most important and must be done. Bs are done when you have completed the As or have time because you have planned well! Cs should be reconsidered for their value. Do they really need to be on the list, or can they be delegated to someone? Perhaps a C will become

UNCLEAR GOAL	CLEAR GOAL
RESIDENT Will accept long-term care placement Will understand importance of diet	RESIDENT Will verbalize interest in facility activities Will state two positive results of low salt diet
NURSING ASSISTANT Will know correct handwashing procedure Will know fire safety procedure	NURSING ASSISTANT Will demonstrate aseptic handwashing technique Will list procedure steps in fire safety plan
FIRST-LINE MANAGER Will know facility medication policy Will understand responsibilities of managing a unit Will recognize importance of good communication	FIRST-LINE MANAGER Will demonstrate facility procedure to document narcotic administration Will list six major tasks of first-line manager Will demonstrate use of effective communication skills

TABLE 14–1   Sample Goal Statements

a B or an A on tomorrow's list. Do not discard it; there was a reason to put it on your list today.

Consider these three tasks: (1) an a.c. blood glucose check, (2) a gastrostomy tube dressing change, and (3) supplemental nourishments for four residents. All three should be done now! The blood glucose check is an "A" because the blood sugar needs to be evaluated before the meal. The dressing change is a "B" because it is not as urgent and can be fit in at a more convenient time. At this time, supplemental nourishments will become a "C," and delegated to a nursing assistant.

The ABC ranking can be used to organize a daily schedule, or for a week or month in long-range planning. When beginning a new job you may write a more detailed list to include all routine activities. As you gain more experience, and become accustomed to the routine of the facility and resident unit, you may write only the top-ranking tasks as priorities change.

Maslow's Hierarchy is a useful tool to use when setting priorities. You have used this guideline when planning care. A person's physiological needs must be met before other needs can be addressed. When setting priorities for the best use of your time, those which are life-threatening or urgent are always Priority #1.

Factors That Influence Priorities.

Schedules, Policies, and Procedures. In any workplace, there are established schedules that provide parameters. These are as simple as the scheduling of lunch and break times. In health care facilities there are routine times of medication administrations; treatments and therapies also have specific times scheduled. Knowing these established times assists in planning resident care and team work, figure 14–2.

Rules, regulations, and policies will influ-

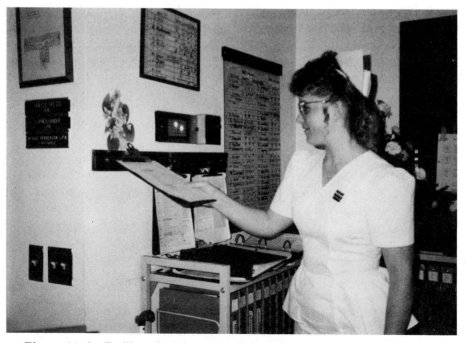

Figure 14–2 Facility schedules and policies influence organizing your time.

ence planning. External influences are those regulations established by agencies of the state or federal government. Internal policies are developed by the long term care facility. For example, a state health department regulation may state meal trays are to be served within five minutes of arriving on the unit. A facility rule may state that residents are to be dressed in street clothes when eating in the dining room.

Time to Complete Tasks.   Most nurses have not timed themselves on specific tasks. It is when new responsibilities are added, the "out of control" alarm rings, or when other motivational activity occurs that nurses take a look at time-on-task.

In your nursing education, steps identified in nursing procedures were prioritized for efficiency as well as for the safety and comfort of the patient. Recall one of your first labs. Bedmaking! The clean linen was placed in order; the first piece to be placed on the bed, the mattress pad, was on the top. You did not waste time sorting through the linen looking for the correct item. You were also instructed to complete the bedmaking on one side before finishing the second side. You saved time-on-task by eliminating unnecessary trips from one side of the bed to the other side.

The length of time to complete a task will vary among individuals as well as between the new graduate and the experienced nurse. The approximate time-on-task, as well as the questionable safety of leaving a resident during a procedure, assists in combining tasks. Measuring temperature, pulse, and respiration does not take more than a few minutes and could be interrupted. However, catheterizing a resident takes more time, cannot be interrupted, and the resident should not be left unattended.

Most people underestimate the amount of time it takes to complete an activity or project. They measure by "ideal time" and do not consider interruptions and other factors. Remember that "on-the job" is not the same as "in-the-laboratory."

Health Status of Resident.   The acuity of the physical and mental status of the resident influences priorities by changing the frequency and duration of tasks. The vital signs of a stable resident may be taken weekly. The resident experiencing a fall in his bathroom will have his vital signs, including perhaps a neurological check, assessed every four hours. Weekly vital signs can be a "B" priority and taken at a convenient time during the day for the nurse and resident. The every-four-hours vital signs are a top priority "A" and need to be done on time.

Between-meal nourishments are often a "B" priority, or a task delegated to a nursing assistant. However, if the resident is demonstrating signs of dehydration, the nourishment becomes an "A" priority with this individual because you will need to make hydration and nutrition assessments when you are encouraging fluids.

Resident Preferences.   Throughout your nursing education, part of the preparation of the care plan has been to include the patient in organizing his care. This is important in long term care facilities because it is the resident's home and he has already lost a degree of independence and decision making; you want to maintain some independent living.

Many resident requests relate to their lifelong lifestyle. Perhaps they were early risers, or maybe they preferred to "sleep in." Imagine the adjustment to long-term care of a resident who worked the night shift his entire working life!

How and when a person has taken medications for a chronic disorder influences planning. Persons with emphysema often have a time and routine for taking their bronchodilators. They feel better and are less anxious if this schedule is followed.

Not every resident preference can be met, considering the 30 residents, 4 caregivers, and the length of the workday. When organizing your time and prioritizing lists, there will be more time to meet these requests. It will also become clear which requests can and should be met. Figure 14–3 illustrates prioritizing the task of administering medications to four residents.

First-line Manager Experiences and Values. During your nursing education you may have felt that there was only "one way" to do a skill or complete a procedure; your instructor's way! Your education has been designed to meet nursing standards of practice. With experience, nurses learn how to be flexible within a scope of practice. When to use clean or sterile technique is an example.

An individual's personal values and life experiences play a role in prioritizing tasks. Values and experiences reflect on the degree of importance and the length of time devoted to a task. A nurse whose grandfather died of complications of diabetes may feel the need to spend extra time with diabetic foot care. Perhaps another nurse's mother died of cancer. This nurse may devote more time to assisting a resident and family members through the grief process.

Within the framework of organizing the best use of time, there will be variables with each nurse. You will have to work with a plan and determine what works best for you.

Delegating Tasks. **Delegating** is the act of appointing or assigning a specific task or project to an individual or group. Student nurses have delegated part of the care or treatment to the patient, but usually have not had the experience of delegating to other caregivers. The objective of delegating part of the patient care is to promote patient independence and unit effi-

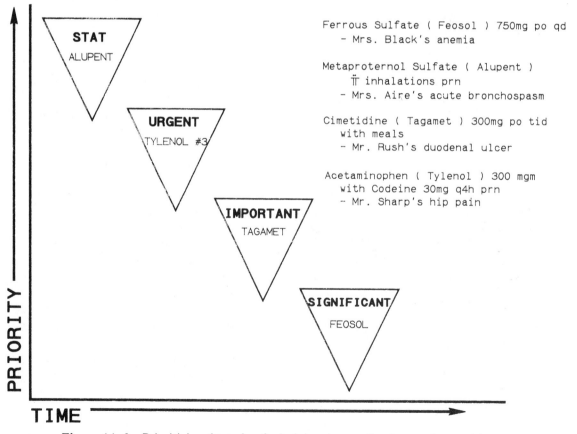

Figure 14–3 Prioritizing the tasks of administering medications to four residents.

ciency, not to help the nurses get their work completed.

An important part of organizing your time is deciding what to delegate to others. It is an unrealistic goal for the first-line manager nurse to be able to meet all the needs of a group of residents. What tasks can be delegated depend on the job description of the caregiver and the health status of the resident. A nurse cannot delegate the task of administering a resident's PRN pain medication to a nursing assistant. If it is the policy of a long term care facility for nursing assistants to take vital signs, that task could be delegated. However, if a resident's condition is unstable, it is not advisable to delegate this task to a nursing assistant because additional assessments other than the vital sign measurements need to be evaluated. Figure 14–4 summarizes skills to assist in organizing your time. It is important to remember when delegating a task, especially to an unlicensed caregiver, that the nurse is still accountable for the task.

Your Organization in Action

The Nursing Process as a Framework

Organizing your work and workday is more comfortable when you use a method or model that is familiar. The Nursing Process has been a convenient tool for nurses to plan and problem solve care. It is also a good tool to use in making the best use of your time.

Assessing Use of Time

Assessment, the first step in the Nursing Process, includes data collection and analyzing the data to determine a nursing diagnosis. In organizing your time, the data collection is your "To Do" list. Analyzing data becomes prioritizing your tasks and the nursing diagnosis becomes goal setting. Delegating tasks fits into analyzing and prioritizing the "To Do" list. This decision becomes a part of the goal setting process.

ORGANIZING YOUR TIME

- Establish Goals
  - Realistic
  - Acceptable
  - Simple, clear, and concise
  - Measurable
  - Motivational
- Set Priorities
  - Develop "To Do" lists
  - Rank in order of importance: A, B, C,
  - Factors influencing priorities: schedules, policies, procedures time to complete task health status of resident resident preferences first-line manager experiences and values
  - Short-term goals: accomplished in a day or week
  - Long-term goals: accomplished in weeks or months
- Delegate Tasks
  - Determine according to scope of nursing practice
  - Determine according to job descriptions
  - Determine according to resident health status
  - Nurse is responsible for tasks delegated

Figure 14–4 Nursing skills to assist in organizing your time.

Planning Use of Time

The planning step of the Nursing Process identifies the actions and time frame to meet the goals set in the assessment step. To make the best use of time in the workday, the first-line manager needs to have a basic plan for the activities of the day. This is not carved in stone! Priorities may change one hour into the workday, but a basic plan assists in rearranging tasks if events indicate the necessity.

Planning Ahead.   Perhaps you have heard the planning slogan, "Plan Ahead: It wasn't raining when Noah built the ark." It is helpful to make general mental or written notes before the workday begins.

Notes can be made at the close of the day summarizing the day's activities and projecting for the next day. You can leave work knowing where the starting point will be the next day. Some people prefer to make mental or written notes enroute to work on the bus, in the car, or walking.

Planning ahead is not intended to be an extensive mental or time-consuming activity. It should assist you to leave work responsibilities at work and permit leisure activities to leave you refreshed for the next workday. Planning ahead should prevent your arrival at the workplace with the thought, "Where should I start?"

Blocking Out Time.   Planning your tasks within time frames of two or three hours sets mini-goals for timed tasks and helps keep you on task. It will also aid you in problem-solving time management problems. These blocks of time could also be arranged according to your unit routine: report until break, break until lunch, lunch until 2 p.m. medication administration, and wrap-up of activities before report.

Organizing the Tools.   Organizing the equipment you will need to complete the day's activities is a time-saver must. The first tools are those required of nursing students: watch, bandage scissors, and pens that work! A small notepad to fit in your pocket is also a good idea. Instead of saying, "I must remember to . . . ," you can make a written note and make the best use of your time.

Many first-line manager nurses are assessing residents at the time of medication administration. A medication cart is often used with, or without, a unit dose system. These carts should include a stethoscope, blood pressure cuff, thermometers, flashlight, tape, and other "tools" to save time and steps. When nurses become acquainted with the needs of the resi-

dents there is not as much "guesswork" to determine supplies. Remember the courtesy of replacing depleted supplies for the oncoming staff. It helps them make the best use of their time.

Gathering the tools for procedures is equally important. You have experienced this in your nursing education. It takes only a few minutes to think through the procedure and gather the necessary supplies, figure 14–5. Recall completing a sterile dressing change when everything went like "clock work"! It was done correctly, and you were efficient and "in control." Planning pays off!

Determining Energy Levels.   Are you a morning person? A night person? Are you the first one on task with a project? Thinking about your own energy levels may help you to determine if you would like to work during the day, evening, or night. It will also help you in planning your work time. Some persons have a high energy level during the beginning of the work time. Others peak toward the end of the workday when most tasks are completed and there is time to concentrate.

There are times in the workday that are not scheduled for medication administration, treatments, or other routine activities. You may need to complete some monthly documentation, spend some time getting acquainted with a new resident, or review a procedure on new equipment. You will have to determine the energy level expected by these intermittent tasks. Combine the tasks with your energy levels during the day, and plan accordingly.

Implementing Your Plan of Organized Time

A first-line manager in long-term care needs to fine-tune the skills of data collection for resident care. Prioritizing the "To Do" list for organizing time will enable the nurse to oversee the care of the 30 residents. To fine-tune the efficiency of the workday involves putting your plan into action and continually evaluating and revising. You may implement methods of expe-

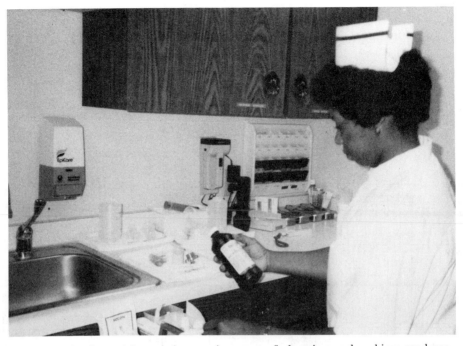

Figure 14–5   Organizing equipment is a part of planning and making good use of time.

rienced nurses, but what works for another nurse may not work for you.

Work Sheets.   Using work sheets, or developing your own, is helpful when following your plan. Recall the one or two patients assigned during your clinical experience. Work sheets to note patient information were provided by your instructor or the clinical facility. As a first-line manager nurse you will not have work sheets for 30 residents!

When you are new to a position you will be taking more written notes during report. These will be by room number and will include information about residents requiring special treatments or additional assessments. Information about stable residents can be obtained from the kardex or medical record. In long-term care, as the nurse becomes acquainted with the residents, notes are taken on change of status, new orders, and new admissions. In addition to sequential notes by room number, work sheets by time or task may be helpful, figure 14–6.

Expect Interruptions.   You can expect interruptions when implementing your time plan. Many of the interruptions in your time are anticipated events; you just do not know when they will occur! Residents' families telephone with questions; a resident becomes acutely ill and needs additional time with care; or a resident needs to be transferred to a hospital. Another time a nursing assistant may experience an injury and an incident report must be completed.

There will be times when you will feel you have encountered more interruptions than scheduled activities. It may be difficult to get back on track. However, if your time is organized, you can return to your plan and continue or revise as necessary.

Evaluating Your Work Time

You have experienced evaluating the efficiency as well as the quality of your nursing care. In caring for your assigned patients, you

SAMARITAN BETHANY HOME
BRAIN BOARD

ADMISSIONS	DIABETIC/URINE/BLOOD CHECKS				NEW ORDERS & CHANGES
	NAME	7	11	4	HS
DISCHARGE & DEATHS					
RESIDENTS OUT	ELEVATED TEMPS				
HOSPITAL PATIENTS					
CLINIC APPOINTMENTS	WEIGHTS				
BLOODWORK & X-RAY PREP	BLOOD PRESSURE				CARE CONFERENCES

N13 R0590

Figure 14–6   Sample work sheet for organizing time (Courtesy of Samaritan Bethany, Inc., Rochester, MN)

measured your time use and quality of care against procedures practiced in the learning laboratory in school. During performance appraisals scheduled with your instructor, accuracy and efficiency were discussed.

As a first-line manager nurse you will need to evaluate the efficiency and quality of your work. You will also need to evaluate the resident care on the unit for which you are responsible.

First, were you ready for report at the end of the workday? Did you meet all your goals for the day? If you were efficient, did you feel good about the quality of your work? Take time to pat yourself on the back for a workday that went well and made you feel good!

Not every day is going to run smoothly. Health care is not a business of robots programmed to work with nuts and bolts. The caregivers and those receiving care are people who are continually changing. You will need to be flexible to meet the frequent changes. Organizing your time will provide you a plan which allows changes.

If smooth running days are not occurring in your workdays, it is time to find out why. You will need to review your "To Do" list, prioritizing, delegating, and goal setting. One way to evaluate your use of time is to keep a log of your actual activities. It takes only a few seconds every 15 to 30 minutes to note your activities for that time period. Be honest with yourself. At the end of the workday, or several days of keeping a log, analyze your activities. You may begin to see a pattern of inefficient use of time during particular activities or times of the day. Figure 14–7 is a sample tool for logging your time.

After reviewing your goals, look at your interruptions. Are they time-wasters? Putting things off, and expanding the time with interruptions, may be two time-wasters you are facing. Socializing with co-workers after report and not being able to say "NO!" to residents and staff when you are busy are other potential interruptions.

Organize your time to help avoid setting aside the more undesirable tasks; you have outlined a method to tackle them. Keep interruptions, such as telephone calls, to the point, especially on busy days. It is important to have a therapeutic rapport with residents and their families. However, a busy day is not the time to inquire about a daughter's rose garden! Figure 14–8 summarizes the use of the Nursing Process in organizing your time.

Communications in Organizing Your Time

Pleasant, accurate verbal and written communications are the framework for positive interactions in any situation. They are the foundation to well-organized team work and safe resident care.

Verbal Communication

In other courses in nursing education you have learned the value of therapeutic communications in planning and implementing patient care. Many models are based on Carl Roger's client-centered therapy. As a psychotherapist, he was reflective and non-directive in his approach to clients. His belief of unconditional positive regard and empathetic understanding of clients is a basic principle of nursing care.

It is important for the nurse to continue to use this approach with residents and other caregivers in the role of the first-line manager. A sample of effective communication techniques, with examples adapted to interactions with a nursing assistant, is shown in figure 14–9.

Remember that part of this verbal communication is the message cues given by the tone of voice. The pitch of your voice, the placement of pauses, or the intensity of specific words influences your message. The person with a habit of ending a comment or question with a nervous giggle sends a confusing message. A blind resident may interpret this as an affront.

TIME MANAGEMENT LOG

TIME	ACTIVITY	REVIEW COMMENTS
7 - 7:30	Received report from noc shift. Made assignments for NA	
7:30 - 8	NA. Showed me & brought pictures to group - took 15" Made rounds on unit	Should have postponed til coffee break
8 - 8:30	Breakfast tray up. Cleaned up spill on carpet	Should have called housekeeping
8:30 - 9	Evaluated chest pain Mr. Adams. Finished picking up tray. Started treatments	Needed to be a priority. — delegate to NA
9 - 9:30	↓ Took 2 phone calls from resident families.	Could have returned calls after treatments were finished
9:30 -10	Rechecked Mr Adams. Coffee break 9:30 to 9:45 finished morning treatments	
10-10:30	Documented treatments. Documented episode of chest	Should have done earlier while info fresh.
10:30-11	pain on Mr Adams. Made rounds on unit. Took phone call from pharmacy	
11-11:30	Postponed performance appraisal of NA. Mr Adams c/o chest pain again. Evaluated, Documented, Called Dr.	Resident needed to be the priority
11:30-12	Lunch break	
12-12:30	Lunch tray up - assisted c̄ distribution and feeding	Could have been delegated to NA.
12:30 -1	Dr to see Mr Adams - transcribed new orders for new meds	
1 - 1:30	Began afternoon treatments ↓	
1:30 - 2	Performance appraisal for NA. done but interrupted x2 by phone calls	Should have asked that message be taken
2 - 2:30	Made rounds with ANP - Did not get all orders transcribed	Should have been a priority.
2:30 - 3	Completed documentation for afternoon	Should have been done earlier while info was fresh -
3 - 3:30	Reported off to eve. shift - 5' late for report.	Report needs to be on time for on coming shift.

Figure 14-7   Sample tool for problem-solving use of time

ASSESSMENT

Patient Care	*Use of Time*
Data collection	"To Do" list
Analyzing data	Prioritizing, delegating
Nursing diagnosis	Goal setting

PLANNING

Nursing Interventions	Nursing Action
To address patient problems, meet goals	Plan ahead
	Organize tools
	Determine energy levels

IMPLEMENTATION

Follow nursing orders, complete medical treatments	Put plan for unit workday into action:
	Use work sheets
	Expect interruptions

EVALUATION

Evaluate results of nursing intervention	Evaluate efficiency and quality of own work
Were goals met/progress towards goals achieved?	Problem-solve: time-wasters
Return to data collection	Pat-on-back for job well done
	Revise "To Do" list

Figure 14–8   Using the nursing process to organize time

Think about answering a patient's call light, "Is there something I can do for you?" Repeat the question using different voice cues. What message are you sending with each cue? As a first-line manager nurse you will also be sending voice cues to nursing assistants and other caregivers.

To make the best use of your time, the use of clear, concise verbal communication is a must. In addition to communicating one-to-one with residents, nursing assistants, and other staff members, you may be speaking in small groups of people. Examples are resident care conferences and networking committees within the long term care facility.

Communication Within Small Groups. When nurses are responsible for planning a resident care conference, they first must identify who needs to be included in the group. Those who may be involved could be the resident, family members, social worker, dietitian, physical therapist, nurse practitioner, and family physician. The nurse should use the skills of organizing time when preparing topics to be

BEGINNING THE CONVERSATION

Objective: To encourage comfortable verbal interactions

- Broad Opening Statements — provides receiver with an opening to share ideas or feelings.
  "Your new uniform looks very nice on you."
  "You seem more quiet today."

- Rephrasing Statements — encourages receiver to continue with thoughts.
  "You said you have a headache?"

- General Leads — encourages receiver to expand thoughts.
  "Tell me more." "Oh?"

PROMOTING THE CONVERSATION

Objective: To encourage continued sharing of thoughts

- Acknowledge Thoughts — provides receiver with assurance that his views have value
  "It must be difficult to work around the P.T. schedule."

- Silence — time for sender and receiver to collect thoughts

- Shared Observations — encourages receiver to continue sharing ideas and observations.
  "The new ADL schedule is working well."

- Selecting Rephrasing — key words or phrases encourage the receiver to continue with a specific thought.
  "Never?" "Always?" "Not fair?"

- Provide Information — presents facts, avoids rumors
  "The new policy states all residents must be dressed in street clothes to eat in the dining room."

CLARIFYING THE CONVERSATION

Objective: To assure that information exchange has the same meaning to sender and receiver.

- Clarify — assures clear understanding, unmistakable
  "Please repeat that for me."

- Validate — Confirms the message was understood
  "All the temperatures you took were under 98.6?"

- Verbalize Implied Messages — verify hints, indirect comments
  "You feel I'm not being fair with my requests?"

- Promote Feedback — encourages ongoing intermittent responses to identified ideas, thoughts, feelings
  "Let me know by next week how you feel about the new disposable washcloths."

Figure 14–9 Effective communication techniques

addressed. Speaking slowly, using skills of effective communication, will assist in completing the conference with minimal gastrointestinal "butterflies" for the new nurse! Standing in the group, regardless of the arrangement of people, is more formal. However, this may be necessary at times to maintain control or direction of the group; it also helps to avoid interruptions.

Telephone Communications. The first-line manager nurse in long-term care has many tasks that include telephone communications. You will be providing resident information to the physician more often by telephone than at the resident's bedside. In long-term care, telephone communications will be more frequent with persons such as the pharmacist, attending or consulting physician, and the resident's family, figure 14–10. There will also be interdepartmental telephone communications with food service, housekeeping, maintenance, and other services.

Telephone etiquette is important in representing yourself, your profession, and your employer. This courtesy benefits organizing time by guiding the conversation to the reason for the telephone call in an efficient pleasant manner.

As a first-line manager nurse you will need to know the facility's telephone policy for your position. First, what is the preferred message when answering? "Highrise Manor, Mary Jones, third-floor charge nurse speaking," is an example. You will also need to know what resident information can be given to the family. You may tell Mrs. Witzel how her mother tolerated dinner last evening, but can you tell her the results of the blood work drawn yesterday morning? What types of questions need to be transferred to administration? The second- and third-line managers will provide guidelines for you to screen telephone calls.

When communicating by telephone, make the best use of your time by determining the reason for the call if it was not stated. Keep information and questions directed specifically

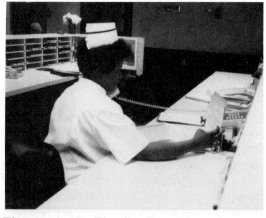

Figure 14–10   The first-line mananger nurse consults with physicians and others via the telephone.

to that concern. Use techniques of effective communication to validate the objective of the conversation. Before the call is concluded clarify if a follow-up call is needed.

Nonverbal Communication

The nonverbal messages people send are often called "body language." Facial expressions, and body posture and movement, send out positive, negative, or neutral messages. These may enhance verbal statements or send conflicting messages. Nonverbal messages make a greater impact and are remembered longer than verbal communication. No doubt you have heard "actions speak louder than words."

The interpretation of nonverbal messages has many variables including: individual perception, geographical location, culture, primary language, and age. If you have lived in other communities or a different geographical region you may have noted some of these differences.

As a first-line manager nurse your body language will be interpreted by the 30 residents on the unit, their families, the nursing assistants, the second-line manager and other staff in the facility. You want to be certain that the messages received are those you intend to send personally and professionally. You will also be reading the nonverbal messages of those with whom you come in contact, figure 14–11. Use effective communication techniques to clarify and validate verbal and nonverbal messages.

Written Communication

Written communication must also be clear and concise. In your nursing education, written communication related to patient care has been primarily charting. Written communication also includes interdepartmental requisitions, order forms, anecdotal notes for second-line managers and oncoming staff, performance appraisals, and other documentation. The health care delivery system continues to review more frequently the nurses' documentation. Nurses are becoming more aware of the legal accountability of documentation.

In writing memos for care conferences or other communications, one guideline to follow is the journalistic "who, what, why, where, and when." The use of medical terminology in memos and other written communication will depend on the background of persons who are to read the information. Determine if there is a form to be used and, if not, what format is recommended. Nurses are accustomed to dating chart entries and should continue this practice and date all written communication. Remember, when in doubt, document in writing.

The neatness of the writing as well as the use of correct grammar and spelling will reflect on the credibility of the nurse. The dependability of the first-line manager is directly related to communication skills. Second- and third-line managers generally rely on those who relate well with others. Figure 14–12 is an example of a clear and concise interdepartmental memo.

Blocks to Communication

Blocks to effective communication may be intentional or unintentional. Sometimes people do not want to deal with the content of a conversation. A verbal approach is to change the subject. A nonverbal approach is to walk away.

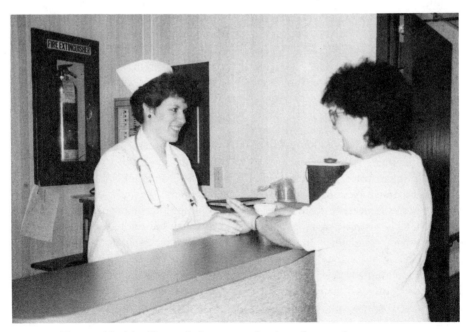

Figure 14–11 Nonverbal communication also sends messages

NURSING MEMO

TO: _Bill Smith, Maintenance_

FROM: _Sue Jones, LPN — 2 North_

DATE: _March 4_

SUBJECT: _Malfunctioning electric bed N205A_

The head of the bed in N205A will not raise when the electric control is used. All other functions seem to be working properly. The resident is usually out of bed between 9am and 1pm. It would be helpful if it could be repaired during these hours.

Figure 14-12   Interdepartmental communication must be clear and concise.

During patient care you may have observed a patient turn his head or look out a window when the conversation became uncomfortable. Voice cues and body language can block effective communication.

As an inexperienced student nurse you may have blocked therapeutic communication to the patient because you did not feel secure in your role. Perhaps you were apprehensive about not having the right answers. After gaining some experience, you may feel more comfort-able in answering questions and giving information about basic care. Experience assists in preventing blocks to communication, but everyone stumbles occasionally. It is important for the first-line manager nurse to be able to identify blocks to communication to avoid problems in the organization and flow of team work.

Examples of Communication Blocks. How a question is framed can block communication. Leading questions tend to direct the answer. "You know the routine here, do you mind taking an extra assignment?" Questions that begin with "Why" are uncomfortable to most people. "Why don't you want to be assigned to Resident Group A?" Requesting explanations often follows, which also may be uncomfortable. Interrupting answers with another question blocks communication. This, unfortunately, is a bad habit busy nurses can develop.

Responding with stereotyped comments or reassuring cliches are other easy bad habits to develop. "You'll do just fine," or "TELL me about it!", or "There's nothing I can do about it," or, "That's the way we've always done it here," would not allow the resident or nursing assistant to express their feelings or concerns.

Agreeing or disagreeing and approving or not approving may jeopardize effective communication. Agreement focuses on ideas or judgement and approval focuses on an action. Quick agreement and approval makes it difficult for either party to change an idea or decision. Disagreement or disapproval without rationale may lead to withdrawal or anger. Mrs. Sanchez tells the nurse that her family never visits her. The nurse responds, "Oh no, I'm sure they come whenever they can." Will Mrs. Sanchez express those feelings again? Probably not.

Giving advice interrupts the person's problem-solving process. This is not the same as providing information. Many times people verbalize a situation and may or may not be seeking advice. The first-line manager may provide information that could assist in decision making. Answering a question with another question directs the person to review their thoughts. "Have you thought about this before?" "What do you think you should do?"

Rumors can be a block to communication by reducing verbal communication or increasing ineffective nonproductive communication. **Rumors** are gossip or hearsay with no confirmed information. In any workplace, they are time-wasters. They reduce productivity as some people are using time to circulate the rumor, and others are using time to dispel the rumor and provide facts.

In long-term care, the first-line manager will be confronted frequently with rumors. This nurse practices in close proximity to residents, nursing assistants, and service staff. The facility is the resident's home. They are concerned with all activities, and there is opportunity for conflicting information. There are many unlicensed staff members who do not fully understand the nature of confidentiality in health care settings.

To dispel rumors, the first-line manager needs to be an active listener. Accurate information which will clarify any misunderstandings must be provided promptly. If the information is of a confidential nature it should be stated, "The information you have is incorrect. I cannot comment any further as the situation involves resident confidentiality." Detailed explanations are not necessary to dispel rumors.

Communicating effectively in the workplace is not easy. This is especially true in health care where the process and the product involves people. The first-line manager cannot expect to be a perfect communicator. However, being aware of some of the many influences in communication can assist in continual improvement and effectiveness.

Organizing Time in Managing the Resident Unit

The challenge for the new graduate and new first-line manager is to transfer the skills of organizing the care of a few patients to managing the care of approximately 30 residents in a long term care facility. The role commands the ability to have many activities or tasks in process at the same time. It is like a juggler who manages to keep many balls in the air at the same time. He must practice to know how high to toss them, how far apart to keep them, and how to be ready to catch them at the right place and time. It's all in the timing! Like the juggler, the nurse at the end of the workday wants all the activites in control, figure 14–13.

An example of organizing your time in the implementation of the care of two patients is shown in table 14–2. In this situation, Mr. O'Brien, 48, is hospitalized for a herniated lumbar disc. He is on bedrest with bathroom privileges and goes to physical therapy twice a day.

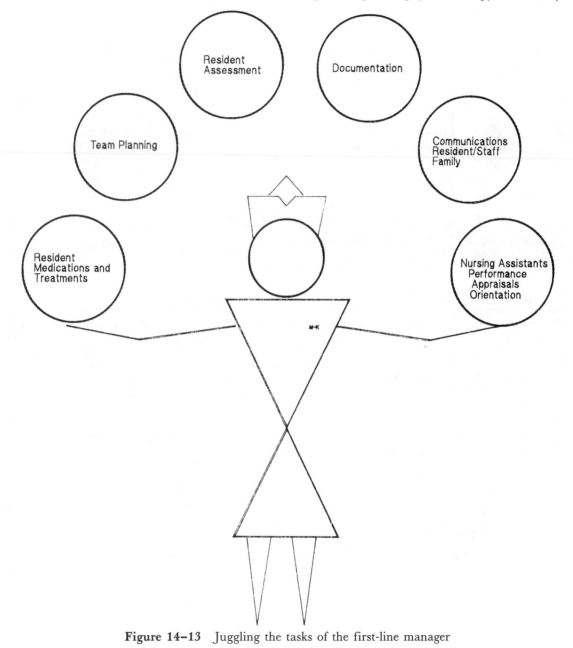

Figure 14–13 Juggling the tasks of the first-line manager

Miss Bookletter is a first-day-post operative cholecystectomy. She is NPO until bowel sounds are present, and has an IV, foley catheter, and abdominal dressing. She is to ambulate in the hall four times a day.

Compare the implementation of care of the two acute care patients with organizing time in a 30 resident unit, table 14–3. It illustrates a two and a half hour block of time in the schedule of the first-line manager nurse, including

TIME	MR. O'BRIEN	MISS BOOKLETTER
7 a.m.–7:30	team report check kardex	team report check kardex
7:30–8 a.m.	check: V.S., circulation; set-up meal tray	check: V.S., IV rate, abdominal dressing, indwelling catheter Post-Op Day 1 assessments; walk in hallway
8 a.m.–8:30	review chart assist with oral care, set up bath	rest
8:30–9 a.m.	assist bath: wash back, legs, backrub	check status (sleeping)
9 a.m.–9:30	rest (nurse break)	(break 15 min.) review chart
9:30–10 a.m.	check patient status (resting) 10 a.m. meds	deep breathing exercises; set up oral care, bed bath
10 a.m.–10:30	to Physical Therapy make bed, room order	assist with bath: back, legs, backrub; IM analgesic, rest
10:30–11 a.m.	chart returned from Physical Therapy, check extremity circulation	check patient status (resting) deep breathing exercises, assist to chair, make bed
11 a.m.–11:30	check status (resting)	walk in hallway back to bed; check: V.S., IV, dressing, catheter; update I&O
11:30–12:00	V.S., check circulation update I&O update charting check patient status report to primary nurse	chart check patient status report to primary nurse

TABLE 14–2 Organizing Time to Implement Morning Care

TIME	SELF	N.A.	RESIDENTS	OTHERS
7 a.m.	Receive report Plan assignments	Give resident assignments	Six unstable: evaluate status	Call kitchen: diet changes
7:30	Document: unstable resident condition	Serve/feed breakfast Observe resident response		Call maintenance: broken bed
8 a.m.		A.M. cares Observe residents/ N.A.	Reassess: unstable resident condition Administer meds	Call housekeeping: spill on carpet Call P.T.: resident condition report
8:30	Document: phone calls		Treatments; decubiti, GT feeding, dressing change	Call M.D.: resident in unstable condition Call family: changing condition of resident
9 a.m.		Prepare residents: M.D. examinations	Administer meds, V.S. on unstable residents	
9:30	Accompany M.D. resident examinations			

TABLE 14–3   Organizing First-Line Manager Use of Time on a Residential Unit

the responsibilities for tasks involving self, nursing assistants, residents, and other individuals.

Using the Nursing Process can again assist you; put it to work in your timing. As part of the data collection, use your sense of vision, hearing, and touch. Sharpen these skills to make more prompt, yet accurate, judgements. You will not be able to return to the resident's room every 15 or 30 minutes to verify an observation or make additional assessments. It may require an on-the-spot decision. Depending on the acuity of the resident, you may need to delegate ongoing observations to the nursing assistant and request periodic reports. For example, "Sally, Mr. Tinucci says he doesn't feel well. He looks flushed and his skin feels warmer than usual. Will you please take his temperature and let me know the amount of his liquid intake for breakfast?"

Intuition becomes a tool for the experienced nurse and first-line manager. It is the ability to perceive or know something without a conscious problem-solving decision. Perhaps you have observed a nurse with a puzzled expression say, "There's something not quite right with Mr. Bradford, but I don't know what it is." Often the intuition is on target as more concrete symptoms become evident. You will develop intuition in managing a resident unit as you put your nursing education in practice and gain experience.

Cost containment has become a part of nursing management. As costs of health care rise and payers of that care look more closely at those costs, nurses have become more involved. Nurses are the primary users of facility supplies. Disposables are often costly and are not used as exclusively in long-term care as they are in acute care. One example is the use of washable cotton pads in place of disposable bed protectors.

Most long term care facilities expect the first-line manager to be conservative with supplies and demonstrate cost containment measures to nursing assistants. This is as simple as taking only the linen you need into a room. Extra linen would have to be rewashed before it is returned to the linen storage area.

Long term care facilities do not have generously stocked central supply rooms. Supplies, such as sterile dressings or gastrostomy tube feeding equipment, are usually ordered in large quantities for individual residents. You will learn to improvise since stock supplies are often limited. Determine if clean or sterile supplies are appropriate. Organize a procedure to use only the necessary supplies and think through your actions to avoid contamination of supplies.

Your first position as a first-line manager nurse will seem overwhelming. There will be a period of orientation to guide you in becoming acquainted with residents, staff, policies, and procedures. However, you will need to plan for the first time you are responsible for the unit alone. Keep in mind basic principles of your nursing education, which include patient safety and comfort. Start with observation of appropriate activities of daily living for the residents, administration of medications and treatments, and required documentation. Do not promise residents and nursing assistants "extras" until you are comfortable with completing the "As" on your "To Do" list.

Legal Considerations for the First-Line Manager

Nurses practicing in any setting must be aware of the legal aspects of nursing practice. First, all nurses must be licensed in the state where they are practicing. It is the nurse's responsibility, not the state or employer, to apply for licensure and to follow renewal policies. Some states require continuing education classes for nursing license renewal. It is becoming a wider practice by Boards of Nursing and/or employers to require refresher courses for all nurses who have not been in active nursing practice for several years.

Second, nurses should be aware of the

Nurse Practice Act in their state of practice. *Nurse Practice Acts* are nursing laws enacted by state governing bodies. Boards of Nursing are the usual agencies implementing the laws, approving schools of nursing, licensing nurses, and monitoring the practice of nursing.

The scope of nursing practice within a Nursing Practice Act may vary to some degree from one area to another. *Scope of practice* means how nursing is practiced in a community or geographical area. A nurse in a rural area may have a broader scope of practice, and a nurse in large research hospital a higher technical level of practice. This is reflected in the job description. In legal questions concerning nurses, the authorities usually look at scope of practice and *reasonable care.* This means expected action by most nurses in a given setting and situation.

Third, nurses should obtain a job description before accepting employment. The job description is the employer's expectation of the position. Nurses are accountable for the identified responsibilities and should inform the employer if additional education is required for some tasks. For example, a new graduate may not have had any experience with gastrostomy tube feedings. Inservice education can usually be arranged.

Nurses practicing as first-line managers in long term care facilities need to be aware of special considerations in this practice setting. First, as discussed in previous units, the acuity of residents has increased dramatically in recent years. Long-term care nurses are providing post-operative care as well as high-tech care for residents with chronic disorders.

Second, these nurses are providing this level of care with no on-site physician. There are no daily physician "rounds" to monitor the medical conditions of the residents. Nurses practicing in this setting need to develop sharp observation skills. They also must have guidelines regarding when to call the physician. However, nurses should not hesitate to call a physician with a resident concern.

Unlike acute care settings, long-term care nurses cannot call a "Code Blue." There are no anesthesiologists, critical care nurses, and others to respond. Some long term care facilities use the "911" telephone emergency number in a Code Blue situation. Nurses must know the DNR/DNI (do not resusitate/do not intubate) wishes of the resident and the facility's policy for emergency situations.

In all practice settings nurses are responsible for their actions and for the care they provide. First-line managers in long-term care are responsible for the residents on the unit to which they are assigned. Nursing assistants are providing some of the basic care. This means that the first-line manager must provide clear directions and ask clear questions that result in direct answers. You are accountable for the tasks you delegate. Nursing assistants are not licensed caregivers. In long-term care, nursing assistants are educated through a federal government training program and placed on a registry in the state where they are working.

One key in the first-line manager position is to know your practice limits. This means to consider your nursing education, your license, your experience, and your job description when making nursing practice decisions.

Long term care facilities have expectations of the first-line managers that reflect on the legal aspects of nursing. They expect nurses to practice within the guidelines of Nurse Practice Acts and facility job descriptions. They also expect nurses to follow lines of authority in decision making. Confidentiality in all aspects of nursing care within the facility is a top priority with all employers. Every resident has the right to expect that information in the medical record will be kept completely confidential.

Nurses are expected to keep current in practice by reading periodicals, and attending workshops and inservice education as well as other educational opportunities. Using good judgement will also guide you in your role of first-line manager nurse. Do not hesitate to have your questions answered by your employer, Board of Nursing, or professional organization.

Summary

Adapting and expanding patient care skills to organize your time is a continuous and challenging experience. To be successful as a first-line manager in long-term care will take a conscious, dedicated effort.

Organizing your time includes establishing goals, setting priorities, and delegating tasks. Establishing goals is patterned after patient goals in care plans. They should be realistic, simple, and measurable.

Prioritizing time places tasks in order of importance. An A,B,C model assists in ranking tasks. Recall another ABC priority model: the Airway, Breathing, and Circulation priorities in cardiopulmonary resusitation; the airway must be open before any other activity can begin. Factors that influence ranking of priorities include: (1) schedules, policies, and procedures; (2) the time to complete the task; (3) the health status and preferences of the resident; and (4) first-line manager experiences and values.

Delegating tasks involves assigning tasks for which you are responsible to nursing assistants. The decision-making process focuses on job descriptions and the acuity of resident health.

The Nursing Process is a framework for putting organization of time into action. "To Do" lists, prioritizing, and delegating are analyzed in the assessment phase of organizing time. Approaches to the planning phase include: (1) planning ahead, (2) blocking out time, (3) organizing the tools, and (4) determining the energy levels of the first-line manager nurse.

The implementation phase can flow smoothly with the use of work sheets to guide a timely completion of tasks. Expect interruptions; health care involves people and events, and priorities are continually changing.

Evaluating your use of time is necessary to improve efficiency. Just feeling good about the flow of the day's activities is a sign of effective organization. When the workday does not flow smoothly for a period of time, it is wise to evaluate your use of time in a more structured manner.

Continual organizing may seem time consuming. You may think, "I don't have the time," or "What's in it for me?" Taking a few minutes to plan well saves time in the end. What's in it for you is enjoying your work more by feeling in control and "on top of things." Your efficiency is cost containment for your employer and may be reflected in advancement in salary or position for you.

Effective communication skills influence organization of time. Nurses can adapt effective communication skills used in patient care to interactions with residents and staff in managing a resident unit in long term care.

Nurses will use effective communication techniques in one-to-one interactions with residents, family members, nursing assistants, and other staff members. Additional opportunities to adapt these techniques are in small group meetings and with telephone communication. The first-line manager will find an increase in the percentage of the workday involved in telephone and written communication.

Nonverbal communication or "body language" as well as voice cues influence the verbal message. They may enhance a statement to "make a point," or send a conflicting message to confuse a situation.

Blocks to communication may include the type of question asked or how it is framed. "Why" questions are uncomfortable to many people. Stereotyped comments, agreeing, not agreeing, approval, or disapproval have the tendency to close a conversation very quickly. As a result, residents or nursing assistants will not share their thoughts or feelings; they may respond with anger or withdrawl. Rumors are also nonproductive communication.

Written communication is becoming increasingly important in all aspects of managing resident care. First-line managers must be clear, concise, and accurate. Knowing your audience will determine if you can use medical terminology in the communication.

Organizing and implementing the care of a 30 resident unit is a challenge for the first-line manager nurse. It becomes a skill in balancing tasks and time. This unit focused on the first-line manager nurse, but did not intend to isolate this caregiver. You need to grow into a more independent autonomous caregiver. You will have the support and assistance of the second-line manager, inservice or staff development nurses, and the third-line manager director of nursing service. Ask for their guidance. It is the nature of nurses to guide all people to their greatest potential.

Finally — the "bottom line." Safe resident care must be practiced within the guidelines of Nurse Practice Acts. You are responsible for your license to practice nursing; value it and protect it. Job descriptions should reflect your level of licensure and the scope of nursing practiced in your community, and be within guidelines of the Nurse Practice Act.

For Discussion

- During your next clinical assignment use a time management log to record your activities.
  - Critique your time use: make a star by blocks of time that demonstrated good use of time and circle blocks of time that indicate time-wasters.
- Make a list with columns identified by A, B, and C. Review your clinical assignment and place tasks in columns by degree of importance. Compare the A's with your actual implementation on your time management log.
- In a group discussion share two positive signs of organizing your time and one area that needs work.
- Listen to staff nurses give reports and exchange information with team members. Identify techniques of effective communication.
- Choose a setting other than health care to observe nonverbal communication. Watch facial expressions and body language, and listen for voice cues in messages that are conveyed.

Questions for Review

1. List two components of effective use of time. *goals - priorities - delegate task*
2. Explain how the Nursing Process can be used as a tool to put your organized time into action. *Organization of time in action 'plan*
3. Identify four effective communication techniques. *concise, accurate 2 block*
4. Identify three blocks to effective communication. *clear, pleasant 3 Org. tools*
5. Discuss how nursing management is involved in cost containment. *4 Energy*

4. rumors, answer question with a question, giving advise, agreing or disagree s reason

5. Disposibles, time

Unit 15
Managing Human Resources

Objectives

After reading this unit you should be able to:
- Identify characteristics of effective leadership.
- Identify own abilities in effective leadership.
- Describe the process of managing a resident unit.
- Discuss the role of the first-line manager in the orientation of peers and nursing assistants.
- Identify objective techniques in appraising the performance of nursing assistants.
- Discuss personal growth outcomes of work for caregivers.

Human resources include the nursing skills and personal talents that each staff member contributes to the efficient functioning of the resident unit. It is part of the role of the first-line manager to seek out these abilities and include them in the implementation of the management of the unit. For example, one caregiver may demonstrate exceptional patience working with residents practicing rehabilitative skills learned in physical therapy and speech therapy. Another nursing assistant may have talents with hair and nail grooming which increases resident self-esteem.

This unit will focus on characteristics of leadership for the role of the first-line manager nurse. First, transferring characteristics of leadership that are developed from patient care into skills for managing a resident unit will be identified. Next, leadership characteristics will be viewed from the role of the nursing assistant. What does the nursing assistant expect from the first-line manager nurse?

To be an effective caregiver and first-line manager, the nurse first must learn self management. No one can be 100 percent in areas of self management and leadership. However, realizing generally accepted characteristics and knowing one's own strengths and weaknesses guides individuals in their roles.

There are role expectations for all levels of caregivers. The awareness of one's own role expectations as well as other caregiver roles is part of the team process. Delegating tasks is within the role expectations of the first-line manager; this nurse must be knowledgeable of roles of other caregivers.

The long term care facility human resource network includes the first-line manager nurse. Functions new to this nurse include presenting part of the orientation process to some new employees, and preparing the performance appraisals of the nursing assistants directly observed by the first-line manager. Techniques that result in accurate and fair appraisal will be presented.

How work meets the personal growth needs of an individual will complete this unit. Surprisingly, money or income is not usually the top priority when people are asked what they want out of a job. The paycheck is necessary to meet the physiological and security needs as identified by Maslow. Meeting social needs, self esteem needs, and self-actualization needs in the workplace are other desired outcomes and are often higher priorities in job satisfaction.

Characteristics of Leaders

Reflect on someone you feel is a good leader. Perhaps it is someone you knew when you were younger, such as a scout leader, a softball coach, or a youth director in church. More recently, you may have had another career or job where you were directed by someone you felt was a really a "good" leader. What were some of the characteristics or attributes of that person that made you feel that way? Would these attributes fit a "good" nursing leader?

Managing Staff

Who are you? In other nursing courses, such as interpersonal communications or mental health, you may have explored personality development and looked inward to see who you are. You were studying people because that is

the nature of health care. Understanding yourself contributes to the helping contract and trust relationship with patients. Now you want to reflect on your personal attributes in light of how they will fit into characteristics of leadership and managing a resident unit.

Self-awareness or **self-concept** is how individuals view themselves. It is a verbal picture that includes physical appearance, learning ability, beliefs, and feelings. It also reflects on your interactions with others. Although there are hereditary factors in personality, much of our self-concept is developed through life experiences, figure 15-1.

Most people will have positive and negative items on the list of who they are. These pluses and minuses will fluctuate from time to time. It is the positives we build on to grow in experience and self-worth. The minuses we work on

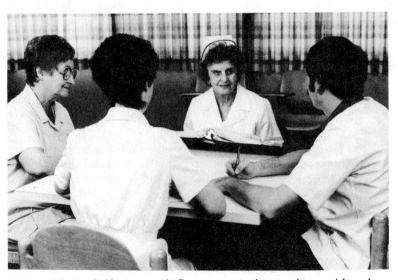

Figure 15-1 Self-concept influences our interactions with others (From Hegner and Caldwell, *Assisting in Long-Term Care*, copyright © 1988 by Delmar Publishers Inc.)

with or without the help of others. Sometimes we just leave the minuses alone! It is when the self-concept has more negatives or becomes more negative that self is threatened and becomes dysfunctional.

A positive or healthy sense of self is important in the role of the first-line manager nurse. You will send a signal of confidence and support to residents and other caregivers. The knowledge and skills learned in your nursing education will strengthen your view of self as a nurse.

Individuals with a weakened sense of self experience stress, and have a difficult time in implementing resident care, as well as managing a resident unit. Unless the self-concept can be strengthened through course work or therapy, the nurse will probably not be successful in the role. This nurse may even leave the position.

Closely tied to a positive self-concept is **assertiveness**. Assertive behavior displays a confident or positive position on beliefs and ideas. This is not the same as aggressive behavior, which may be a forceful or an attacking type of behavior.

First-line managers need to be assertive in effective communication to express the needs and direction of the resident unit. Individuals who are successful with assertiveness gain the respect of residents and caregivers. Passive behavior would allow someone else to assume the leader role. Recall your first clinical experiences in your nursing education. Perhaps you did not feel confident in your role or with a particular patient. Did the patient start directing his care?

Aggressive approaches may promote anger or withdrawal in residents and nursing assistants, depending on their self-concept. Neither anger nor withdrawl are healthy in the efficient functioning of a resident unit.

Stress became an everyday word in the 1980s. Most everyone began to move in the "fast lane," or at least a fast-er lane. The rapid advancement of technology brings services into our homes at a dizzy pace. Likewise, it seems that we expect that we should also move and produce results faster. This is true in health care as in other workplaces. All these outside influences that produce physical stress are called *stressors*.

You have studied stress in anatomy and physiology as well as in other course work. Many conditions studied in medical and surgical nursing indicate that symptoms are exacerbated by stress. Perhaps you also know what stress and accompanying anxiety do to productivity. If you had many stressors related to school, work, family, or friends, how effective was your studying? Anxiety interferes with clear thinking when taking an exam. Most students have had that experience at one time or another.

There are stressors in the role of first-line manager. You will be responsible for many residents and tasks. You will also be responsible to other caregivers and the facility. Organizing your time and planning the management of the resident unit will prepare you to deal with the stressors.

It is important for the first-line manager nurse to take measures to avoid stress and anxiety which could result in dysfunctional behavior, when you could no longer be in control of self or the resident unit. The result could be poor judgement regarding time use, resident care, and interactions with nursing assistants and other caregivers. Other results could include ineffective, nonproductive communications. Stress, anger, and fatigue tend to precipitate inappropriate message cues. A sharp voice tone, unkind remarks, or negative facial expressions yield nonproductive communications.

Recall stress management techniques. Take care of yourself! Good nutrition, adequate rest, exercise, and leisure activities are a good start. Avoid excessive stressors by planning your workday. In your role of first-line manager, control relates to your decision-making responsibilities. Anxiety and stress will interfere with this control. When this happens, stop and "take a deep breath." This means to take a few minutes in a quiet area to review or revise your work plan before resuming the day, figure 15–2. The day will improve.

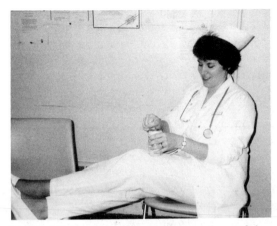

Figure 15-2   Taking a break during the workday is a part of stress management techniques.

Feeling good about yourself is important to your success. Managing self is a continual, progressive, and insightful process.

Strengthening Leadership Characteristics

Characteristics that occur naturally in a person are nurtured through life experiences and practiced in directing patient care. These characteristics need to be strengthened for the role of the first-line manager nurse in directing activities of the resident unit. Leadership characteristics are defined and applied to patient care in Figure 15-3.

Not every person can be skillful in every area. Our individuality allows some of us to be more creative, and others to be able to have a greater depth of understanding in specific areas of knowledge. A successful first-line manager requires some degree of skill in each of the characteristics. This nurse needs the ability to tap the talents of other caregivers which adds strength to one's own management.

Knowledge.   Knowledge may be defined as an accumulation of facts that has been learned or grasped by the mind. It usually relates to a topic or an area of study. In a broad sense, you have a basic knowledge of gerontology. For a more specific reference, you have a general knowledge of physical signs of aging.

Your nursing course work provides information for decision making in patient care. You retrieve this stored information and apply it. In many situations you use psychomotor skills when you implement a nursing procedure such as applying a sterile dressing.

The first-line manager nurse needs to use and strengthen knowledge related to: (1) nursing in general, and nursing related to the elderly in particular; (2) effective communication techniques; (3) use of time for self and others; (4) interpersonal skills; (5) facility policies and procedures; and (6) basic functioning of the health care delivery system, particularly related to long-term care.

Demonstrating a degree of knowledge influences your credibility with others. People also respect those who are willing to say, "I don't know," and seek the answer. Those who bluff, or mislead, or continually say, "I don't know," do not gain the confidence of residents and caregivers.

Judgement.   Judgement is the ability to make comparisons and then decisions. "Using good nursing judgement" is a phrase often used to describe patient care decisions based on nursing theory and experience. Good nursing judgement is "good common sense" in the everyday practice of decision making.

In the role of the first-line manager nurse responsible for a resident unit, you will be making decisions regarding the care of the 30 residents. You will also be making decisions regarding some of the actions of the nursing assistants and the general flow of activity of the unit. Nursing knowledge and skills of time management and communication will assist you in making good nursing judgements.

Residents and nursing assistants will depend on you to make judgements that apply particularly to residents' activities of daily living. Many times decisions will need to be made almost instantly. Experience will help in making these decisions.

Awareness.   **Awareness** is a state of being alert to surroundings and interpreting the information collected through sight, sound, touch, and taste. It is like having an antenna to receive signals. Perhaps at some time you felt that your mother or a teacher had "eyes in the back of her head," or ears "a mile long"! Their sense or awareness of activity was very keen.

For the first-line manager in long-term

- KNOWLEDGE
  - is an accumulation of facts, usually related to a single topic, learned or grasped by the mind
  - is nursing course work that provides information for decision making in patient care
- JUDGEMENT
  - is an act of decision making, ability to compare and decide; often stated as "good common sense"
  - is use of knowledge from nursing course work in problem solving and decisions related to patient needs
- AWARENESS
  - is an alertness or quickness in thought to interpret information collected through sight, sound, touch, and taste
  - is nursing knowledge "at-the-ready" to collect clues from patient and environment
- CREATIVENESS
  - is the ability to be productive through imagination or inventiveness
  - is adapting nursing knowledge to meet individual needs
- FLEXIBILITY
  - is the ability to modify; adjust to change
  - is rearranging nursing care as indicated by change in patient status, schedules, or environment
- CONCERN FOR OTHERS
  - demonstrates interest and importance of well-being of fellow human beings
  - is relating to patients as individuals
  - is demonstrating interest in the uniqueness of individual worth
- SELF-DISCIPLINE
  - is the ability to control or direct one's actions
  - is using nursing knowledge to provide efficient safe patient care in a professional manner
- ATTITUDE
  - is nonverbal communication that projects one's thoughts, feelings, moods, or opinions
  - is presenting a positive therapeutic self to patients and other health caregivers
- POSITIVE ROLE MODEL
  - is demonstrating or imitating the standard of excellence of a specified group
  - is representing health; good physical, mental, and social well-being

---

Figure 15–3   Leadership characteristics in patient care

care, this awareness must be developed to have a sense of what is going on in every corner of the unit. The awareness must be there at the same time as the isolated concentration of preparing and administering medications. Efficient planning to set up your workday will assist you in being in control or "on top of things." This will keep the signals clear and your "awareness antenna" working.

Creativeness. **Creativity** is the ability to be productive through imagination or inventiveness. In nursing it is often adapting equipment or supplies to complete a procedure or meet a patient's need. Everyday examples include using a box, chair, or wastebasket turned on its side to elevate a patient's feet when a footstool or wheelchair extensions are not available.

In a long term care facility there are many opportunities for the nurse to be creative. The facility is isolated in the sense that there is usually no on-site central supply and in some situations no on-site laundry. Pharmaceuticals and supplies for treatments have to be ordered from an outside source and may take 24 hours or more to arrive.

Perhaps you have already heard the phrase, "you'll have to improvise." In making a bed you may have used a bath blanket for a mattress pad or a folded flat sheet for a draw sheet when linen is in short supply. This is improvising. Using nursing judgement will help you decide if the substitute materials are acceptable for the job. Resident safety and comfort must be met.

Flexibility. **Flexibility** is the ability to modify plans and adjust to the changes without the process becoming a stressor. In nursing practice it is rearranging nursing care due to changes in a patient's health status, schedules, or the environment. You have experienced this in your clinical assignments. A patient's physician orders an x-ray that interrupts the morning care, a patient is unexpectedly scheduled for surgery and preoperative routines must be completed, or a wound has become infected and the patient must be placed on isolation precautions.

This flexibility is needed by the first-line manager in long-term care as the residents health status changes, activities within the facility are rescheduled, new resident's arrive, or staffing patterns change. Having a daily plan gives you a base for changing and rearranging. How flexible you are in your personal life will give you a clue as to how flexible you will be in the workplace.

Concern for Others. **Concern for others** is the amount of interest and importance a person places on the well-being of other persons. This is measured subjectively and objectively. A person may feel and think they have this concern, but not project it in a manner perceived as concern by others.

In nursing, concern for others is perhaps the highest priority in a personal attribute. Nurses must be "people persons" to be successful. They must relate to patients as individuals, demonstrating an interest in the uniqueness of individual worth. Those who are interested in health, but are uncomfortable working so intimately with people, can practice in research or other areas of health care.

It is particularly important in long-term care for the nurse to have a deep concern for others because of the nature of the care setting. Residents usually are admitted for permanent placement; this is their home. The nurse will be more involved with families of residents. Some nurses state that they care for a family as well as a resident.

Self Discipline. **Self-discipline** is the ability to control or direct one's actions. In nursing, this is using nursing knowledge to provide efficient safe patient care in a professional manner. This covers a wide scope of practice. For example, it means sticking to your plan of care to complete tasks on time. It means not projecting your values on a patient with values different from your own. It means maintaining your composure when a patient verbally strikes out at you with profane language. He probably is disturbed over his situation, not angry with you. It means responding in pleasant respectful tones when other caregivers seem to bark commands amidst frustrations.

Self discipline is tied closely to concern for others in the long term care facility. It takes an even temperament to work closely with the same residents and nursing assistants on a continual basis. It may not be easy, but it is a leadership characteristic expected of the first-line manager.

In addition to the interpersonal skills required, disciplining yourself to adhere to the work plan for the unit and keeping everyone on task is expected. Rethinking the situation and your actions while counting to 10 is a start in control and self discipline. Sometimes you may need to count to 1000!

Attitude.   Attitude is the nonverbal communication that projects one's thoughts, feelings, moods, or opinions. An attitude can be expressed in verbal message cues by tone of voice or other cues. Persons presenting a positive attitude are a part of a therapeutic environment. Everyone around this person feels good about themselves and their work.

For nurses this begins with personal hygiene and uniform. A neatly groomed nurse with a clean, properly fitted uniform and polished shoes presents the image expected of nurses and nurse leaders. People who are responsible, dependable, and punctual demonstrate attitudes expected of nurses. The nature in which nurses complete their tasks demonstrates their attitude. Willingness to help others, trying alternative measures to meet patients' needs, seeking challenges in nursing, and applying a smile and pleasant tone of voice are examples of a positive attitude. These attitudes need to be nurtured in long-term care as the first-line manager sets the tone for the activity of the resident unit.

Positive Role Model.   A *positive role model* demonstrates or imitates the standard of excellence of a specified group. There are cultural and societal expectations for every role: parents, teachers, politicians, athletes, lawyers, nurses, and physicians.

Nurses as well as other health caregivers represent health. Health is physical, mental, and social well-being. A role model sets a good example. The public questions why some doctors and nurses smoke. They wonder about obese health careworkers who should know the health risks.

In long term care facilities, as well as other health care settings, nurses represent themselves, the nursing profession, and the facility where they are employed. Exhibiting characteristics of leadership instills confidence in the nurse, and projects this confidence to other staff, residents, family, and the employer.

Projecting Leadership Characteristics

The nursing assistant in long-term care follows the directions of the first-line manager nurse. Leadership characteristics expected of this nurse by the nursing assistant are outlined in figure 15-4.

Representing nursing as a good role model is perhaps one of the most important characteristics the first-line manager can present to the nursing assistant. From this model, the nurse can build personal credibility and team unity in the resident unit.

Nursing assistants want to be valued in their role and desire respect as persons and caregivers. They want first-line manager nurses that care about people. They want nurses who are willing to help them, willing to answer questions, and make decisions. Nursing assistants are willing to be productive caregivers for nurses who are fair and consistent with decisions regarding resident care and the caregivers.

In long term care facilities, like other workplaces, productivity will depend on interactions of managers and workers. The first-line manager nurse needs to be aware of expectations of the nursing assistant as well as those of the resident, family, and employer.

Clarifying Roles in Managing a Resident Unit

Part of the managing of the resident unit is clarifying the roles of the caregivers. A *role* is a set of expectations. In the long term care facility these are established in the job descriptions, policies, and procedures. However, caregivers do not thumb through job descriptions daily to review their tasks and the expectations of employers. These expectations are shared verbally and on work sheets in the process of developing work relationships.

The roles do need to be defined in the job description and shared with caregivers at the time of employment and at other appropriate times. When the role is defined, and the expectations shared, there is a committment to that

---

- KNOWLEDGE
  - about the residents and their health problems
  - about the facility policies and procedures
  - to answer questions appropriately; with respect and acknowledging nursing assistants desire to learn

- JUDGEMENT
  - to be willing to look at situations and make decisions
  - to initiate action or produce outcome for a justifiable problem or complaint

- AWARENESS
  - to needs of the resident unit; residents and caregivers
  - to share information with nursing assistants as caregivers

- CREATIVENESS
  - to suggest different approaches to resident care

- FLEXIBILITY
  - to be open to changing assignments
  - to accept nursing assistant suggestions in planning workday

- CONCERN FOR OTHERS
  - to accept nursing assistants as caregivers in nursing care
  - to respect the nursing assistants and their caregiver role
  - to be willing to assist nursing assistants in caregiving
  - to be fair and consistent in delegating tasks

- SELF-DISCIPLINE
  - to organize workday in resident unit
  - to promote efficiency in caregivers and unit activity

- ATTITUDE
  - to project a positive atmosphere in resident unit
  - to encourage others in a positive attitude

- POSITIVE ROLE MODEL
  - to represent nursing as public envisions
  - to instill in nursing assistant the desire to model nursing behaviors

---

Figure 15–4   Leadership characteristics expected of first-line managers by nursing assistants

role. As the person identifies more with the role and becomes more committed, security increases along with productivity. If a job description is revised, or other changes occur that affect the role, the process of defining and establishing expectations should again be initiated. If this does not occur, the caregivers are uncertain of their role and tasks and the working foundation of the resident unit becomes shaky.

The need for redefining roles will occur in the rapid change and growth of the health care delivery system. Rules, regulations, procedures, and techniques are changing almost daily. In this process it is easy for information to fall through a gap in the communication system. Information may not be shared with all caregivers. It becomes important to get appropriate items verified and the activity of the resident unit back on track.

Leadership and planning go hand-in-hand. The planning promotes a proactive rather than a reactive direction to managing a resident unit. *Proactive* means planning or deciding what tasks will be done to meet a goal. It is like planning a family reunion. The decisions are made for the time, place, food, music, games for all ages, and alternate plans for inclement weather. A *reactive* response would be to wait until everyone arrived and then decide what you are going to do with all these people!

You may have heard a reactive approach to managing expressed in phrases such as "crisis management," or "putting out fires." Because health care involves people in every situation, the outcomes are often uncertain or unclear. Therefore, proactive planning will not always work and reactive measures will have to be taken. A plan will provide the framework for change. As the first-line manager nurse gains experience, some events are anticipated and priorities are more easily established.

Team Planning

The caregivers in a resident unit need to be coordinated to accomplish the tasks in the workday. Successful coordinating involves identifying the goals for the resident unit. This includes the "what" needs to be done. The "who" is determined by the roles of the caregivers. The "how" is nursing procedures and facility policy established for resident care. All of this requires the interpersonal and nursing skills of the first-line manager in the development of working relationships.

In addition to the potential of uncertain roles in team planning, role conflicts can occur. These may occur because of individual values. Our *values* are strong beliefs that guide us in our lives. Some are unconscious; we are not aware of them. Some are private and we do not want to talk about them. Other values we talk about; and some are such a deep part of us that they are demonstrated in our behavior. These conflicts can occur because of different values between people, or a conflict between a person's values and the task that is required of the role.

When resolving conflicts between your own values, or conflicts between people, use a problem-solving approach. First, obtain the facts. Look at the facts to determine the issue that is creating the conflict. Obtain additional information needed from the second-line manager, references, or other appropriate sources. Then consider possible actions and the resulting outcomes. Finally, choose the course of action.

This process can be followed in personal or group conflicts. Perhaps there is a conflict within a group of nursing assistants. The first-line manager can assemble those involved, and direct the group through the problem-solving process to resolve the conflict.

Delegating Within the Resident Unit

The first-line manager most often delegates tasks to nursing assistants. After the nursing assistant has been identified as the level of caregiver to complete the task, the next decision is which person should be delegated the task.

There are many considerations in selecting an individual for a task: (1) does the task involve an assigned resident or other workday assignment; (2) does the time involved fit in the current work load; (3) what is the amount of experience the person has with the task; (4) will individual personality fit the task; (5) has the individual managed the task successfully in the past; and (6) is the individual dependable?

Delegating the task must include clear and complete directions, figure 15–5. An example of unclear direction is: "Sally, please distribute the morning nourishments." A more clear direction could be: " Sally, please distribute the 10 a.m. nourishments. This is the list of residents. The starred names may need some assistance. Give me the list before lunch and note how much each resident drank and if there were any problems. Do you have any questions?"

The first-line manager nurse also must give the nursing assistant authority over the task. In giving authority, the nurse sets this task aside until the nursing assistant reports the results. Authority is not given with the task when there is a continual "checking up" on the nursing assistant, such as suggesting steps to complete the task. The nurse may want to complete part of the task; this no longer is giving authority.

When there are problems in delegating authority, the first-line manager should problem solve the situation. Is it personal in wanting to maintain authority over the task, or was it an uncertainty with the person to whom the task was delegated? Evaluate the process of delegating as well as the outcome desired from the task itself. First-line manager nurses often demonstrate tasks to nursing assistants and then turn over the authority to complete them in the future. Table 15–1 presents a guideline for demonstrating a new task to a nursing assistant.

Discipline

There are occasions when workers must be disciplined. It is not usually comfortable for either party; the person doing the disciplining, or the person receiving the discipline. Providing necessary and appropriate discipline is a role

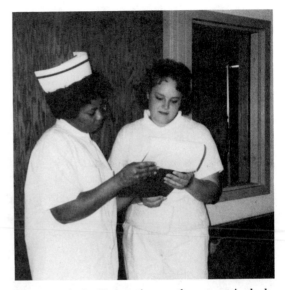

Figure 15–5 Delegating tasks must include clear, complete directions.

responsibility of a manager. The first-line manager nurse in a long term care facility is responsible for some disciplinary measures with nursing assistants.

Disciplinary action is usually required when a facility policy or procedure has not been followed. For example, a resident or family member may voice a complaint about quality of care. The objective of discipline is to correct the problem and improve the performance of the nursing assistant, not to "punish" the nursing assistant.

To make the process somewhat comfortable for the first-line manager nurse, the problem-solving process should be followed. First get the facts independently from all parties. Mrs. Schmitz states, "I just don't like the care my mother is getting." The nurse should encourage conversation to learn about Mrs. Schmitz's specific concerns. After reassuring her that she will receive an answer, the nurse will procede to ask the nursing assistant to recall events related to the situation.

KEY POINTS	REASON
• Review facility procedure manual or nursing skills textbook	• Directions should be accurate; consistent
• Explain why procedure is done; possible outcomes for resident	• Increases commitment to task; accuracy
• Assemble appropriate equipment and supplies	• Promotes adherence to standards
• Explain activity to resident	• Obtain resident permission; reduces apprehension
• Use aseptic technique; safety and comfort measures	• Promotes adherence to standards
• Demonstrate steps slowly, in correct order	• Provides time to grasp information
• Ask for questions	• Determines if task was explained clearly
• Request return demonstration; determine appropriate time	• Determines ability to complete task
• Identify specific outcomes of task to report to nurse	• Promotes continuity of care; efficiency in resident unit

TABLE 15–1 Guidelines for Demonstrating a New Task to Nursing Assistants

Follow through the problem-solving process. Be sure to use facility policies and procedures as your guideline. Perhaps part of Mrs. Schmitz's complaint was that her mother got breakfast at 8 a.m. when she was accustomed to eating at 6 a.m. This is a personal preference and perhaps a more thorough explanation of the meal schedules would be helpful.

Another part of the complaint was that the resident did not get denture care. This is part of the procedure for daily care and should be evaluated. If disciplinary action is to be taken, the usual process involves a verbal warning for the first offense. Part of the process should be reviewing the procedure to ensure the nursing assistant clearly sees what is expected behavior.

Guidelines to assist the first-line manager in initiating a verbal warning are: (1) discipline in private; (2) provide a clear explanation of the offense; (3) provide time for the nursing assis-

tant to respond specifically to unsatisfactory behavior; (4) provide an explanation of expected behavior according to facility standards; and (5) set a time to re-evaluate the situation.

Remember, this is disciplining the person's behavior as measured by the role expectations of a nursing assistant. It does not mean you attack the nursing assistant as a person. Discipline should take place as soon as the facts are obtained and the problem-solving process is completed. Discipline should be fair and consistent. Similar offenses should have similar disciplinary actions. All nursing assistants should receive the same discipline for the same offense. Be firm once your decision has been made. Avoid being manipulated or influenced by excuses. Do not avoid discipline with the idea that the problem will correct itself. You also do not want to initiate the process of a verbal warning if you feel angry or frustrated. Keep a clear focus on the behaviors expected of the role and by the facility.

First-line manager nurses should follow the facility procedure for disciplinary actions. Usually a clarification of a policy or procedure is the first step. Next is the verbal warning. If the unsatisfactory behavior continues, a written warning is next. At this point in the disciplinary process, the second-line manager becomes responsible for the decisions and actions.

The first-line manager nurse should write an anecdotal note or use the facility form for written warnings. The complaint and resulting actions should be identified for the second-line manager nurse. Be clear and concise with facts, and avoid interjecting personal opinions.

Although the responsibility of disciplining is not welcomed, following the guidelines discussed will be helpful. Keep in mind that the objective is for behavior to change, which will result in improved performance by the nursing assistant.

Participating in Staff Orientation

The orientation process is not new to you. During your nursing education you probably have had many hours devoted to the process of becoming acquainted with schools, courses, and clinical sites. At times, the hours and information probably seemed endless. However, if you had not received some information to help you become familiar with the environment, you would have had to ask questions for every decision and action. You would have been frustrated, and would have had difficulty adapting to the environment or situation.

Orientation continues to be an important beginning in the workplace. The nurse becomes involved in a part of orienting peers to the role and responsibilities of the first-line manager. Monitoring tasks during the orientation of new nursing assistants may also be a responsibility of the first-line manager nurse.

Orientation Overview

All staff members of a facility will receive an orientation. There are usually three basic areas of orientation: the building and grounds, employee policies and procedures, and department information. You have been included in at least a basic building orientation for your clinical assignments. It may begin with a history of the facility, and then a tour of resident areas and resident service areas. Usually your interaction with areas or departments, such as physical therapy, medical records, or housekeeping, is presented briefly during a tour.

General facility policies include a considerable amount of information and paperwork. This includes fire code and disaster plan information; accident or incident reports applicable to residents, visitors, staff, and self; parking permits; and location and availability of meals during working hours. Facility policies provide information about dress code, time cards, vacation and scheduling requests, employee benefit packages, and other general policies and safety rules. Some facilities have a handbook printed with brief descriptions of facility policies and procedures.

No one expects a new employee to remember every detail. The philosophy of the facility and the degree of importance placed on particular areas is set in the general tone of the orientation. One policy that has surfaced in recent years is the smoke-free environment. The facility policy is usually stated at the time of the first interview to inform potential employees.

The orientation to the department is specific to the staff member: nursing, medical services, support services, or business office. The nursing department information will include: the organization of the nursing service and philosophy of nursing as practiced in the facility, emergency procedures, overview of charts and other documentation, and the pharmacy and medication administration systems. Other information relating to residents would include: admission, transfer, and discharge routines, and state laws regarding Resident's Bill of Rights and adult abuse.

Orientation for new nurses is usually five or more days. For two or three days classes are held in a conference room. The information on policies for employees and the benefit package are presented and government and facility employment forms completed. Some facilities include back exercise classes to promote good on-the-job body mechanics. CPR classes or refresher courses may also be included in an expanded orientation. The remaining two or three days are spent with nurses on the resident unit.

In larger facilities several departments will be involved in the orientation process: administration, pharmacy, and nursing, including inservice or staff development. In a smaller facility, the director of nursing service may complete most of the orientation.

In two to four weeks, the nurse will be expected to be, for the most part, independent in assignments. Before this time there may be additional orientation classes or individual guidance with procedures that are not familiar to the new nurse. Facilities usually have a three to six month conditional employment period. During this time, nurses are observed for abilities in all aspects of their nursing practice.

Orientation to the Resident Unit

Orientation to the resident unit for the new nurse is often completed by the first-line manager nurse. Many facilities use the "buddy" system, permitting the new nurse to accompany the first-line manager throughout the workday activities. When orientation is your responsibility, remember that you do not have a second chance to make a first impression. The first-line manager nurse is representing the manner in which nursing is practiced in the facility.

After you are informed you will be assisting with the orientation of a new nurse, you will have some time to plan the day. Use skills of organizing time to plan an efficient tour of the unit and clear explanations of procedures. This makes the activity convenient for you, and more

understandable for the new nurse. There usually are orientation checklists to note the procedures you will need to explain or demonstrate. Be prepared for questions about the facility and its policies. Many times questions surface when the nurse is involved directly in the work setting. If you do not have the information, contact the staff member responsible for the orientation.

Another important part of the orientation process is the welcoming or socialization of the new nurse. This decreases the anxiety and helps the new nurse feel like a member of the staff and part of the facility. A sense of job satisfaction begins to emerge before any individual responsibility is assigned.

When new nursing assistants are being oriented to the resident unit, the first-line manager nurse may be responsible for observing the accuracy of some procedures. Examples are methods of transferring residents, including the Hoyer lift, and correct placement and securing of restraints.

Appraising Work Performance of Nursing Assistants

Performance appraisals are completed periodically with workers in nearly every workplace. Some appraisals are the basis for merit or salary increases, or position promotions. However, the major objective of the appraisals is to assist the person in improving some area of work responsibility and to offer praise for areas of excellence.

Nursing students are familiar with performance appraisals as a part of the clinical experience portion of nursing education. A comparison can be made between the student experience and the workplace appraisal as both reflect observations of on-the-job skills.

First, there is a tool for defining expected behavior for effective performance. In education, learning objectives are identified with appropriate steps for achieving a specified degree of skill. In the workplace a tool is also necessary to identify facility expectations and to serve as a guideline for appraising performance. Some facilities have a combined job description and performance appraisal tool. If they are separate documents, the performance appraisal should reflect expectations outlined in a job description.

Second, only behaviors expected in the role or position of employment are evaluated. This was discussed in approaches to disciplinary action by the first-line manager nurse. Figure 15-6 illustrates the concept of separating behaviors of an individual as a person, from expected behaviors in a variety of roles. Heredity and experience influence who we are as a person.

Our personality and changes in environment influence our behavior in roles such as parenting or nursing. Your nursing instructors appraised your performance according to behaviors expected of a student nurse. You were not being evaluated for your behavior as a parent, a volunteer firefighter, or a member of a rock band. Those are other roles you may have, but they are not part of the performance appraisal of a student nurse.

Sometimes people become defensive during a performance appraisal interview because they respond to remarks about their performance as "personal" rather than role behavior expecta-

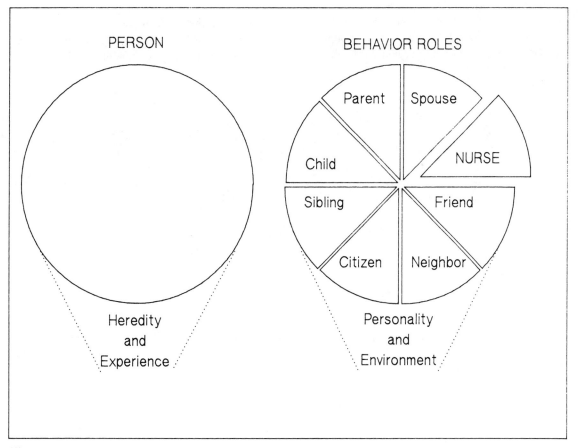

Figure 15-6 Performance appraisals should evaluate the individual's performance as a nurse separate from other aspects of personality.

tions. That is easy to do as our work, particularly the nature of nursing, is tied very closely to who we are as a person. The first-line manager nurse must keep focusing on behaviors expected of a nursing assistant, and make that evaluation clear, when completing a performance appraisal and interview.

Third, performance is usually divided into categories of expectations. In nursing education three general areas are knowledge, skills, and attitude. Knowledge is the facts learned and most often evaluated by pencil and paper tests. Skills are evaluated by watching a person perform tasks. These are psychomotor activities as they combine the knowledge about the tasks and the ability to complete them accurately. Attitudes are difficult to appraise because attitude behaviors often are not well defined. Those expected by nurses may include compliance with a uniform and grooming code, attendance

policies, willingness to be a member of the team, and other interpersonal skills.

The first-line manager nurse can consider a similar grouping of abilities when appraising the performance of nursing assistants. The knowledge expected is based on the required training and testing for the position. The skills are those listed on the job description. Facility procedure manuals will have appropriate steps and outcomes identified. Attitudes expected by the facility will be outlined in employee policy handbooks and in the job description or performance appraisal tool. These guidelines will not make completing a performance appraisal a "snap," but should give the first-line manager nurse a starting place. Figure 15–7 illustrates behaviors expected of nursing assistants.

Finally, the performance appraisal should be objective and not subjective. It means the same as when you are charting resident infor-

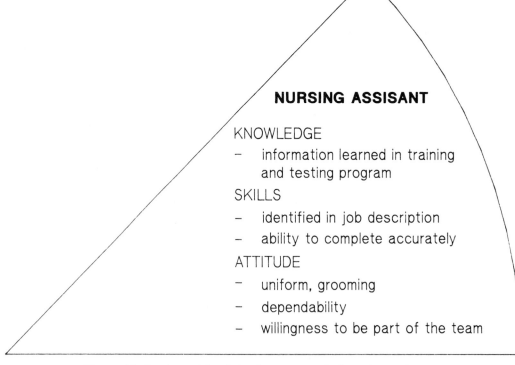

NURSING ASSISANT

KNOWLEDGE
- information learned in training and testing program

SKILLS
- identified in job description
- ability to complete accurately

ATTITUDE
- uniform, grooming
- dependability
- willingness to be part of the team

Figure 15–7   Appraising behaviors expected of nursing assistants

mation. You must document what you see and hear, not what you think or feel. This is factual information, not opinions. Examples of subjective and objective performance appraisal comments are identified in Table 15–2.

The second-line manager nurse will provide you with written or verbal directions to complete the facility appraisal form. You may receive the names of the nursing assistants a week or two before the performance appraisal is to be completed. This will give you several days to observe more closely and clarify any uncertainties in performance. The appraisal should be your objective comments, not a summary of comments and views of others. It is not good practice to ask the peers, other nursing assistants, for input into a performance appraisal. Full-time first-line managers in larger facilities are often given three performace appraisals to complete every month.

Ranking of performance on an appraisal tool may be numerical with numbers five through one representing performance from excellent(5) to unsatisfactory(1). Other tools may rank performance "good," "fair," or "needs improvement." The form should explain the expected level of performance for each ranking. The facility may also indicate at which level formal action must take place to guide the nursing assistant in improving performance. Individual entries or sections of the form usually provide a space to add written comments. Some, but not necessarily all, of these areas should include subjective comments. It makes the appraisal more meaningful to the nursing assistant and also demonstrates that you took some time in the preparation.

A sample performance appraisal and facility guidelines for completing the appraisal are presented in figure 15–8. The nursing assistant has been employed by the facility for several years and this is a routine six months review.

Some facilities require anecdotal notes or critical incident reports to be made and filed during the period between performance appraisals. These notes are to represent both outstanding and unsatisfactory events in the nursing assistant's work day. They are to be shared at the time they are written, and included in the scheduled performance appraisal.

The performance appraisal interview is the time when the first-line manager nurse shares the completed performance appraisal tool with the nursing assistant. Approximately 10 to 20 minutes should be scheduled at a time conve-

SUBJECTIVE COMMENTS	OBJECTIVE COMMENTS
• She always looks sloppy.	• Uniform is often soiled and wrinkled; shoes unpolished
• He's a good aide.	• Dependable: has called in sick one day, never tardy
• Is always safe.	• Uses brakes and safety devices consistently; uses gait/transfer belt with all residents
• Is usually disorganized.	• Frequently forgets necessary supplies; interrupts bath to search for linen, equipment
• Knows what she's doing.	• Follows facility procedures for resident care; completes activities independently
• Is often crabby and irritable.	• Displays sharp tone of voice to residents; does not respond verbally to staff questions; shrugs shoulders

TABLE 15–2   Examples of Subjective and Objective Comments on Performance Appraisals

SOUTHVIEW ACRES HEALTH CARE CENTER

PROCEDURE FOR COMPLETION OF JOB DESCRIPTION/EVALUATION FORM

1) Form is initiated by the Personnel Department according to pre-determined schedule and sent to appropriate Department Head.

2) The Department Head or his/her designee will evaluate the employee in each of the areas listed under "functions/standards" according to the rating system listed below.

3) The evaluator will list any comments that are appropriate and will also list specifics to explain and/or clarify the particular rating given.

4) The evaluation process also includes a conference between the evaluator and the employee. At this time, any growth areas and goals along with general comments should be discussed.

5) Attached to the actual evaluation form will be statistical information regarding the employee from the Personnel Department. Be sure to use this information in giving the employee a rating in the appropriate area(s), including the overall rating (XI).

6) The evaluator will sign the form(s) where appropriate including his/her title.

7) The employee will also sign and date the form(s) where appropriate. Remind the employee that their signature signifies the fact that they have read this material. It does not mean they agree with it. If they do disagree they have the right to submit a written rebuttal.

RATING SYSTEM FOR EMPLOYEE EVALUATION

For each "function/standard" listed on the evaluation form, rate the employee, using the following numerical scale (0 thru 5). Remember that the purpose in evaluating employees is to summarize and discuss their weaknesses and strengths and to assist the employee in establishing an appropriate self-improvement plan.

0 - not applicable-employee was not required to perform function/standard during the time period being evaluated.

1 - poor-not meeting standard-unsatisfactory performance-requires frequent and regular supervision.

2 - fair-meets moderate amount of standard-below average performance-requires frequent supervision and/or guidance.

3 - average-meets standard-typical performance-requires medium amount of supervision and guidance.

4 - good-meets most aspects of standard-above average performance-requires occasional guidance or coaching.

5 - excellent-meets all aspects of standard-extremely good performance in all aspects-requires little or no supervision.

Figure 15-8 Sample performance appraisal and sample facility guidelines for completing a performance appraisal (Courtesy of Southview Acres Health Care Center, West St. Paul, MN)

SOUTHVIEW ACRES HEALTH CARE CENTER
NURSING ASSISTANT JOB DESCRIPTION AND EVALUATION

NAME *Martha Lansing*   START DATE *3/31/84*   RATE _____

Primary Function: Provides direct patient care services and other assigned
                    duties, under the supervision of the Director of Nursing,
                    according to the philosophy, policies and procedures of
                    Southview Acres Health Care Center.

Qualifications: Must have good mental and physical health, be of good
                    moral character, able to see and hear well, able to use
                    hands and body well enough to perform basic functions.
                    Should be 16 years of age or older. Successful completion
                    of previous nursing assistant training and able to success-
                    fully complete or test-out of the AVTI curriculum (MN
                    Statue 144.A61 - Supp 1977).

FUNCTIONS/STANDARDS	RATING	COMMENTS
I. Helps to maintain a clean/safe comfortable environment for the patient/resident.		
A. Uses correct medical asepsis.		
1. Washes hands frequently and uses correct technique.	4	
2. Handles supplies and equipment using proper technique.	4	Remember to carry all equipment & touching uniform
3. Cleans and sanitizes patient unit and equipment.	4	
B. Prevents hazards of immobility.		
1. Uses elbow and heel protectors.	4	when Required
2. Uses sheepskin and alternating pressure mattress.	4	
3. Uses footboards and cradles.	4	
4. Follows positioning and turning schedules using correct procedures.	3	Remember all residents must be repositioned ē 2 hrs.
C. Provides for patient and employee protection and safety.		
1. Uses siderails and safety devices, as directed by the nurse.	5	
2. Adjusts the bed height.	4	when Available
3. Recognizes and removes environmental dangers.	4	
4. Provides easy access to the signal light.	4	
5. Answers signal promptly, without regard to whose patient it is.	3	Remember good teamwork- Answer lights regardless of whose patient when able

Figure 15-8   (Continued)

Nursing Assistant Job Description   -2-
and Evaluation continued

FUNCTIONS/STANDARDS	RATING	COMMENTS
6. Doesn't leave patient alone in tub or shower.	5	
7. Recognizes known hazards, common in a health care facility providing long term care.	4	
II. Patient Care		
A. Assists patients with basic personal care.		
1. Gives baths according to routine and as directed.	5	
2. Gives backrubs as directed.	4	Remember to do c daily cares
3. Cares for patient's hair.	5	does very well c this
4. Assists with, or gives oral hygiene and denture care.	4	
5. Gives perineal care as directed.	4	
6. Gives nail care as needed with weekly bath per accepted procedure.	3	all residents nails must be trimmed c ea. w/p, notify nurse if too long or thick
7. Gives skin care according to routine procedure.	4	
8. Assists patients with dressing/undressing as needed.	4	
9. Shaves patients as needed.	3	Remember our female residents require this Also
10. Changes bed linen according to schedule and as necessary.	4	
B. Assists patients with special care as directed by the nurse.	4	
1. Gives special skin care to treat or prevent skin breakdown.	4	
2. Uses support garments or stockings or Ace bandages correctly.	5	
3. Takes vital signs as directed.	NA	
III. Assists in providing nutrition and fluids.		
1. Prepares patients for meals.	4	
2. Serves correct tray to correct patient promptly-- checks tray card.	4	
3. Checks tray for correct food and accessories, sets up tray/food as needed.	4	

Figure 15–8 (Continued)

Nursing Assistant Job Description   -3-
and Evaluation continued

FUNCTIONS/STANDARDS	RATING	COMMENTS
4. Feeds patients when necessary.	4	
5. Reports changes in patient's appetite and intake to nurse.	4	
6. Records intake and output accurately, as directed.	4	
7. Oversee dining room as necessary.	4	
8. Supplies fresh water to patient at least two times per shift and as necessary.	3	reminder - fresh water to be given @ beginning of shift, as well as before leaving
9. Provides pleasant, social environment for patients in dining room at meal-times.	4	
IV. Assists patients in elimination needs.		
1. Places patient on bed-pan properly when necessary per accepted procedure.	4	
2. Offers urinal to male patients when necessary per accepted procedure.	4	
3. Assists patients with proper use of toilet.	4	
4. Follows established bowel and bladder retraining schedules.	NA	no resident on such schedule @ this time.
5. Collects routine urine and stool specimens.	NA	all specs obtained by nurse
6. Reports changes in patient's elimination pattern to nurse.	4	
V. A. With patients.		
1. Uses terminology, manner or speech, and non-verbal techniques appropriate to the individual's level of understanding.	4	
2. Shows awareness of sensory deficits by: a. establishes eye contact and speaks directly to the patient.	4	
b. uses low tone of voice.	4	
c. provides for quiet environment during conversations.	4	

Figure 15–8 (Continued)

Nursing Assistant Job Description   -4-
and Evaluation continued

FUNCTIONS/STANDARDS	RATING	COMMENTS
3. Explains actions and plans to patient before starting.	5	very good re: this
4. Treats patient information with confidentiality.	5	
5. Maintains a calm, pleasant manner.	5	is very professional
6. Uses touch as a means of communicating concern and comfort.	4	
7. Never, under any circumstances, abuses patient, physically or mentally.	5	
8. Reports changes in patient's responses to the nurse.	4	
B. With staff and supervisors.		
1. Maintains calm, pleasant and cooperative manner with staff.	4	
2. Handles complaints or grievances according to department procedure.	4	
3. Treats personal information about staff with confidentiality.	4	
4. Reports pertinent patient information to staff as necessary.	4	
5. Participates in the development of patient care plans.	4	
6. Willingly gives assistance, when possible, to fellow workers, who need help.	4	if unable, please tell them why. Remember how important team work is.
7. Treats fellow employees with consideration, tolerance and respect.	4	
8. Respects and follows chain of command.	4	
VI. Provides activity and exercise for patients with attention to safety and good body mechanics.		
1. Uses good posture and body alignment for self.	4	
2. Moves and lifts patients according to the nursing department procedure.	4	
3. Positions patients properly and turns them or repositions them every two hours and as often as necessary.	4	
4. Transfers patients with pivot transfer technique when appropriate.	4	

Figure 15-8   (Continued)

Nursing Assistant Job Description   -5-
and Evaluation continued

FUNCTIONS/STANDARDS	RATING	COMMENTS
5. Uses safety devices and transfer belts properly and when appropriate.	5	
6. Assists patients with exercises when directed:	3	please check list of Ambulatory residents
a. walking		
b. range of motion	4	
VII. Assists patients to deal with psycho-social needs.		
1. Helps patients deal with losses.	4	
2. Able to accept feelings and behavior of patients in a sensitive manner.	5	offers very effective communication
3. Displays patience in dealing with patients displaying angry and hostile behavior.	5	
4. Uses reality orientation techniques on all patients who are confused.	4	when indicated
5. Assist patients with transportation to scheduled activities/treatments provided by ancillary departments.	4	
6. Treats all patients as adults.	5	
VIII. Maintains good personal hygiene and grooming.		is always very neat et professional in appearance
1. Follows established departmental dress code.	5	
IX. Continuation of job knowledge.		
1. Attends accepted number of general inservice and unit meetings.	5	
2. Attends pertinent out-of-facility seminars, on a voluntary basis.	NA	
3. Keeps current with posted information in home-base lounge.	4	
4. Responsible for information posted on official and scheduling bulletin boards.	4	
5. Realizes knowledge or performance limitations and seeks appropriate assistance and retraining.	4	

Figure 15-8   (Continued)

Nursing Assistant Job Description   -6-
and Evaluation continued

	FUNCTIONS/STANDARDS	RATING	COMMENTS
X.	Is familiar with all established personnel and staffing policies/ procedures as outlined in the Personnel Manual. See attached reports.	4	
XI.	Overall rating in comparison to other employees in similiar position.	4	

GROWTH AREAS AND GOALS:

① Though Martha is very thorough c̄ residents ADL's, needs to concentrate on making sure nail care et showing, is also done on residents @ appropriate times.

② Martha is generally very pleasant c̄ all staff et residents, however have noticed a slip in amt of team work being done, c̄ more concentration on own assigned group. Please remember importance of team work. If there is a problem c̄ any of the other staff, please feel free to speak to one of the nurses re: your difficulty.

GENERAL COMMENTS:
    Martha is always very pleasant c̄ staff et residents. She displays excellent communication c̄ residents et treats them all c̄ respect et dignity. Her assigned residents always look very nice et are very happy. She is a very enjoyable person to have on staff. Keep up the good work, Martha!

Rated by: _Shelley A Raak_   _LPN_
            NAME   TITLE

This evaluation has been discussed with me.

_____   _____
EMPLOYEE SIGNATURE   DATE

Figure 15-8 (Continued)

nient for both persons. It should be scheduled in advance and not be a surprise encounter. The facility should have a small conference room to provide privacy for the meeting, figure 15–9.

Use effective communication techniques to help the person feel more comfortable initially and throughout the interview. Use broad opening statements about the resident unit or an area of personal interest to the nursing assistant. Next, clarify that the objective of the performance appraisal is to assist the person to do the best job that can be done. The appraisal tool should be reviewed, addressing both strengths and weaknesses in performance. Using the problem-solving approach, assist the person in outlining a specific plan for improving behavior. Have the person write down the steps to place more commitment in the plan. Close the interview with praise and set a future meeting time if there are plans or activities to review before the next performance appraisal.

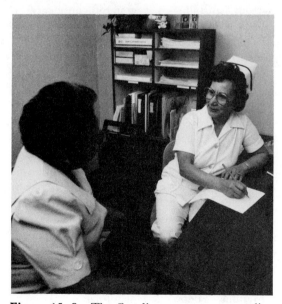

Figure 15–9 The first-line manager nurse discusses a performance appraisal with a nursing assistant (From Caldwell and Hegner, *Nursing Assistant*, 5th edition, copyright 1989 by Delmar Publishers Inc.)

If the appraisal interview becomes unproductive, it should be terminated and rescheduled. Excessive defensive behavior or anger does not result in an objective review of performance. The goal of the interview will not be met. The first-line manager nurse should set a new time to assure the review will be addressed and not avoided. At this time a decision can be made regarding the inclusion of the second-line manager in the next interview.

Preparing your first performance appraisals will probably be a stressor to you. It is an important responsibility to be fair and consistent in observing behavior, documenting it objectively, and presenting it verbally. Follow the steps discussed and seek advice and direction from the second-line manager.

Developing Personal Growth in the Workplace

In every workplace people want and need to have an identity; to be recognized for their contributions. A part of recognition is continual self-growth. When an athlete receives an award for a particular achievement, he must strive to improve on his record. He will not get ongoing applause for meeting the same goal every year. But his award motivates him to train more and beat his own record.

The same concept applies in the workplace. An individual wants and needs recognition; a pat-on-the-back or "thumb's up," a verbal "way to go," or a letter expressing a job well done, figure 15–10. For this recognition to be more than a one time event, the individual must be motivated to compete with past achievements, and strive for continual improvement and praise. It is the responsibility of the first-line manager nurse to recognize, praise, and motivate the nursing assistant.

Maslow's hierarchy, used in prioritizing resident needs, can also identify how a job meets the needs of the worker. The paycheck

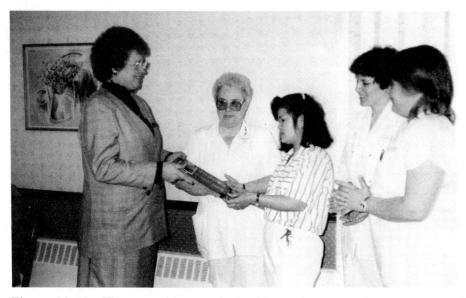

Figure 15–10 The recognition received with employee awards meets personal growth needs in the workplace.

helps meet physiological and security needs. It helps provide food and shelter and other basic needs. The employee benefit package that includes insurance and health care also meets the physiological and security needs. Other benefits that could apply relate to credit unions, profit-sharing, and uniform allowances.

The social, self-esteem, and self-actualization needs are met in other ways in the workplace. Social needs are met by being a member of a group. For the nursing assistant in a long term care facility, it is being a member of the resident unit on second floor, a member of the facility nursing assistant group, and being identified as a staff member of the facility as a whole. Another part of the social need is to be recognized, called by name, and accepted as a contributing worthwhile member.

Self-esteem needs will be met when the nursing assistant has a healthy self-concept nurtured by the first-line manager nurse and other facility staff. The result will be confidence in daily tasks and a good feeling about accomplishments. Such a positive impression can be "con-

tagious," instilling a degree of confidence in others. When self-esteem needs are met with a healthy self-concept in place, it will make the process of handling difficulties more manageable. When residents are irritable, other caregivers uncooperative, or unexpected problems surface, this nursing assistant will have a stronger coping mechanism in place.

Self-actualization may be accomplished in the nursing assistant role when the individual feels a broader sense of accomplishment. This sense of self-worth relates to meeting the needs of an elderly population group and contributing to the philosophy of the long term care facility. For many, this is a real sense of self-fulfillment and a feeling of contribution to society. For some, self-actualization means obtaining more education in nursing or other health related programs. Figure 15–11 summarizes the personal growth needs of the nursing assistant that are met in the workplace.

In managing a resident unit, the first-line manager nurse should be aware of personal growth needs of the nursing assistant caregivers.

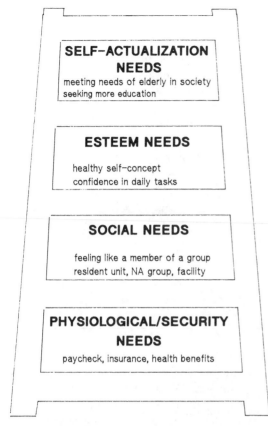

```
┌───────────────────────────┐
│    SELF–ACTUALIZATION     │
│          NEEDS            │
│  meeting needs of elderly in society │
│  seeking more education   │
└───────────────────────────┘

┌───────────────────────────┐
│      ESTEEM NEEDS         │
│                           │
│  healthy self–concept     │
│  confidence in daily tasks │
└───────────────────────────┘

┌───────────────────────────┐
│      SOCIAL NEEDS         │
│                           │
│  feeling like a member of a group │
│  resident unit, NA group, facility │
└───────────────────────────┘

┌───────────────────────────┐
│  PHYSIOLOGICAL/SECURITY   │
│          NEEDS            │
│  paycheck, insurance, health benefits │
└───────────────────────────┘
```

Figure 15–11 Meeting the personal growth needs in the workplace

Part of this awareness will be to learn about the individual's personal goals related to work and determine how they can fit into the resident unit goals. Learning the nursing assistants' likes and dislikes will assist in putting their talents to work to promote self-esteem and unit productivity. Ask for, and include, their suggestions for improving the unit activity. Nurturing personal growth needs reaps many benefits.

Summary

The process of managing human resources in the daily activities of a resident unit is an exciting challenge for the first-line manager nurse. Human resources are identified as the nursing skills and personal talents of each staff member. The first-line manager nurse must remember self as the resource that can ignite the talents of others.

Being able to manage one's self is a key ingredient for a successful first-line manager nurse. This includes a sense of self-awareness and a healthy self-concept. Developing a degree of assertiveness is important in maintaining the direction or working goals of the resident unit. Interferences in managing self are usually related to stressors that produce anxiety which result in nonproductive behavior. Due to the nature of health care, everyone needs to initiate stress management techniques.

Leadership characteristics applied to patient care can be adapted to the role of first-line manager. Those characteristics are: (1) knowledge, (2) judgement, (3) awareness, (4) creativity, (5) flexibility, (6) concern for others, (7) self-discipline, (8) attitude, and (9) positive role model. Nursing assistants view nurses as leaders with abilities to direct them. At the same time they desire to have their role valued and respected. As a positive role model, nurses represent themselves, the profession, and the facility where they are employed.

The roles of caregivers must be clarified for the most efficient functioning of the resident unit. The job description helps in defining the roles. Task lists may be developed from the job description to assist in day-to-day assignments.

Team planning coordinates the roles of the caregivers in completing the activities in the resident unit. Delegating is part of team planning. Personality traits and individual abilities are considered in the decision-making process. This assists in determining the right individual for a task.

Conflicts can occur between caregivers or between the caregiver and a task required of the role. The conflicts are usually related to personal values or beliefs. The first-line manager nurse needs to use a problem-solving approach to assist in resolving conflicts.

Providing appropriate disciplinary action

for the nursing assistant is part of the role of the first-line manager nurse. Discipline is usually required when a facility policy or procedure has not been followed. The objective of discipline is to correct unsatisfactory behavior and not to punish the individual.

An orientation program is necessary in every workplace. In long-term care the first-line manager is involved in this process with peers; it usually involves orienting a new nurse to the resident unit. The first-line manager nurse represents nursing as practiced in the facility and assists the new nurse to become acquainted with the residents and staff.

The first-line manager nurse completes performace appraisals for nursing assistants.

Some facilities incorporate a combined job description and performance appraisal. Most forms have a ranking system to evaluate performance and provide an opportunity for written objective comments. Knowledge, skills, and attitude behaviors expected of the role are appraised. A private interview time is scheduled for the first-line manager nurse and the nursing assistant to review the performance appraisal.

Finally, most people want more out of a job than a paycheck. Personal growth outcomes are needed for the person to experience recognition and self-worth. It is part of the role of the first-line manager nurse to nurture the nursing assistant to meet social, esteem, and self-actualization needs.

For Discussion

- Make a list of 10 phrases that describe you. Share the list with a classmate. Identify the attributes that are leadership characteristics.
- Recall clinical experiences with patient assignments. What characteristics of leadership did you implement to complete your assignment?
- What stressors have you seen in licensed nurses that have interfered with their management of patient care?
- Identify personal growth outcomes you are experiencing in your nursing education.
- Recall performance appraisals you have received in workplaces before your nursing education. What were your positive and negative feelings about the experiences?

Questions for Review

1. List four characteristics of successful leaders.
2. Define proactive planning.
3. Identify two points to consider when delegating a task.
4. When is disciplinary action appropriate?
5. What document clarifies role responsibilities?
6. What is the role of the first-line manager in appraising the performance of nursing assistants?
7. What are two responsibilities of first-line managers in orienting peers to the resident unit?
8. What are two personal growth outcomes in the workplace?

Unit 16
Additional Influences on Nursing Management

Objectives

After reading this unit you should be able to:

- Describe geographical influences on nursing practice in long term care facilities.
- Discuss the impact of facility ownership on nursing practice in long-term care.
- Identify first-line manager leadership characteristics expected by long term care facility management.
- Discuss the public's expectations of the first-line manager nurse.

The practice of nursing is so comprehensive that it is almost impossible, in any health care setting, to define borders of impact. The influence of your patient care and teaching travels far beyond the patient's bedside. Nurses make statements that are valued by their patients and the public. Perhaps you have heard someone say, "My nurse said I should put my feet up when I'm sitting." Families and visitors listen intently to your comments. Your style of nursing is reflected in your interpersonal skills. It sends a clear message, "The nurses at Highrise Manor are really nice." The community also sends signals that influence the practice environment of the nurse.

In this unit the discussion will focus on factors outside of the resident unit that influence its functioning. This includes the geographical setting of the long term care facility, Midwest or Southwest, urban or rural. The ownership of a facility, whether church, community, or government, will also influence the flow of activity in the resident unit. The administrative management, nursing management, and particularly the management style of the second-line manager directly affect the functioning of the resident unit.

The influence of these outside factors on the activity of the resident unit is primarily in the atmosphere or general tone of the environment; it affects the spirit, mood, and social aspects of the resident unit. The scope of geographical influence is so broad that only a sampling will be identified in this unit.

Understanding the complex nature of owning and operating a long term care facility is not expected of first-line manager nurses. Examples of ownership factors will be presented for you to see how they influence your responsibilities as a first-line manager nurse.

Environmental Influences on Nursing Practice

Where you have chosen to complete your nursing education is an environmental influence on your clinical experience as a student. The setting may be a metropolitan area or a small community. Your acute care experience may be scheduled in a large research hospital or a 100-bed community hospital. The long-term care assignments may be in a 250-bed corporate facility or a 30-bed community facility, figure 16–1.

The first-line manager nurse in a long term care facility will find the atmosphere of nursing practice influenced by the geographic setting of the facility. The nurse who has lived in a neighborhood or community for a long time and practices in that area may not realize the environmental influences. It is when the nurse relocates to another community that the effects of life styles, traditions, and other factors become evident. This situation could also occur with a resident. For example, a woman in North Dakota may choose to live in a long term care facility in Los Angeles to be near her son and family. The lifestyle of southern California living would be reflected in the long term care facility. This may be a new experience for the North Dakota woman.

Primary language may be an influence with residents or other caregivers in the facility. Young people who emigrated with their families

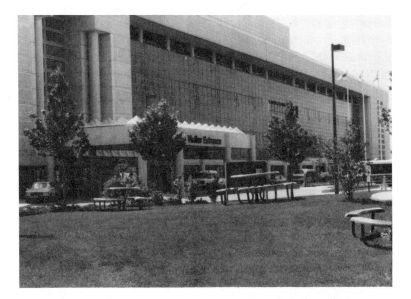

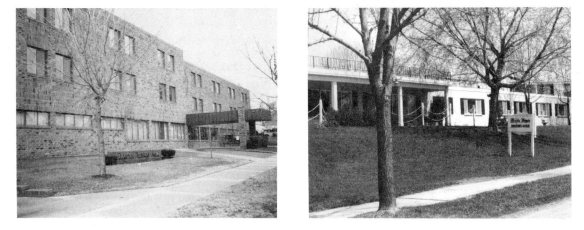

Figure 16–1   The setting and size of the facility will influence the management of the resident unit.

from Southeast Asia in the 1970s are now in the work force. Most of this population became Americanized quickly and learned the English language. Some had finished school in their native country and may not be as fluent in English.

The primary language influence may be reflected in many communities. Remember, some residents nearing the century mark may be first generation immmigrants. They may not have needed to develop sophisticated language and communication skills to be successful in their productive years. Long term care facilities in particular regions of the country, or in ethnic neighborhoods, may have a group of residents that prefer to speak the language of their native home. The flow of the resident unit may be smoother if some caregivers live in the community and are more familiar with the language and traditions of the residents.

The style of English usage varies from region to region and from generation to generation. If all the nursing assistants are young people, the residents might not understand current accepted language expressions. However, no one should underestimate the desire of some residents to be "hip," "cool," or whatever the current operative phrase may be. The bottom line, of course, is to be sure the message is clear by using effective communication skills.

Food preferences and meal planning may be another influence on the functioning of the resident unit. The first-line manager is not directly responsible for diets or meal planning, but is responsible for monitoring weight, hydration, and general nutritional status. Most elderly in long term care facilities established eating patterns when meals were "plain" meat, potatoes, vegetables, and bread, each in a special corner of the plate! Today's variety of Americanized ethnic food may seem "exotic" to some residents. Pizza may become a more welcomed meal when you are the elderly population!

Meal planning in a long term care facility generally reflects the preferences of the neighborhood or area. A resident who lived most of

his life in another region may not enjoy the local menus or seasoning. The first-line manager nurse must keep alert to the environmental influences when developing a resident care plan.

The sense of community and availability of family are important influences on the resident unit. These factors are difficult to discuss in relation to geographical region or urban and rural settings. The rural community has a tendency to "adopt" residents; most have probably lived in the community during all their adult life. The churches and community groups include the residents in their activites, visit them on a regular basis, and may take them into their homes for a meal. The first-line manager nurse incorporates this sense of community into the unit plan. Families and visitors will be part of the daily activity.

This same sense of community can occur in an older established neighborhood in a large city. The opposite can also occur. Because of the size of the city, undefined neighborhoods, or absent family members, the residents can be more isolated. Community service groups, scout groups, and others can provide programs and entertainment, figure 16–2. However, some resi-

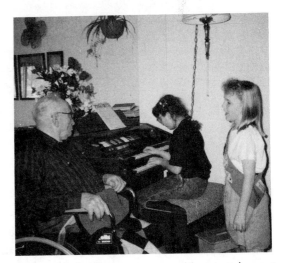

Figure 16–2 Scout troops provide entertainment and include residents as part of the community.

dents are not comfortable if they do not personally know members of the service groups. In these situations, the nursing staff becomes family to this resident.

The family unit will play a dominant role in the planning and functioning of the resident unit. Their preferences, requests, degree of participation, response to resident placement, and other concerns will be reflected in the resident care plan. The first-line manager nurse may devote almost as much time to the family as to the resident.

The lifestyle of residents, and activities scheduled by the facility, all interact and influence the team planning of the unit. Generally, the resident population will reflect the lifestyle of the area. The residents in a rural facility may be primarily retired farmers and small town merchants. They may prefer scheduled days for fishing at a nearby lake, or to go for a ride to check the progress of the crops. A picnic-type celebration in the facility is enjoyed and careful attention to local news is important.

The resident population group in a metropolitan area may include more retired professional people. A day out planned to see a baseball game, an afternoon symphony concert, or lunch at a sidewalk cafe may be enjoyed. Perhaps these were favorite activities during younger years.

These examples are a sampling of potential influences on the resident unit. To organize time efficiently and implement the unit activity smoothly, the first-line manager must be aware of the practice setting and the family and community influences on daily planning. Figure 16–3 summarizes geographical influences on nursing practice in a long term care facility.

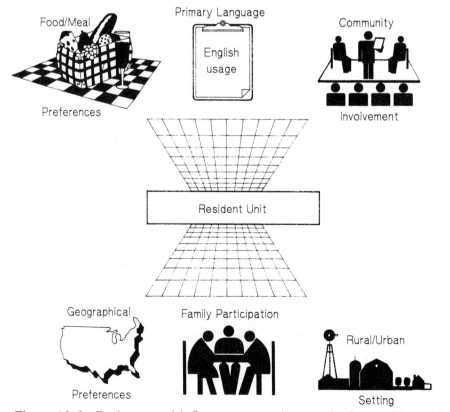

Figure 16–3   Environmental influences on nursing practice in a resident unit

Facility Ownership Influences on Nursing Practice

To the new first-line manager nurse, the ownership and business management of the facility does not seem to be related to the nursing management of a resident unit. However, there are many direct and indirect influences of owner philosophy and policy on the atmosphere and functioning of the unit. Having a basic understanding of these factors assists the nurse in planning resident unit activity.

In a small community facility the owner/administrator may be visiting residents almost on a daily basis, figure 16-4. In a large corporate facility, perhaps only a few staff members have met an owner or member of the board of directors during an on-site visit.

Requests for equipment may be channeled through the appropriate departments and to decision makers in a few days in a smaller or locally owned facility. In a corporate system,

similar requests may have to be sent to the home office or submitted for annual budgets. Ordering resident supplies may follow a similar procedure. In some facilities a local pharmacy may process orders, and in others a large amount of supplies are ordered monthly from a wholesale distributor.

In a large corporate facility the forms for resident records, employee files, interdepartmental memos, and other communication may be uniform throughout the system. Every facility uses the same documents. In smaller facilities, there may be more flexibility in the format for paperwork. Standard forms, purchased from office supply companies, may be implemented. When the nursing staff proposes a change in a chart format in the smaller facility, it may be adopted fairly quickly. The process to channel a change through committees and departments is a less complex project.

These are a few examples of how the ownership and the system of operating a facility could

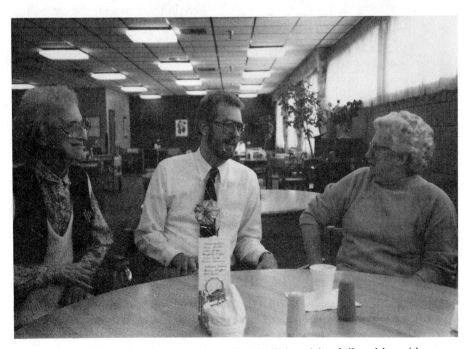

Figure 16-4 The administrator of smaller facilities visits daily with residents.

influence the functioning of the resident unit. The first-line manager may need to do more long-range ordering of supplies in one facility than in another. When you are employed as a first-line manager in a facility, it will be helpful to develop a basic understanding of the general operation of the facility.

Government Influences

Nonprofit and for-profit facilities must be licensed by the state in which they are located. Each state sets standards for regulations and periodically conducts surveys of facilities. It may be the state health department that is responsible for the rules and regulations that implement the law. Survey teams evaluate the quality of care by reviewing resident records, infection control, and safety procedures; they observe nurses during resident care, and visit with residents. The quality of care evaluated is the outcome of all the policies and procedures of the facility.

The state licenses facilities for skilled and intermediate care. *Skilled* care means the resident's acuity and level of dependence require the skills of licensed nurses to assess and monitor the resident's condition. *Intermediate* means that the resident has a degree of independence, and does not need continual monitoring by a licensed nurse.

An example of federal government influence on caregivers in a long term care facility is the directive to employ nursing assistants who have completed minimum training requirements. In the 1980s many states began to require a basic course which taught personal care tasks. These were 30 or more hours of class with or without a skill test. More recently the federal government mandated a 75-hour course for nursing assistants working in long-term care. This is a nationwide directive providing for a uniform level of competence.

Any facility that participates in federally financed programs (Medicare and Medicaid) is required to be certified for these programs.

Under federal guidelines the state surveys and regulates the facilities. Resident acuity and the appropriate care required are major concerns of these programs.

In the ongoing cost containment goals of the healthcare delivery system, the Medicare and Medicaid guidelines are in a continual review and revision process. The first-line manager nurse needs to be aware that some supplies will be covered and some will not under these programs. The resident or family may need to make a decision as to whether they want to purchase a supply that is not reimbursed by a funding program. In some situations the facility may be required to cover the cost of supplies ordered by the nurse, but not covered by government or private insurance programs.

The first-line manager nurse may feel this is all very complicated. It is! It is the responsibility of the second- and third-line managers and other facility staff to have an in-depth understanding of payment systems. As a first-line manager nurse you will need to ask questions that relate to your responsibilities in directing the care on the resident unit.

Types of Facility Ownership

Examples of ownership of a facility are non-profit, for-profit, and government owned. An example of a nonprofit facility is one that is owned by a church. Two types of for-profit are ownership by an individual or family, and ownership by a corporation. The federal government operates long term care facilities through the Veterans Administration.

Nonprofit Facilities. Churches are the major owners of nonprofit long term care facilities. Ownership may be in the form of a single community church or a large denomination owning several facilities throughout the country. If a corporation has been formed by the denomination, any assets remaining after expenses are placed in a trust to upgrade or replace facilities. A board of directors who volunteer their time govern the policies of the facility.

Residents in this facility may be affiliated with the religious preference of the sponsoring denomination, but are not limited to this group. The attitude and philosophy of the church are reflected in the atmosphere of the facility; a chaplain may be a member of the staff, figure 16–5. The church may have an auxiliary and other volunteer groups to service social and spiritual needs of the residents.

For-profit Facilities. A for-profit long term care facility may be privately owned by an individual or family. The owner is often the administrator and family members may comprise a majority of the governing board. Two or three people from the community may be on the board to provide expertise in finances or government operations.

The atmosphere may be family oriented in a small facility. It may be less formal than a corporate for-profit facility. The owner may grill hamburgers for a resident picnic and dance with residents at the Valentine's Day Ball. The personality of the owner and family will be reflected in the day-to-day functioning of the resident unit. Concerns and suggestions expressed by the first-line manager may at some time be heard directly by the owner/administrator.

Corporate for-profit facilities may be owned by a business group within a state or by a very large organization with facilities in several states. Today, corporations are diversified and many own a variety of businesses in which the services or products are not directly related to one another. The governing boards of these long term care facilities represent a wide variety of expertise. Board members may or may not be salaried. Stockholders would receive dividends on their investment in this for-profit facility.

Policies are usually uniform throughout the corporation's long term care facilities. Nursing staff may see corporate consultants assisting with policies and procedures. Perhaps a corporate staff development person designs inservices to be implemented in each facility. A dietitian

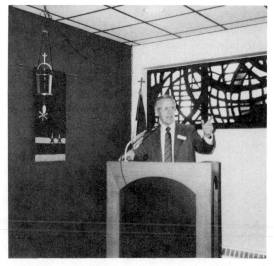

Figure 16–5 Chaplains are staff members in church owned facilities.

may be employed to oversee meal planning in several facilities. Although the first-line manager may feel encumbered with less flexible policies, the expertise of corporate consultants may be of great value in organizing time and managing the resident unit.

Government Owned Facilities. Long term care facilities can be operated by all three levels of government: local, state, and federal. The community or locally controlled facility is owned by the city and governed by the city council. This group functions much like a board of directors. Federal and state program funds as well as local taxes may support this facility. The citizens may have a lot of pride in this facility and make it a community effort to provide for the needs of older community members. In decisions that require a vote by the community, there may be a considerable amount of time and energy involved in the decision-making process.

Nurses responsible for the resident unit in a community facility must be aware of community attitudes and beliefs regarding the facility. Civic and volunteer groups servicing the facility may feel a sense of ownership. Residents may have been members of these service groups in their younger years.

Individual states may have long term care facilities operated with federal and state funding programs and state taxes or other state sources of revenue. A commission of appointees from the public and private sector are responsible for the policies governing the facility.

Some state facilities have resident units comprised of elderly with behavioral problems. These residents may have physical conditions such as chronic brain syndromes that have resulted in violent behavior. They have not responded to therapy and pose a potential safety threat to themselves, other residents, and staff.

Nurses practicing in state facilities need to be aware of operating policies that affect planning resident care. This population group of residents may not all be from the community. Some residents may need placement in a facility hundreds of miles from their home. Civic or fraternal groups often support these residents with programs, services, and one-to-one visiting.

The federal government operates long term care facilities through the Veterans Administration. Federal funds support the health needs of veterans. Guidelines for policies and regulations are developed and implemented by the Veterans Administration. They inspect facilities for compliance with regulations.

Facilities for aging veterans are located regionally. Some residents may be a long distance from their homes and families. Service groups such as the Veterans of Foreign Wars (VFW), Daughters of the American Revolution (DAR), and others give support to the residents of a Veteran's Home.

Nurses employed in these facilities are employees of the federal government. Employment practices, salary schedules, and other benefits are uniform throughout the system. As caregivers in these facilities, nurses need to remember the life experiences of this population group. The physical and emotional trauma of

military service may compound the general aging process.

Nursing Practice and Facility Ownership

The nurse applying for a position should read the philosophy statement of the long term care facility. This is often stated in public information brochures as well as in employee orientation packets. Your beliefs and personality will need to blend with that of the facility. A large corporate facility may feel overwhelming and not be the warm cozy atmosphere of your small town experience. Perhaps a church affiliated facility makes you feel uncomfortable because it is a faith different from your own. If you cannot adapt and enjoy your working environment, perhaps you should seek employment in a facility where the philosophy and atmosphere are a closer fit to your own.

This overview of some influences of facility ownership on the functioning of the resident unit will assist the first-line manager nurse in planning the functioning of the resident unit. How the ownership of a long term care facility influences management of the resident unit is shown in figure 16–6.

First-Line Manager Leadership Qualities Expected by Facility Management

The first-line manager nurse interacts most frequently with upper level management through the second-line manager nurse. Second-line managers in long term care facilities must place a considerable amount of trust in the first-line manager. Many second-line managers are responsible for several resident units. To manage their time efficiently, this nurse must delegate the role and authority of first-line manager to the nurse in that position. The trust occurs in believing the tasks will be implemented accurately and efficiently. In addition, it is expected that

NONPROFIT FACILITIES
- Churches are major owners: single church or a denomination
- Monies remaining after expenses are used to upgrade or replace facilities
- Governed by board of directors who volunteer their time
- Philosophy of church reflected in facility atmosphere
- Residents may be affiliated with, but not limited to, religious preference of ownership denomination.

FOR-PROFIT FACILITIES
- Privately owned: individual or family
  - Business providing income for individual or family
  - Governing board mostly family members; owner is often the administrator
  - Atmosphere may be family oriented, reflecting the personality of the individual or family
  - Residents may be from neighborhood, or adult children may live in the area
- Corporate owned: local business enterprise or large corporation owning many facilities
  - Profits disbursed to stockholders in dividends on their investments
  - Governing boards represent a variety of business expertise; may be local or national board
  - Atmosphere may reflect local control and tradition, or national uniform corporate policies
  - Residents may be from community; corporate policies are reflected in daily care

GOVERNMENT OWNED FACILITIES
- Community or locally owned: a business for the community
  - Supported by local taxes plus federal and state programs
  - Governed by the city or community council
  - Atmosphere reflects the community's sense of ownership; citizen volunteers may be involved in daily activity
  - Residents are usually members of the community; they personally know staff and volunteers
- State owned: a business for the state
  - Supported by state taxes or other revenue plus federal and state programs
  - Governed by appointees from public and private sector
  - Atmosphere may reflect local traditions; civic or fraternal groups may be involved in activities
  - Residents may not be from immediate area; families may have frequent or infrequent involvement in care
- Federally owned: services for government and military employees
  - Supported through federal funds and programs
  - Governed primarily by the Veteran's Administration
  - Atmosphere reflects that of large facilities in a government operation
  - Residents are long distances from home; have comradeship of other veterans, support from service groups

Figure 16–6   Summary of ownership influence on the resident unit

the second-line manager will receive appropriate information and feedback, figure 16–7.

Characteristics of leadership are considered when the second-line manager appraises the performance of the first-line manager nurse; it is an ongoing assessment of leadership abilities. Second-line managers' expectations are also based on the months or years of experience a nurse has accumulated in a leadership position. They are willing to assist nurses with ongoing development in leadership responsibilities.

Knowledge

Knowledge expectations begin with the theory base and procedure skill ability acquired in nursing education. First-line manager nurses are expected to use references to verify observations or procedure steps. They need to inform second-line managers when there is a procedure new to them which may require a demonstration or supervision by the inservice nurse. The first-line manager is expected to attend inservices, workshops, and read periodicals to keep current in practice.

The first-line manager is expected to learn federal and state regulations that apply to the functioning of the resident unit. Many procedures have been developed from regulations that meet the laws. The Resident Bill of Rights is an example.

Meeting regulations includes documenting specific information at identified time intervals on resident records. There are safety regulations for residents, staff, and equipment. Examples include restraint orders, temperature of facility water heaters, and the use of transfer or gait belts. Although procedures are usually developed by other levels of management, the first-line manager must be aware of regulations and report compliance or problems.

Regulations also apply to the complex funding of resident care. The first-line manager becomes involved when ordering supplies and medications, or scheduling therapies or appointments for residents. An example may be in scheduling appointments at the facility beauty

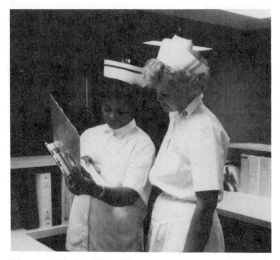

Figure 16–7 First-line manager confers with second- and third-line managers when appropriate.

shop. Haircuts and weekly shampoos are usually included in the charge for the resident's room. A permanent wave is an example of an extra charge. This nurse must know if the resident or family will pay for this service. The facility management may tell you, "Don't order it until you find out who will pay for it!" This is the decade of cost awareness! The second-line manager expects you to have a general understanding of procedures and the wisdom to verify situations with facility policy and procedure manuals.

Skill

Being able to make decisions regarding resident care and the functioning of the resident unit is expected of the first-line manager by the facility management. The decisions are good judgements based on nursing education and experience. Second-line managers evaluate quick thinking and problem solving abilities to determine how the first-line manager will respond in a time of crisis. The nurse is expected to respond in a calm and professional manner that conveys confidence and reassurance.

Skills of organizing time and prioritizing tasks are expected. This also includes having foresight and intuition to anticipate needs of the residents and unit. It is being proactive rather than reactive; the skills should be self-directed. Second-line managers do not want to have to supervise every task of the first-line manager.

The first-line manager nurse is expected to have the self discipline to direct and control the resident unit activity. When unplanned activity occurs that could threaten that control, the second-line manager expects the nurse to request help to maintain control.

The facility management expects the first-line manager to utilize effective communication techniques with residents, all staff and departments, family members, and visitors. This nurse is a major link between the resident and the facility, and the resident and the community. Effective communication influences residents' care, efficiency in the functioning of the facility, confidence of the resident's family, and the reputation of the facility.

Attitude

The owner and the administration, of the long term care facility expect an attitude of loyalty. The first-line manager nurse, like other employees, is a representative of the facility. This means being faithful and supportive to the philosophy and efforts of the facility. Loyalty means being proud to be an employee, sharing in service to the elderly in the community.

Like families, long term care facilities will have problems because of all the people involved in the operation of the facility. The management expects loyal employees to work out resident, employee, and facility problems through problem-solving channels, not to speak derogatorily of the facility in public.

Long term care facilities, like all health care facilities, expect strict resident confidentiality. First-line manager nurses must be aware of this demand as it is a responsibility of all nurses in any practice setting.

The second-line manager observes the attitude and response of the first-line manager regarding dependability and responsibility. It is expected that the nurse is motivated and self-directed to demonstrate this behavior and maintain the level of trust necessary for the role. Being a positive role model for nursing assistants and presenting a positive image to the public is expected. Residents and nursing assistants feel confident in the nurse that creates a sense of authority.

Long term care facilities expect the first-line manager to have an attitude of productivity in being meaningfully occupied when there are free moments. Being aware of this expectation assists the first-line manager nurse in delegating tasks, and guiding the nursing assistant to utilize time in a productive manner.

An example of guiding the nursing assistant in utilizing time wisely is in organizing tasks into blocks of time. This provides time to accomplish short-duration tasks. One block of time completes residents' personal care; the next block includes activity surrounding the residents' lunch. Some nursing assistants may gather near the nurses' station after the personal care is completed to wait for the meal trays. The first-line manager can guide the nursing assistant to make use of this time by ambulating residents, checking linen supplies, or reading birthday cards to a resident.

The knowledge, skills, and attitudes expected of the first-line manager nurse include a wide variety of abilities. To be successful in the position, this nurse must maintain effective communication with the second-line manager. Figure 16–8 summarizes the long term care facility's expectations of the first-line manager nurse.

Public Expectations of the First-Line Manager

The families of residents have a great need to develop trust in the first-line manager nurses who are reponsible for the care of a family

KNOWLEDGE

- General knowledge of nursing theory and procedure skills
- Know own limits: verify observations and procedures with nursing references, seek assistance from second-line manager
- Increase nursing knowledge through inservices, workshops
- Learn basic concepts of federal and state regulations, and funding sources related to resident care
- Learn facility policies and procedures the influence the functioning of the resident unit

SKILL

- Ability to complete nursing skills and procedures accurately and safely
- Ability to organize time and prioritize tasks
- Ability to make and implement decisions based on good nursing judgement
- Ability to be self-directed and self-motivated
- Ability to be self-disciplined to control unit activity
- Ability to use effective communication skills

ATTITUDE

- Displays loyalty to the facility
- Displays willingness to address problems through facility problem-solving channels
- Demonstrates resident confidentiality in all situations
- Displays dependability and responsibility to facility
- Demonstrates positive role model behavior for nursing assistants; positive nursing image to the public

Figure 16–8   The facility's expectations of the first-line manager

member. Families expect this nurse to be able to answer questions regarding the current activity and health status of their relative. This means keeping updated with the resident's chart and other references, not commenting, "Well, I don't know, I wasn't here yesterday."

The trust level is needed because the family has made the decision to make the long term care facility the home of their parent or other family member. Other units have discussed the difficulty people have with this decision. The family expects a considerable amount of dedication to their relative from the nursing staff, figure 16–9.

Residents and visitors expect the first-line manager to be able to answer general questions about the facility. This includes schedules, routines, and directions to departments and other staff in the building. You are not expected to know all the details, but to be willing to locate the information. Remember, to protect resident privacy and confidentiality, be sure you determine the name of the individual and his relationship to the resident.

Families also expect the first-line manager nurse to have a general knowledge of facility policies and procedures that affect the resident. This may include services to care for the resident's personal clothing, the procedure for having a birthday party in the facility, or how to arrange for transportation services.

You are expected to have the knowledge and skills in nursing to answer health questions and give directions to residents and family members. If a resident is able to leave the facility for a few days to celebrate a holiday with the

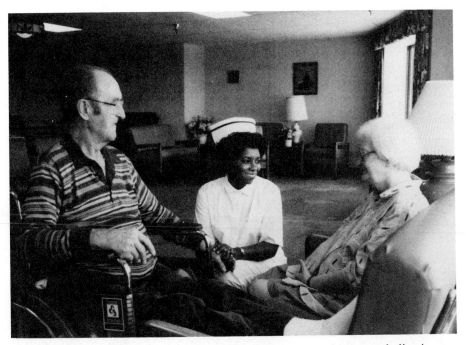

Figure 16–9   The family trusts the first-line manager and expects dedication to the elderly.

family, her treatments will need to be continued; medications and supplies for treatments are sent with her. The family expects the nurse to give clear, simple directions.

Families, in particular, expect the first-line manager to be in control of the resident unit. Most people can evaluate this control just by watching and listening to nurses. Residents are very candid in explaining resident unit activity to family members. Families also expect the first-line manager nurse to be responsible for all activities on the unit, including actions taken by nursing assistants.

The public, family, visitors, community groups, and others coming to the long term care facility expect the first-line manager nurse to demonstrate social etiquette and professional ethics. These are the same principles you have discussed in other nursing courses relating to patient care.

Remember that instilling confidence and trust in families and visitors is always an effi-

cient use of time. Avoiding a confrontation or dismissing a complaint may require additional hours in days ahead to reestablish confidence. The trust level may never return. A sampling of the many individuals having a variety of expectations of the first-line manager nurse is illustrated in figure 16–10.

Summary

Many factors outside of the resident unit influence the directing of unit activities by the first-line manager nurse. The geographic location of the facility will affect the atmosphere of daily activity. The region of the country and the metropolitan or rural setting will reflect the traditions of the area and the earlier life styles of the residents.

A sense of community in the neighborhood or town will be reflected in the visitors and volunteer groups that service residents. They

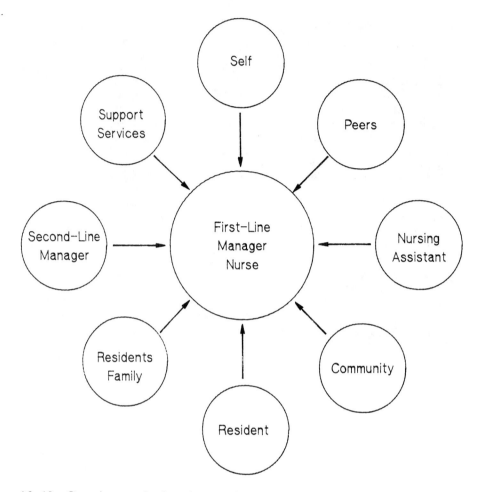

Figure 16–10   Caregivers and others have differing expectations of the first-line manager's role.

may assist with religious services, holiday parties, and other events. The first-line manager nurse needs to consider this sense of community in daily team planning. These events have great significance to residents and visitors.

The extent of family participation with the activities of an individual resident or a resident unit will influence time management and implementation of care. There will be time planned to answer questions and arrange for family activities.

Who owns the long term care facility will influence the activity of the resident unit. Facil-

ities are organized as nonprofit or for-profit and may be individually or corporately owned. The funding of the resident's care has perhaps the greatest influence on the first-line manager nurse's directing of the resident unit. Funds are provided through the state and federal government when facilities meet regulations. The nurse must gain a basic understanding of funding sources and reimbursement guidelines. It is particularly important in documenting care, ordering supplies, and making arrangements for resident care.

Another influence of facility ownership on

the resident unit's functioning is the interaction of administration in the daily activity. Requests for new equipment or changes in procedures may occur quickly in a small family-owned facility, but take longer in channeling through a corporate structure. First-line manager nurses in large corporations may benefit from consultants in education, management, or other specialties.

Long term care facility management expects leadership qualities in first-line manager nurses. Expectations of the first-line manager nurse by the second-line manager and other administrators include: (1) knowledge of nursing theory and skills; (2) knowledge of facility policy and procedures; (3) basic understanding of state and federal regulations and funding of resident care; (4) ability to organize and prioritize tasks and make decisions; (5) ability to function independently; (6) use of effective communication with residents, all staff, families, and visitors;

and (7) ability to be a good role model for nursing and represent the long term care facility. The second-line manager places a considerable amount of trust in the first-line manager nurse and delegates the authority to manage the unit.

Families of residents, visitors, and other community members also have expectations of the first-line manager nurse. They need to develop a high level of trust in those providing care for their relatives. Nurses who answer questions directly, are willing to problem solve, and project genuine interest in the elderly will be respected by the public.

The topics discussed in this unit may not seem to relate to resident care and all the skills and procedures you have studied. When you look at the far-reaching influences of your nursing practice, and the complex nature of the community where you practice, these factors do affect your resident care and responsibilities for directing the resident unit.

For Discussion

- Identify environmental factors that influence the care of your assigned residents.
- Interview a nurse employed in the position of a first-line manager nurse in a long term care facility. Determine some aspects of facility ownership that influence the directing of the resident unit.
- Interview neighbors or friends who have a family member living in a long term care facility. Ask them what qualities they expect in the nurses responsible for their relative's care.

Questions for Review

1. What are four geographical factors that influence directing the care in a resident unit?
2. What are the three types of ownership for long term care facilities?
3. What are two situations where the first-line manager nurse needs a basic understanding of methods of funding for resident care?
4. What are six qualities that second-line managers expect in first-line manager nurses?
5. What are two qualities the public expects in first-line manager nurses?

Unit 17
Styles of Management
for the Resident Unit

Objectives

After reading this unit you should be able to:

- Describe a participative style of management.
- Describe a directive style of management.
- Describe a motivational style of management.
- Discuss how group dynamics is involved in managing a resident unit.

Styles of management explain the relationship between people and their work. Management, as defined in the beginning of this section, is the act of controlling, arranging, or directing an activity. How that activity is directed and controlled is the style of managing and is the technique or process used to direct the activity.

There are many variables in the choice of management style. A person's personality and method of dealing with daily activities will influence the management style in the workplace. The types of tasks to be accomplished, the experience of the workers, and the external and internal regulations in the workplace are additional factors that influence the style of management. For example, a fire emergency would require directive style management in implementing fire code policies.

Three basic styles of management can be observed in the long-term care setting. All three are useful in selected situations. The success in directing a resident unit is not in the exclusive use of one, but in the blending of the three.

A *participative* or democratic style distributes responsibility and authority to all members of the group. This means that in the resident unit, the nursing assistants would take an active part in the problem-solving and decision-making process of resident care.

A second style of management is the directive approach or autocratic management. The *directive* style of management keeps authority and decision making with the manager. This style does not permit team members to be involved in the problem-solving process related to resident care.

The *motivational* style is people oriented and based on the belief that a person's attitudes and feelings about work are directly related to performance. This style of management is also known as the laissez-faire style. The style promotes self-direction in work with ongoing positive comments regarding productivity and results. Giving nursing assistants frequent or daily compliments and encouragement is part of a motivational style of managing.

The first-line manager nurse needs to have a basic understanding of management styles to determine which approach is the most appropriate to complete a task or direct a resident unit. Being aware of styles of management assists in problem-solving nonproductive situations within the unit. For example, a nursing assistant having considerable autonomy in a previous job may resent a consistent directive approach by the first-line manager nurse. The nurse will explain to the nursing assistant the need for the directive approach, or examine the unit activity for a possible change in management style.

Group dynamics are the energies in individuals that make members of the group function as a whole to meet a goal. These energies may be physical or emotional, strong or weak, creative or passive, verbal or nonverbal. The group needs to be interdependent.

This unit will present an overview of the basic ideas of these three styles of management. You will be able to determine what styles you have used in other work, organizations, or volunteer groups. This discussion will provide you an opportunity to think about a style that may work best for you. Reflecting on your membership in a variety of groups will assist you in understanding group dynamics.

Participative Style

A participative style of management promotes a distribution of responsibility and authority throughout the workplace. It utilizes the group in solving problems to complete tasks and meet goals.

Two approaches to the participative style are formal and informal methods of directing activity. The formal approach involves meetings, written goals, and identifying tasks to meet the goals. Members of the group volunteer for specific responsibilities or are delegated tasks by the leader. The leader coordinates the efforts of the group and schedules additional meetings to review progress and make necessary changes in the plan.

Formal Participative Examples

Your participation in scouting, or other groups when you were a youngster, is an example of this style of management. A leader organized the efforts of the group for a fundraising activity, and members volunteered or were assigned publicity, collecting money, canvassing neighborhoods, and other tasks. Charts monitored progress and problems were addressed in meetings. The success was celebrated, positive and negative events were discussed, and recommendations made for future fundraisers.

In long-term care, an example of formal participative style management is in the safety or infection control committee. Representatives from the resident unit, nursing management, housekeeping, maintenance, administration, and other departments meet on a regular basis to address policies and problems related to the safety of residents and staff in the facility. The staff member responsible for safety or infection control is the leader of the group. Other members are responsible for information or activities that relate to their department.

On a resident unit a meeting of team members or a resident care conference encourages a participative style of management. Resident care plans are revised with team members providing information about their part of resident care and offering suggestions for change, figure 17–1.

This formal method of participative management can be time consuming. It requires time for meetings and documentation in addition to the time on task for each member's responsibilities. However, the method is goal oriented and time limited. This means a project will not go on forever! It forces a group to work together and progress can be measured.

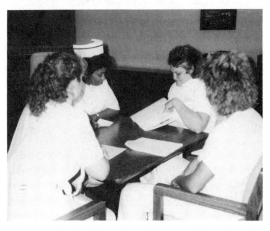

Figure 17–1 The first-line manager implements participative management during a team meeting.

Informal Participative Examples

An informal style of participative management is a practice style. This does not require written objectives and is useful in daily tasks in the workplace. Meetings may be informal brainstorming. *Brainstorming* is a technique of group problem solving that encourages creative thinking and spontaneous participation.

In the long-term care setting this informal participative management occurs daily as resident care problems are solved. Perhaps a resident requiring oxygen and gastrostomy feeding equipment is admitted. The first-line manager nurse and nursing assistants assemble in the resident's room. Nursing assistants will discuss the placement of furniture and equipment for their convenience in resident care. The first-line manager nurse evaluates the plan considering policies and procedures for administration of oxygen and other treatments.

The informal participative style encourages group members to seek their own solutions. Team members are inspired by the process and they experience a trust and respect for their involvement. This method is quick and spontaneous, and in long-term care takes very little time away from resident care.

A concern with decision making in the informal style of participative mangement is the potential of communication problems. If all team members are not present, there must be a method for all to submit their views and to have the decision communicated. Sometimes bulletin boards or team notebooks are methods of communication in this informal style. There also must be a method of informing the second-line manager. The participative style of management is illustrated in figure 17–2.

Directive Style

A directive style of management often assumes that there is one "best way" to complete tasks. The way is directed to a group by the manager or leader. The style focuses on the work method rather than the worker; it is product rather than process or people oriented. It does not permit input from team members. Autocratic leadership in this style has the manager dictating to workers. The tasks and methods to complete the tasks are identified. Directive style management is rigid, with the manager making all the decisions.

If you have been involved in team sports you may have been a part of directive management. The coach illustrates game plays and each position knows when and where there will be action.

The military approach to management is mostly directive in nature. In battle or other conflicts members need to follow orders. Time does not permit participative problem solving. In "MASH," Hawkeye and B.J. shout orders over the roar of helicopters in triage situations. They are very directive in managing emergency situations!

In long-term care, as in other health care settings, there are situations where directive style management must be used. These are in emergency or crisis situations. Procedures for a Code Blue and disaster situations such as storms, fires, or accidents require directive management. These situations expect people to follow orders and not ask questions, figure 17–3.

In workplaces today, the directive management style is considered outdated for most activities. It is looked upon as a traditional style because it was developed many years ago during a time of rapid growth in industry. Today, workers want to be part of the process and decision making to make the product or meet the goal.

Directive style management requires a leader that can and will make decisions. The first-line manager nurse must make daily decisions regarding nursing assistant assignments and other scheduled activities. When a crisis occurs this nurse must be ready to implement a directive management style. For example, if a resident is found unconscious, immediate deci-

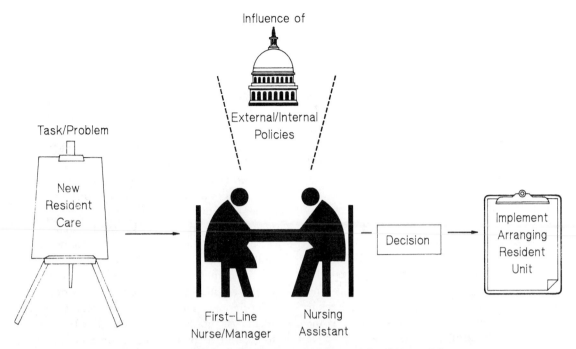

Figure 17-2   Using participative style in task/problem solving

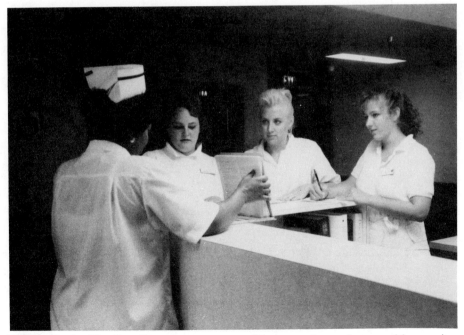

Figure 17-3   The first-line manager nurse directs nursing assistants with morning assignments.

sions must be made. The nurse will stay with the resident and begin assessments while directing the nursing assistant to bring a blood pressure cuff and additional help.

Routine tasks often require a directive method. However, if all decisions are made by management, there is no challenge to the worker. If the first-line manager nurse uses the directive approach a majority of the time, nursing assistants will not be able to share ideas, and will probably not be as productive. Figure 17–4 illustrates the directive method of management.

Motivational Style

A motivational style utilizes forces that influence people to control their activity and make their own decisions. The focus is on the worker, believing the key to productivity is the worker rather than the work method. This style believes in a strong relationship between a person's attitude toward work and the level of performance.

The participative and motivational styles are different. The participative method focuses on the product or goal; members provide input to achieve the goal. In the motivational method, the focus assures job satisfaction in the worker; this will ultimately achieve product goals. Praising specific tasks, providing recognition for exceptional work, increasing job responsibility, and providing opportunities for advancement are examples of assuring job satisfaction. The motivational method also includes a satisfactory work environment and reduced levels of supervision.

A motivational style of management does not require a special worker; it requires a special manager. The manager needs to be alert to the abilities and activities of the worker and offer frequent comments, praise, and encouragement. A "no comment" leader will fail in a motivational management style and the group will not succeed in productivity.

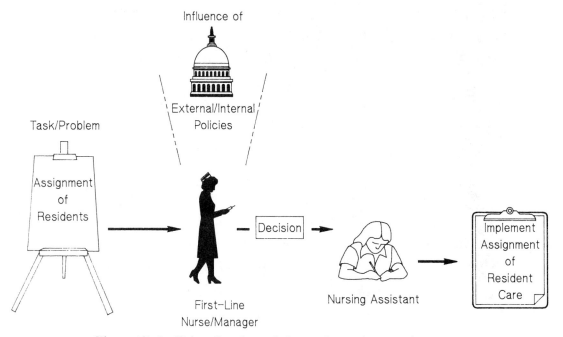

Figure 17–4 Using directive style in nursing assistant assignments

In a long term care facility the motivational style will be successful in many situations. The first-line manager nurse needs to keep alert to this method of productivity. During the busy daily activities it could be very easy to overlook the need to provide a verbal "good job," or other motivating compliment.

An example of motivational management on the resident unit may be in resident grooming. Hair and nail care is part of routine hygiene procedures. However, nail polish, hair combs, and appropriate jewelry are often neglected extras. A nursing assistant may have a special talent and interest in this area and take the time to assist assigned residents. The first-line manager nurse can offer compliments on ability and effort of the nursing assistant, and the positive psychosocial response of the residents. Results of this motivational management may be that the nursing assistant includes a manicure hour every week for interested residents. This event could be initiated and planned independently by the nursing assistant, figure 17-5.

The motivational style appears to make everyone feel good; the resident, nursing assistant, and the first-line manager nurse. This nurse is the leader and is responsible for inspiring team members and giving them praise. Like most plans, however, there have to be limits. The motivational method needs to be included in some type of structured plan. Members of the group will know where they stand; there needs to be a benchmark. The basic ideas of the motivational style of management are illustrated in figure 17-6.

Blending Management Styles

The success in managing a resident unit is not in the exclusive use of one management style, but in the blending of the three styles. As first-line manager nurses gain experience and practice management styles, it will become more apparant when and where to use each method.

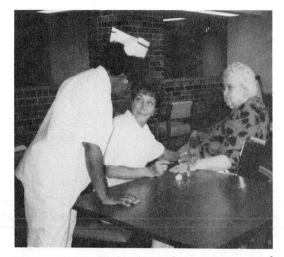

Figure 17–5 Praise is an important part of motivational management.

Long term care facilities are unique health care settings for a practicing nurse because it is a permanent home for most residents. For many nurses the residents and staff will remain relatively constant. This provides the first-line manager nurse with the opportunity to gradually put management practices in place and to evaluate results. Like nursing procedures and skills, management skills also need practice; you need to know the objectives and goals to be successful.

An example of blending management styles on the resident unit is in implementing the resident's care plan. The directive style is needed for implementation because of the format and sequence of the nursing process, and federal, state, and facility guidelines and regulations. The participative style can be used in the individualization of care plans. Nurses and nursing assistants can brainstorm to plan the approach for each resident. The first-line manager nurse uses the motivational method to compliment and encourage the nursing assistant in specific aspects of the care plan.

Factors to consider when choosing a management style for a task or in directing the resident unit include the experiences of the nursing

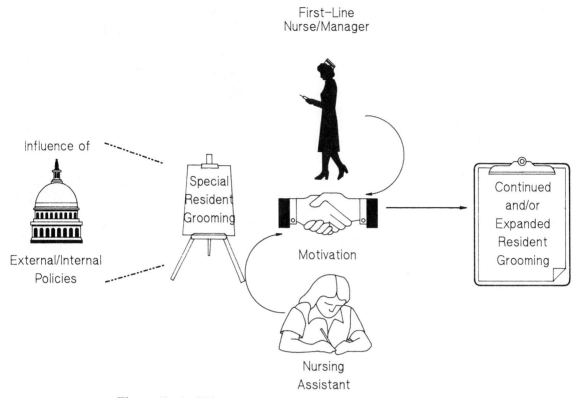

Figure 17–6   Using motivation for encouraging positive actions

assistant, the time of day, and the organizational structure of the facility. A directive style may be more appropriate with a new nursing assistant who has just completed the required training classes. With no previous experience, this team member may have some difficulty with the participative and motivational styles of management.

This situation is similar to your beginning nursing education. Your instruction in class, learning laboratory, and beginning clinical assignments were primarily through the directive management approach. As you progressed through your course work and clinical assignments your instructors' implemented more participative management. With some experience you could offer suggestions in planning patient care. Throughout your education positive

responses from instructors, classmates, and staff nurses have motivated you to continue!

Long term care facility management may prefer particular styles of management throughout the facility to fit with the owner's philosophy. You will need to honor those preferences and learn what degree of flexibility you can implement within the style. If you feel productivity could be improved, work through problem-solving committees in the facility to make changes.

Group Dynamics in the Resident Unit

Group dynamics is how members of a group work together to accomplish the tasks of the group. Part of this working together includes the roles individuals play within the working group. If the group dynamics are dysfunctional in some way, the result will be decreased productivity, unmet goals, and unhappy team members.

Nursing assistants and the first-line manager nurse on a resident unit demonstrate the characteristics of a group. This means they need to interact frequently and are dependent to a degree, on each other. They are identified by others as members of the group. This small resident unit team is primarily task oriented. The first-line manager nurse clarifies tasks and goals and each member completes assigned tasks in an atmosphere of interdependence.

For the group to be successful, individuals must have a commitment to the group; a cohesion or "stick-togetherness" that unifies the members. This may be difficult to maintain if team members change frequently. Other problems can occur if a team member is not cooperative, or does not participate in the standard group behavior in some other way. This individual may join another member with similar ideas and the team becomes divided. Problems can occur as a gulf develops between team members. Meeting resident unit goals becomes an unpleasant process. The first-line manager nurse must be assertive and decisive to maintain a cohesive nature to teamwork.

The behavior of an individual as a group member is equally important as the behavior expected in the position of first-line manager or nursing assistant. Often those behaviors are not clearly identified when they are stated "works well with others," or "is a good team member" in a performance appraisal.

Roles or behaviors of a group member often reflect natural abilities or personal goals. You probably have been in a group where clear group personalities have emerged. Perhaps you have been on a "scavenger hunt" at a party. Frequently, it takes only minutes for a leader to emerge. Followers who tag along are soon evident, as well as the negative member who groans, "we'll never get everything, we'll be the LAST team in."

It is helpful if the first-line manager nurse can identify some individual behaviors in group dynamics. This will assist the nurse in directing the resident unit activity. Figures 17–7 and 17–8 are samples of behaviors in a group process.

There are two points to remember when observing team member behavior. First, even positive behaviors that contribute to the completion of a task or goal can become disruptive or nonproductive. For example, the suggestion-giver is valuable in the participative style of management; suggestions are offered to complete resi-

- **SUGGESTION-GIVER:** presents new ideas or an alternative method of approaching a task

- **COORDINATOR:** keeps the group working together, meshes ideas, blends differences

- **INFORMATION SEEKER/GIVER:** seeks more information related to the task; offers facts about previous experience with task

- **MOTIVATOR/ENERGIZER:** motivates group to complete tasks, provides a stimulus or energy, encourages contributions

- **OBSERVER/FOLLOWER:** comments on the group decisions and activity; passive acceptance of decisions and completes activity without comment (this may not promote group productivity if all or most members are followers)

Figure 17–7 Behaviors that promote group productivity

- **ANGRY AGGRESSOR:** expresses anger or negative comments toward most decisions or activities; rarely contributes positive comments or ideas
- **MONOPOLIZER:** dominates group, often with own ideas and methods to complete tasks
- **AVOIDER/BLOCKER:** avoids being involved in decision or activity whenever possible; resists involvement without reason or becomes negative with interactions
- **JOKER/PLAYER:** avoids serious nature of tasks by displaying playful behavior and disruptive activity
- **HELP SEEKER/RESCUER:** gets others to do own assignments by seeking sympathy; do-gooder is continually helpful by trying to do assignments of others as well as own assignments

Figure 17–8   Behaviors that are unproductive in group activity

dent care more comfortably and efficiently. When the suggestions occur with nearly every resident, and on a daily basis, the flow of activity may be confusing and less productive.

The second point to remember when observing team member group behavior is that most of us can amend parts of our behavior, but our personalities do not allow major changes. For example, someone who has a leader style personality can develop self-discipline to be a follower in some groups, but not in every group. A group listener can be encouraged and nurtured to participate more, but will probably not develop into the group "chatter-box."

In the position of first-line manager nurse, you will need to develop your own management style. This will not come quickly or easily. It may take several years; it may take one or two employment settings before you begin to feel that you are developing a style of your own. Remember, it takes practice.

Some key points to remember when practicing management styles is to: (1) know yourself, your strengths and weaknesses; (2) learn the strengths and abilities of the nursing assistants on your resident unit; (3) manage in "small pieces," not the entire workday; and (4) be flexible and exercise patience.

Perhaps you want to select a mentor. A *mentor* is an advisor or coach. This will be a nurse who is an efficient manager and demonstrates the professionalism you admire. Most nurses are very willing to share the organizational skills they have developed during years of practice.

Summary

Management is the energy or dynamic force in every workplace. As a first-line manager nurse, your style of directing a unit will set the tone and affect the way the nursing assistants complete their work. Your management will influence how services are provided.

Styles of management appear to be a complex idea for the role of the first-line manager nurse. When there is a basic understanding of techniques that can be used to direct the unit activity, the nurse can guide team members in a more productive manner. When the first-line manager nurse has a basic understanding of individual behaviors in the group process, the interactions of the group can be directed to a team effort.

A participative style of managing a resident unit distributes responsibility and authority to all members of the group. A formal style has scheduled meetings, written goals, and tasks assigned to members of the group. The informal style of participative management is a practice style where the group may brainstorm to problem solve a resident care situation. Care plans for residents incorporate both formal and informal methods of participative management.

The directive style of managing a resident unit is a rigid method and the first-line manager makes all the decisions. Team members do not have any input. This style does not encourage creative thinking and tends to reduce productivity in team members. In an emergency or crisis situation, the directive style is necessary.

The motivational style encourages team members to complete tasks and achieve goals by promoting positive attitudes. This style believes the management key is in the worker and not the work method. When utilizing the motivational method, the first-line manager needs to be alert to the strengths of the nursing assistant. Frequent compliments, and noting abilities and efforts, encourage the team member to continue independently.

A first-line manager nurse can be successful in directing the activity on a resident unit when the styles of management are blended. This means each is used at the appropriate time to promote accuracy and efficency in accomplishing unit goals.

Group dynamics within the resident unit need to be positive for the team members to accomplish the goals. This means the activities are well planned, and tasks are prioritized for efficiency and team members interact productively. They demonstrate a commitment to the group and the success of the resident unit.

For Discussion

- Discuss management styles of staff nurse team leaders you are interacting with during clinical assignments.
- How has the management style of individual staff nurses influenced your motivation to complete an assignment?
- Describe your feelings or responses to the management styles of supervisors in previous work experiences.
- Observe group dynamics during the next group meeting you attend. Identify behaviors that promote group interaction and behaviors that prevent the group from meeting goals.

Questions for Review

1. What is participative management?
2. What is directive management?
3. What is motivational management?
4. What is group dynamics?
5. What are three behaviors in group dynamics that assist the group in meeting goals?
6. What are three behaviors in group dynamics that prevent the group from meeting goals?

Unit 18
Implementing the
Nursing Management Process

Objectives

After reading this unit you should be able to:
- Recall legal aspects of the first-line manager role.
- Discuss legal terms related to nursing care.
- Discuss guidelines for decision making when implementing the nursing management process.
- Define and use a style of management in a simulated situation.

A workable data base, experience, and practice result in ongoing success in managing a resident unit. This section has discussed and adapted nursing skills for patient care to skills required in managing a resident unit. This is your workable data base. Next is the practice of these skills and gaining experience in your employment.

Recall that it is your responsibility to be legally qualified to practice nursing in the state where you are employed; you must have a current nursing license. The job description for your employment position will summarize tasks and responsibilities. This document will reflect the scope of nursing practice in the community and the situations which will require your problem-solving skills.

Employer expectations of first-line managers include knowledge directly related to legalities in health care. They are knowledge of facility policies and a basic understanding of state and federal regulations. This includes methods of funding for resident care. They also expect that you have a basic knowledge of the legal aspects of nursing practice.

Implementing the management process on a resident unit requires the understanding of some basic legal terms; they influence behaviors

and responses related to policies and communication techniques. This unit will review some of the more common legal terms related to nursing practice.

A review of guidelines to problem solving will be presented to assist you with a clear step-by-step method of decision making in conflicts. Two simulated situations are presented to focus on situations that can be resolved by the first-line manager nurse, and problems that must be reported to a second- or third-line manager or other administrative positions.

Legal Terms Related to Nursing Care

You may have discussed legal terms related to nursing and health care in other course work because of their implications in patient care. Of course, nurses are not expected to have "expertise" in legal matters. You do need to remember that you are responsible for your own actions; you must implement care within your scope of nursing practice, and must document facts, not opinions. This is using "reasonable care" and knowing your own limits. Basic legal terms that affect health care delivery are reviewed in figure 18–1.

- **PROFESSIONAL ETHICS** – standards of behavior and judgement expected of a given profession, such as maintaining patient confidentiality.

- **NEGLIGENCE** – carelessness; failure to use reasonable care. Results in injury to another. Not using "common sense," such as checking the temperature of bath water.

- **MALPRACTICE** – unprofessional treatment; improper practice resulting in injury to another. Not implementing knowledge and skills learned in professional education or practicing skills beyond scope of license, such as not observing a resident having experienced a recent fall, or prescribing medications.

- **DEFAMATION** – false and harmful attack on the reputation of another. *Libel* – written or printed material that is false, malicious, and damaging, such as opinions documented in a chart. *Slander* – verbalization of false statements that are damaging to a third person, such as comments regarding the practice of a physician or other health care professional.

- **VERBAL ABUSE** – threat or unsuccessful attempt to do physical or verbal harm, such as telling a resident he will be restrained if not cooperative.

- **PHYSICAL ABUSE** – the act of beating or pounding, such as striking an uncooperative resident; may also be unauthorized touching of a person, such as implementing an intimate examination without resident consent.

- **INFORMED CONSENT** – obtaining permission from a resident for specific procedures after an explanation has been given, such stating the physician has ordered an indwelling catheter and explaining the purpose and major steps.

- **INVASION OF PRIVACY** – intrusion on a resident's rights of maintaining person and personal information private, such as not using privacy curtains, exposing a body part to someone else without permission, or not holding medical record information confidential.

- **FALSE IMPRISONMENT** – confining or restraining a resident without consent, such as use of side rails or physical restraints. (Facilities usually have responsibility release forms for signatures of those leaving against medical advice [AMA] or those refusing to have side rails raised or restraints applied when a safety risk has been identified.)

- **GRIEVANCE** – a substantiated complaint that involves working conditions or contract violations, such as disciplinary actions or work assigments.

- **CONTRACT** – a legal agreement between two parties which identifies expected activities for both parties, such as salary, vacations, benefits, number of employment hours. (Most nursing contracts with facilities are between a representative union and the facility rather than individual nurses and their employers.)

- **LIABILITY** – legal responsibility for action or inaction that may cause the resident harm, such as administering the wrong medication or not assessing the circulation to a foot.

Figure 18–1   Basic legal terms that influence health care delivery

Nurses asked to testify in a court or at a hearing are directed to verify reasonable care. This relates to what you saw, heard, did, or wrote. The most concrete information is the patient's legal record; the chart. For this reason, charting must be complete, clear, and concise in documenting the facts. Legal proceedings are very slow-moving and may not take place for months or years after the event. The recall of events may be difficult; the focus will be on the patient's chart as a legal document. Poor charting is not a good defense.

In most situations health care professionals are regulated by civil law, which generally provides the legal basis for nursing practice. *Civil law* deals primarily with wrongs committed by one individual against another, and is created by regulations or by evolution through court decisions.

Grounds for licensure revocation or suspension are not always directly related to health care litigation. Boards of Nursing may implement restrictions on a nurse's license because of fraud, physical or mental incapacity, unprofessional conduct, malpractice, or conviction of a crime. Review the guidelines from your state's Board of Nursing to determine specific behaviors requiring action in the state where you practice.

Some states have peer assistance programs for nurses with substance abuse problems. Licenses are conditional or suspended rather than revoked. After completing a recovery program, the license will be reinstated depending on individual circumstances.

You should consider the need to purchase professional liability insurance when you are employed. First, determine if your employer's liability insurance protects you. Some nurses choose to have additional personal liability insurance even if they have employer coverage. It depends on the responsibilities and risks of the job and personal preference. Remember, your employer's insurance covers you only while you are on the job.

Legal discussions related to health care are not intended to alarm nurses. Despite the most prudent nursing care, unfortunate events do occur. You are asked only to do your best and practice reasonable care.

Guidelines for Decision Making

The skills for decision making, organized into a framework for problem solving, can be especially helpful when you are presented with a situation you perceive as a dilemma. Events that can be dilemmas include those in which all choices seems to be equally unfavorable and any outcomes probably will be unpleasant to someone. Sometimes these events are conflicts between personnel, between the resident's family and staff or facility, or between schedules and personnel or tasks. Dilemmas also include infractions related to rules, regulations, and the implementing of reasonable care.

Five steps in a framework for problem solving a situation that will result in the need to make a decision include: (1) obtaining the facts; (2) identifying the issue or problem; (3) consulting resources; (4) exploring the options and making a decision; and (5) taking action. Using a structured process to solve a problem avoids a "rush to judgement" which may be erroneous. A quick decision with little research also tends to focus on a complaint rather than the actual problem.

First-line manager nurses are confronted most often with conflicts between the resident or resident's family and the implementation of care and treatment, or nursing assistants and expected standards of care.

A problem usually surfaces in the nature of a complaint or observation of unacceptable behavior or practice. The first action taken by the first-line manager is to obtain the facts. Each person involved is interviewed to get the facts from each viewpoint. Facts may also be obtained from the resident's chart. You will need to clarify what facts are relevant to the problem.

Identifying the issue places a clear focus on the problem. It may be simple or complex; it often is related to, but not the same as, the original complaint. Issues may reflect personal preferences, personal beliefs, caregiver incompetence, or professional ethics that could result in termination of employment.

Consulting resources includes facility policy and procedure books as well as nursing textbooks and other health care references. Second-line manager nurses are a resource consulted by first-line managers for guidance in problem solving. Talking through the situation often helps put the problem in perspective.

Exploring the options determines what can and should be done, based on the facts obtained, issues identified, and advice obtained. The outcomes of each option and course of action need to be weighed and considered. A decision must follow, even if it is to take no action.

The action taken is based on the previous steps of the problem-solving process and reflects the first-line manager's own values. Job descriptions and responsibilities often influence the action. Personal care and activities of daily living conflicts are often resolved by the first-line manager nurse. Problems where the infractions are related to laws and may indicate termination of employment are responsibilities of higher level management.

Taking action also includes documentation; this may be on a resident's chart, incident report, an anecdotal note for an employee file, or a memo to the second-line manager. Even when the decision is to take "no action," the facts must be documented.

Finally, you have to feel comfortable with your action. You must be able to "live with it." The decisions are not always easy as they often affect relationships. Sometimes you may not see the positive benefits of a difficult decision for weeks or months. Working through problem-solving and decision-making situations is part of your personal and professional growth. Figure 18–2 summarizes steps of the problem-solving process.

The First-Line Manager Resolves a Conflict

Situation

Monday, 10:15 a.m.; first-line manager Janice Black, LPN, is at the nurse's station having just passed the morning medications and completed resident treatments. Her next action was to call the pharmacist with new physician's orders. She sees Mrs. Riley's daughter, Margaret Smith, walking rapidly toward the nurse's station; she appears to be scowling.

Problem Surfaces

Janice: Mrs. Smith, what can I do...
Margaret: My mother's hair is a mess; it's not even combed properly. She's got food all over her face and her bed isn't made either.
   (Jim the physical therapist steps off the elevator.)
Jim: I'm ready for Mrs. Riley in P.T.
Margaret: That's it; I come to take mother to the dining room for coffee and find her in a mess, and then P.T. wants to take her looking like this. If this continues I'm going to talk to the administrator!
Janice: Jim, would you be able to take Mrs. Riley in an hour, just before lunch?
Jim: Sure, that will work out just fine.
Janice: Mrs. Smith, Ann is assigned to your mother's care this morning. I'll have Ann help her and bring her to the dining room. Perhaps we can talk about your concerns before your mother joins us.
   (Janice accompanies Margaret to a quiet corner of the dining room and offers her a cup of coffee. She returns to the desk to talk briefly with Ann before joining Margaret in the dining room.)

OBTAIN THE FACTS
- Interview independently each person involved in the conflict.
- Review the resident's chart.
- Inspect equipment or check other sources to verify facts.

IDENTIFY THE ISSUE
- Focus on the problem.
- Complaints may be the outcome of the problem.
- Determine influence of individual's preferences, beliefs, or practices on issue.
- Identify possibility of infractions of policies or other care or employment regulations.

CONSULT RESOURCES
- Gather information from textbooks and policy and procedure manuals.
- Present the facts and seek advice from the second-line manager nurse or other administrative person.

EXPLORE DECISION-MAKING OPTIONS
- Base decision on facts, issues, and resources.
- Consider outcome of each possible option.
- Make a decision.

TAKE ACTION
- Action will reflect nurse's own values and experience.
- Decision of "no action" is still a decision.
- Verbalize and/or document action.
- Learn to "live with" decision and action.

Figure 18–2 Steps of the problem solving process

Obtaining the Facts

Janice, as the first-line manager nurse, knew she needed to get more facts from Margaret to clarify her complaint and learn about her concerns. The problem, perhaps, would not be solved today, but Janice planned to arrange a time with Margaret when they would discuss the options for changes in Mrs. Riley's care.

The second part of Janice's plan was to talk with Ann, the nursing assistant, to find out about the morning's events with Mrs. Riley's personal care and her room order.

Interview with Margaret Smith.

Background Information. Mrs. Riley has been a resident for just a little over a week. The admission process has been fairly smooth; the nursing assistants have stated that Mrs. Smith has directed them, and sometimes made demands regarding care, when she was visiting. They added that they are learning how Mrs. Riley and Mrs. Smith like personal care and grooming done, and have not minded the demands. Mrs. Smith has not approached the nurses with any concerns and has not demonstrated any anger toward staff members. The initial care plan conference is tentatively planned for Thursday morning.

Interview Data. During their visit in the dining room, Janice gathers more information about Mrs. Riley and her daughter. Margaret states that she is upset because her mother was always neat and well groomed, "She held her head high, and there wasn't a hair out of place." Margaret adds she feels some guilt because she can no longer care for her mother at home.

Margaret says it works best to visit her mother about 10 a.m. before she goes to work. Her mother is more alert to visit at this time, and Margaret is more rested to cope with the lifestyle changes she and her mother are still experiencing.

Interview with Ann.

Background Information.   Ann has been a nursing assistant at the facility for about six months. This is her first employment in a health care setting. She had seemed overwhelmed during the first weeks due to the number of residents in her assignment. Her organization has improved and she demonstrates an eagerness to learn and a willingness to help others. The residents say they like her.

Interview Data.   (At 10:15 Janice spoke briefly with Ann, directing her to check that Mrs. Riley was well groomed and to bring her to the dining room. Janice told Ann she wanted to meet with her in the conference room about 1:30 p.m. to discuss Mrs. Riley's care plan.) During the discussion with Ann in the conference room, Janice collected facts about Mrs. Riley's care that day. This was the first time Ann had cared for Mrs. Riley. She had combed her hair, but did not know how to style it, so made one long braid. Ann had not checked her assignment sheet which noted that Mrs. Riley could feed herself, but was no longer neat, and must have her face and hands washed after each meal. Ann also thought her first priority was completing all the residents' personal care; she did not get Mrs. Riley's bed made until 10:45 a.m. Janice shared Mrs. Smith's concerns with Ann. She reminded Ann to read assignment sheets carefully. She also reinforced standards of care related to providing care to dependent residents.

Identifying the Issue

Janice analyzed the facts she collected and determined that:

1. Mrs. Smith had not liked her mother's appearance that day.
2. Mrs. Smith misses being a part of her mother's care.
3. Mrs. Riley's schedule does not fit her daughter's schedule for visiting.
4. Ann did not comply with the care plan and standards of care when neglecting to wash Mrs. Riley's hands and face after breakfast.

When reviewing the issues, Janice had additional data to use for developing options and making decisions. Mrs. Riley's very long thin hair was difficult for the nursing assistants to manage. Mrs. Smith's concerns were with the style and what it "used to be," not that her hair was uncombed. The fact that she stated she felt guilty because she could no longer care for her mother is reflected, partly, in the demands she made of the nursing assistants. The unmade bed did not seem, at this time, to be an issue; it seemed to have exacerbated other concerns.

Consulting Resources

Resources that assisted Janice in decision making included facility policies and procedures and Mrs. Riley's care plan. Also, facility schedules were part of the problem solving. Nursing standards, facility procedures, and the care plan are indicated in Ann's neglect to wash Mrs. Riley's hands and face after breakfast. Facility policies and procedures direct that resident's beds are to be made by 11 a.m. The physical therapy department is open between 9 a.m. and 2 p.m.; Mrs. Riley's order indicates physical therapy one time daily.

Exploring the Options

The issue of Mrs. Riley's appearance requires review of her interim care plan and planning with her daughter. Janice clarified the care plan with Ann at the time of the fact-finding interview. Mrs. Smith will be consulted regarding her mother's hair grooming. Possible options include: (1) styling her mother's hair during her morning visit, (2) teaching the nursing assistants how to style her mother's hair, and (3) arranging for the beauty shop to style Mrs. Riley's hair. Janice decides she will encourage Margaret to style her mother's hair when she visits; it will involve her in her mother's care.

Janice also decided to contact the physical therapy department to reschedule Mrs. Riley's therapy to avoid the hour her daughter visits. The request will indicate a time after 11 a.m. because Mrs. Smith is concerned about her mother's appearance in "public."

Taking Action

Janice called the physical therapy department and asked if Mrs. Riley's PT could be rescheduled for around 11 a.m. This was confirmed later in the afternoon by Jim.

On Tuesday morning, when Mrs. Smith arrived, Janice asked her if they could meet for a few moments before she had coffee with her mother. Janice had decided she would address four items: Mrs. Riley's neatness, hair style, morning schedule, and the unmade bed.

Mrs. Smith decided she really would like to style her mother's hair when she came to visit. She also wanted to show the nursing assistants how to do her mother's hair in the event she could not come to visit on a particular day. Janice said she would have two or three nursing assistants available at 10 a.m. Wednesday to watch her fix her mother's hair.

Janice explained to Maragaret that her mother's care plan had been reviewed with nursing assistants regarding washing her hands and face after meals. She added other concerns could be addressed at the care conference on Thursday. The rescheduling of physical therapy was shared and Janice assured Margaret she could accompany her mother whenever she wished.

Finally, Janice added that the facility policy states that nursing assistants must have all resident beds made by 11 a.m. Mrs. Riley's care plan would indicate making the bed before 10 a.m. whenever possible.

Margaret was in agreement with Janice's actions. She said she really liked the facility and looked forward to her mother's care conference on Thursday.

Reflecting on the First-line Manager's Problem Solving

Janice utilized participative and directive styles of management in solving this conflict. She implemented the participative style during interviews with Margaret and Ann. The style was also utilized when involving Margaret in the decision regarding her mother's hair care. It was implemented when attempting to rearrange Mrs. Riley's physical therapy schedule.

The directive style of management was implemented on Monday when instructing Ann to assure Mrs. Riley was well groomed and to bring her to the dining room. It was also used during the interview with Ann when reminding her to consult her assignment sheet and verifying care plan information and standards of patient care. Janice also implemented the directive approach when informing Margaret about the facility bedmaking policy.

Janice demonstrated efficiency in problem solving by addressing the problem immediately, and not "putting it off." It was not an emergency issue, or life-threatening, but it was important to Mrs. Smith and the care of her mother.

The First-Line Manager Reports a Conflict

Situation

Saturday, 12:15 a.m.; first-line manager Tom Rosen, LPN, is assisting a resident with a PRN nebulizer treatment. Nursing assistant Barb Jones knocks on the resident's door and says, "Tom, can I talk with you for a minute?" Tom notes tears welling in her eyes and she seems to be trembling.

Problem Surfaces

(Tom tells Barb he will meet her in the

break room in five minutes. When he arrives Barb still appears upset.)

Tom: Barb! What's the problem?

Barb: I just can't handle this! This is the second night I've had to work with her! It's just awful!

Tom: Tell me what you mean. Who is disturbing you and what is just awful?

Barb: It's Paulette. She's so mean! I just can't work with her.

Tom: She's mean? Can you be more specific?

Barb: Well, like just a few minutes ago...she tied Gladys Kiper's restraint so tight that Gladys gasped and then cried. Paulette slapped her face and swore at her.

Tom: Thank you Barb. Why don't you finish your rounds and I'll talk to you later.

Obtaining the Facts

Tom, as first-line manager, realizes that this may be a potential resident abuse situation. He knows he must collect more data which may verify or dispel Barb's accusation of Paulette's caregiving.

Background Information.   Tom recalls that both Barb and Paulette have been nursing assistants for several years. He is not aware of any warnings or disciplinary action of either nursing assistant. Barb, he has observed, seems to spend extra time with residents. Paulette, although a safe caregiver, seems to complete her assigned tasks and spend extra time in the break room.

Interview with Gladys Kiper.

Background Information.   Mrs. Kiper has been a resident for over five years. She has several deficits; she has limited vision and generalized weakness that has resulted in two recent falls at night. She seems alert, but has a vest restraint at night because of the recent falls and occasional confusion at night.

Interview Data.   Tom approached Gladys Kiper who appeared awake and restless. He asked her how she felt. She responded, "OK I

guess." Tom replied, "I understand there was a problem tonight." Gladys was quiet for a time and then said, "It's OK now." Tom then added he would really like to know if there was a problem. Gladys sighed and stated that the aide had pulled the belt and when she cried out the aide hit her and said naughty things.

Tom continued to visit with Mrs. Kiper. She told him it was Paulette who hit her, she recognized her voice. Gladys would not say what Paulette said, adding, "I don't say those kinds of words." Tom asked Mrs. Kiper if he could look at her skin under the belt. He noted some redness on the right lateral waist area; no redness or other marks were noted on her face.

Interview with Paulette   (Tom approached Paulette while she was restocking the supply room. He asked her to meet him in the break room immediately.) Tom confronted Paulette with Mrs. Kiper's statements and told her that they could be confirmed by another caregiver. Paulette burst into tears. She confessed she had swore at Mrs. Kiper, but did not think she hit her hard enough to hurt her. She said that she thought it was just because she jerked the restraint belt that Mrs. Kiper screamed. Paulette continued that her husband had filed for divorce and her kids were sick. "I just don't know how much more I can take," she added.

(Tom thanked Paulette for being honest and asked her to stay in the break room for a few minutes until he returned.)

Identifying the Issue

Tom analyzed the facts he collected and determined that:

1. Paulette's behavior was inappropriate and possibly indicated resident physical and verbal abuse.
2. Paulette's behavior may be subject to disciplinary action, possibly dismissal.
3. Paulette's current stress level indicates she should not be in a caregiver environment.

NURSING MEMO

TO: Joanne Flood RN, Supervisor

FROM: Tom Rosen, LPN

DATE: October 26

SUBJECT: Incident involving resident and NA

Paulette Godfrey was sent home at 1 a.m. this morning after admitting to striking resident Gladys Kiper in the face.

At 12:15 a.m. Burt Jones informed me she had seen Paulette tying Mrs. Kiper's restraint. Mrs. Kiper gasped and cried and then Paulette slapped her face and swore at her.

I visited with Mrs. Kiper and she stated the aide pulled the belt and then she cried. She also stated she recognized Paulette's voice and that Paulette hit her and said "naughty things." Examination of Mrs. Kiper revealed redness on the right lateral wrist area; no discoloration or marks noted on her face.

Paulette appeared visably upset and seems to have family problems that may have influenced her behavior.

Figure 18–3   Sample anecdotal notes for employee file

Consulting Resources

Resources that assisted Tom in his problem-solving process included the Resident's Bill of Rights, Vulnerable Adult Laws in his state, and "reasonable care" in standards of practice. He also consulted the facility policy manual regarding his authority to remove a caregiver from the unit and resident care. Some facilities delegate this responsibility to first-line managers when they assess the situation as unsafe. Other facilities direct the first-line manager nurse to contact the second- or third-line manager; this may mean a telephone call to the individual's home.

Tom approached Mary, the first-line manager for the other resident unit on the floor, and received confirmation of his analysis of the facts. He also conferred with her regarding the amount of adequate staffing required to meet resident needs.

Exploring Options

Tom realizes that safe resident care is the priority. The other first-line manager has assured him that she has adequate staffing with nursing assistants and could share one with him for some resident care. Tom's decision for options for the remainder of the shift include: (1) accompanying Paulette on her rounds with residents, or (2) sending Paulette home and managing the remainder of the night with the available staff.

Taking Action

Tom decided to send Paulette home. He had reviewed the standards of practice and knew that patient safety had top priority. His evaluation of Paulette's behavior in the break room indicated she was under a great deal of stress and not in a position to make sound judgements at this time.

Paulette was informed that the event would be reported to the second-line manager nurse responsible for the unit. She could also expect to be contacted by the nursing office regarding further action on this event.

Tom completed anecdotal notes for the second-line manager, figure 18–3. He submitted them to the second-line manager nurse at 7 a.m.; this nurse now has the responsiblity for any further action on this event.

Reflecting on the First-Line Manager's Problem Solving

The only management style demonstrated in this situation was the directive style. After Barb first brought her concern to her first-line manager, Tom utilized the directive method to obtain more information from her, Mrs. Kiper, and Paulette. He continued to direct Barb and Paulete while gathering additional information. He directed Paulette to leave the facility and to expect further direction from the second-line manager. He arranged for a security person to accompany Paulette safely to her car.

Tom demonstrated efficiency in his problem solving because there was the potential for a threat to resident safety and possible injury. He could not wait for a conference with the second-line manager. He did assure continued resident safety with the available staff.

For Discussion

- In a group discussion, review the situation related to Mrs. Riley.
  - How could this situation have been avoided?
  - Identify other ways Mrs. Smith could be involved in her mother's care.
  - Role play the first-line manager interviews with Mrs. Smith and Ann, the nursing assistant.

- In a group discussion, review the situation related to nursing assistant Paulette.
  — Discuss first-line manager responsibilities and liabilities when the accused nursing assistant is allowed to stay.
  — Discuss first-line manager responsibilities and liabilities when the accused nursing assistant is asked to leave.
  — Role play the first-line manager positions in interviews with Barb, Mrs. Kiper, and Paulette.

Questions for Review

1. What is "reasonable care"?
2. Why is accurate charting important for testifying in court?
3. When are you covered by your employer's liability insurance?
4. What are two situations that indicate a potential dilemma for first-line managers to problem solve?
5. What are the five steps in the problem-solving process?

Glossary

ACTIVITIES OF DAILY LIVING (ADLs) — Daily self-help which includes personal hygiene, dressing, grooming, eating, toileting.

ACTIVITY THEORY — A behavior response to aging demonstrated by maintaining or increasing participation in social activities; a denial of aging.

ACUITY — Unstable physical condition that may be severe, or critical in nature; requires frequent monitoring by professional caregivers.

ADMINISTRATION ON AGING (AoA) — Federal government agency established to implement the Older Americans Act.

ADVOCATES — People who speak or write in support of other persons or causes.

AGE DISCRIMINATION — The unjust treatment of people only because of their age.

AGEISM — A belief that older Americans should not be part of the mainstream of society; they should step aside, or be forced out of jobs and other social roles to make room for younger people.

AGING — Lifelong process of biological, psychological, and sociological change; perceived by many as physical deterioration.

ALTERNATIVE CARE/SERVICES — Health care given outside the traditional settings of hospital, nursing home, or medical office.

ALZHEIMER'S DISEASE — Irreversible dementia of unknown origin described by Alois Alzheimer in 1907. Victims demonstrate progressive loss of cognitive ability; autopsy reveals neurofibrillary tangles in the brain's nerve cells.

AREA AGENCIES ON AGING — Regional offices within a state designated to implement direct services to the elderly; funded through the Older Americans Act.

BABY BOOMERS — Population group born between 1946 and 1964.

BIO-ETHICAL ISSUES — Situations creating ethical conflict due to the use of technology to support or affect life, such as organ transplants and the right to die.

BRAINSTORMING — Group problem-solving technique to encourage creative thinking and spontaneous participation.

BURNOUT — State of being physically and emotionally worn out by the stresses of one's work or other responsibilities.

CAREGIVER — Concerned person, often a family member, who provides the day-to-day care that enables a frail, ill, or disabled individual to live at home. Also applies to nurses or other workers hired to give the care.

CASE MANAGEMENT — Process of identifying specific needs of a person requiring health or social services, and the contracting and monitoring of those services in the home.

CASE MANAGER — Health care worker, usually a social worker or registered nurse who screens and manages health and social services in the home.

CASE MIX — Long-term care payment system of government reimbursement for costs based on conditions and needs of residents.

CATARACT — Aging change in the eye resulting in a yellow and opaque lens; untreated cataracts are a major cause of blindness in the elderly.

CHRONIC ORGANIC BRAIN SYNDROME — Aging dementia of uncertain onset, possibly caused by cerebral arteriosclerosis. Elderly demonstrate gradual confusion and memory loss.

CIVIL LAW — Addresses wrongs committed by one individual against another; created by regulations or by evolution through the court system. The laws affecting most health care problems.

CLIENT — Consumer or purchaser of health services. Term traditionally used by social workers.

COHORT — People born the same year; persons born between specified dates.

CONFUSION — State of mental disorder with the inability to distinguish between things; associated with progressive dementias in the elderly.

CONTINUITY THEORY — A behavior response to aging demonstrated by the adjustment to physical and environmental changes.

DELIRIUM — Short-term episode of altered state of consciousness; often related to toxic systemic conditions. Person is disoriented and unable to cooperate or follow directions.

DEMENTIA — Broad term used to describe chronic brain syndromes that demonstrate gradual progressive loss of intellectual abilities.

DEMOGRAPHY — Study of population groups; numbers of persons with similar characteristics or bonds; vital statistics.

DEMOGRAPHERS — Persons employed or studying demography.

DEMOGRAPHICS — Specific information related to population.

DEPENDENT ELDERLY — Person 65 years or older who relies on another person for assistance in completing some or all personal tasks for daily living; often for the remainder of life.

DEPRESSION — Feelings and expression of sadness, helplessness, hopelessness, dejection, or low spirits.

DIAGNOSTIC RELATED GROUPS (DRG) — A system of classifying general medical diagnoses. Used to determine monies to be reimbursed to hospitals by government payer.

DILEMMA — Event in which all choices seem to be equally unfavorable; any outcome will be unfavorable to someone.

DISCHARGE PLANNING — Process of discussing care and making arrangements with the patient/resident and family about future care to be given after leaving the hospital or other health care setting.

DISENGAGEMENT THEORY — A behavior response to aging demonstrated by withdrawal from previous role responsibilities.

DYSARTHRIA — Aging changes in facial muscles and joints making it difficult to articulate sounds; results in unclear pronunciation of words.

ELDERHOSTEL — Educational opportunities for older adults offered by colleges and universities on campuses during summer months; includes low cost courses on a variety of topics.

ETHICS — Standards of conduct and moral judgement and philosophy; evaluating principles of right and wrong.

EXTENDED CARE — See Alternative Care.

FOLK MEDICINE — Usual treatment of disease by an ethnic or geographical population group, especially involving the use of herbs and other natural substances.

FRAIL — Physically weak and vulnerable to injury or disease; often used to describe dependent elderly.

FUNCTIONAL ASSESSMENT — Interview and examination of person to determine person's ability to manage own activities of daily living.

GATEKEEPERS — Persons in a community that recognize signs of vulnerability for elderly in the community. They report signs to their employers or identified community agencies.

GERIATRICS — Speciality in medicine focusing on old-age related diseases, conditions, and medical treatment.

GERONTOLOGICAL NURSE PRACTITIONER — Nurse specialist having received additional education and credentialing beyond the registered nurse licensure.

GERONTOLOGY — Study of the biological, psychological, and sociological aspects of the aging process.

GLAUCOMA — Condition caused by increase in intraocular pressure resulting from increased aqueous humor; cause of blindness in aging.

GRAY PANTHERS — Political activist group interested in intergenerational activities; founded by Maggie Kuhn.

GREAT DEPRESSION, THE — A period of severe economic hardship for the majority of the people; 1929-1935 in the United States.

GRIEVING — The expression of sorrow or mourning in response to a loss; work, spouse, friends, home, and independence are examples in the elderly. Stages of Dying/Grieving — Denial, Anger, Bargaining, Depression, and Acceptance as identified by Kübler-Ross.

GROUP DYNAMICS — Energies in individuals that stimulate members of a group to function as a whole to meet a goal.

HEALTH CARE DELIVERY SYSTEM — Entire scope of health care including the goods and services for health care, their delivery, use, and the necessary funding.

HEALTH MAINTENANCE ORGANIZATION (HMO) — A type of prepaid health insurance which focuses on preventing illness and maintaining wellness.

HOLISTIC HEALTH — Health care that focuses on the whole individual and interactions with his/her environment.

HOMEBOUND — Unable to go outside of one's home, usually due to a physical limitation, or exacerbation of disease.

HOME CARE — Taking care of the homebound person, including personal hygiene of the individual and homemaking tasks.

HOME HEALTH CARE — Health care provided in a person's home.

HOSPICE — A philosophy of providing care of the dying person and the family.

INDEPENDENT ELDERLY — Persons 65 years and older who continue to complete their own activities of daily living in their usual place of residence; may require minimal assistance from family or community services.

INDIGENT — A person with a limited income; usually considered below poverty income.

INSTRUMENTAL ACTIVITIES OF DAILY LIVING (IALDs) — Ability to complete functions of daily living that require use of equipment and an endurance level such as vacuuming or other light home maintenance chores.

INTERDEPENDENCE — Group dependence on each other as individuals to accomplish a goal; may also be elderly couples with mutual support to maintain their independence.

INTERGENERATIONAL HOUSING — Multiple household dwelling that includes several age groups: young families, single persons, elderly couples. The purpose is to meet each others needs.

INTERMEDIATE CARE — Patient or resident has a degree of independence and does not require continual monitoring by a licensed nurse.

LEADERSHIP — A characteristic of a group member that demonstrates the capacity to guide, and the ability to influence, lead, enable, and inspire for the good of the group.

LIFE EXPECTANCY — Established at birth, the average age a cohort can expect to live; influenced by environment and technology.

LIFE REVIEW — Recalling past experiences to determine meaning and value of own life. Developed by gerontologist Robert Butler.

LIFE SPAN — Length of time a cohort can live under the most favorable conditions.

LONELINESS — Feelings of unhappiness at being alone; a longing for family, friends, or a former life style.

LONG TERM CARE FACILITY — Health care facility providing care over a long period of time, often the remainder of a person's life; most persons are over 65 years of age.

MACULAR DEGENERATION — Aging change in the eye; reduced blood flow to the macula results in loss of center of visual field.

MANAGED HEALTH CARE — Health care insurance term; describes plans or policies that attempt to contain costs by reviewing physicians performance such as charges, quality of care, and location, and suggest physicians called "preferred providers" to subscribers.

MANAGEMENT — Process of controlling, arranging, directing, or supervising an activity; person is not usually an intimate member of the group.

MANAGEMENT STYLES — Approaches to supervising an activity.
- PARTICIPATIVE — Distributes responsibility and authority to all members of a group.
- DIRECTIVE — Keeps authority and decision making in the manager role.
- MOTIVATIONAL — Promotes self-direction with the belief that a person's attitudes and feelings regarding work influence performance.

MANAGER — A person in charge of a group and responsible for the management activities.
- FIRST-LINE — In health care, the nurse working directly with residents; responsible for a group of residents and some other caregivers.
- SECOND-LINE — In health care, the nurse responsible for a floor or nursing unit including all the residents and many caregivers.
- THIRD-LINE — In health care, often the nurse with the title of Director of Nursing; responsible for all residents, nursing staff, and care provided to residents.

MEANS TEST — A measure of income to determine whether a person qualifies for financial assistance or programs.

MEDIAN AGE — Demographic information that indicates the age at which half the population is younger and half is older.

MEDICAID (Title 19, Social Security Amendments) — Provides reasonably complete medical care of the financially oppressed, regardless of age.

MEDICAL JARGON — Abbreviations, acronyms, or code words used by health caregivers to signal expanded information.

MEDICARE (Title 18, Social Security Amendments) — Government health insurance program, intended for persons 65 and older.

MEDIGAP INSURANCE — Supplemental insurance policy purchased by elderly to assist with costs not covered by Medicare.

MIDDLE OLD — Older adults between the ages of 75 and 84.

MINORITY POPULATION — A racial, religious, ethnic, or political group smaller than, and differing from, the larger controlling group such as in a community or nation.

MORTALITY — Proportion of deaths to the population of an area or nation.

NURSING DIAGNOSIS — Actual or potential health problems of people that nurses can identify and treat independently.

NURSING HOMES — See Long Term Care Facilities.

NURSING MODEL — Nursing care intervention focused on patient needs related to tasks of daily living and maintaining health.

NURSE PRACTICE ACTS — Laws relating to nursing practice that are passed by state governing bodies.

OLD — Having lived a long time. Usually a personal perception based on subjective data indicating physical deterioration.

OLDER AMERICANS ACT — Legislation passed in 1965 that created many health and social services for older adults.

— TITLE III — Revision that provides for state and Area Agencies on Aging (AoA) to develop comprehensive services for older persons; includes nutrition programs.

OLD OLD — Older adults; the elderly population 85 and older.

OMBUDSMAN — Someone whose job is to independently investigate citizens' complaints against government agencies; serves as a liaison between the people and the government.

OSTEOARTHRITIS (Degenerative Joint Disease) — Deterioration, especially of weight-bearing joints, that is a leading cause of disability in the elderly.

OVER-THE-COUNTER (OTC) — Reference used to classify medications not requiring a physician's prescription; may be purchased in drug stores and other retail sites.

PATIENT — A person in a state of physical or emotional ill health who is receiving care or treatment from health care professionals. Used historically in hospitals.

PRE-ADMISSION SCREENING — Assessment of elderly persons to collect data to determine if a person can care for self at home independently, with community services, or if long-term care placement is appropriate.

PRESBYCUSIS — Aging changes in the inner ear resulting in hearing loss.

PRESBYOPIA — Loss of visual accommodation during the aging process.

PROACTIVE — Planning and decision making to determine tasks to be completed to meet a goal.

QUALIFIED MEDICATION ASSISTANTS (QMA) — See Trained Medication Assistants.

QUALITY OF CARE — A measure of the excellence of care received; usually evaluated by documentation, interviews, and observations.

REACTIVE — Decision making in response to activities that have occurred.

REALITY ORIENTATION — Activities implemented to increase awareness of time, place, and person; implemented in persons with confusion or other memory impairment.

REASONABLE CARE — Nursing care that is expected action by most nurses in a given setting and situation.

REGULATION — Rules established to implement laws.

REIMBURSEMENT — Payment for services.

— PROSPECTIVE — Payment given prior to services rendered.

— RETROSPECTIVE — Payment given after services are rendered.

RESIDENT — Person, often elderly, living in a long term care facility; usually a permanent home.

RESPITE — An interval of temporary rest; in health care appropriate persons or professionals to relieve usual caregiver.

RETIREMENT — Withdrawal from work because of age; traditionally age 65.

ROLE — A set of expectations or behaviors assigned to an identified person or group.

SANDWICH GENERATION — Middle age

adult caregivers, providing support or care for aging parents, young adult children, and sometimes grandchildren.

SCOPE OF PRACTICE — Extent or range of nursing activities in accepted practice in a community or geographical area.

SENESCENCE — Process of biological changes with increasing chronological aging; see Aging

SENILITY — Old age; outdated term used to describe confusion in aging.

SENIOR CITIZEN — Usually a person 65 years or older; title used by community and retailers to focus on programs and services for this age group.

SKILLED CARE — Frequent assessment and monitoring by licensed nurses because of the acuity of patients or residents condition, or their level of dependence.

SNOW BIRDS — Semi-retired or retired older adults, having permanent homes in northern climates, who live in warmer climates during colder months.

SOCIAL SECURITY ACT — Original federal legislation (1935) providing supplemental income for persons at retirement; many amendments have occurred. See Medicare, Medicaid.

SOCIAL SERVICES — Activities designed to promote the welfare of the group and the individual, such as, counseling, health clinics, other aid for needy or handicapped.

STANDARDS OF PRACTICE — A level of excellence considered acceptable for members of an occupation or profession.

STATE UNITS ON AGING — State office level administering programs funded through the Older Americans Act.

STEREOTYPE — A fixed idea of behaviors or characteristics of a group of people; in older adults behaviors reflecting the aging process.

SUNDOWN SYNDROME — Symptoms of agitation, restlessness, or disruptive behavior demonstrated during late afternoon or eve-

ning hours; persons are usually alert, calm, and cooperative during morning hours.

SUPPLEMENTAL SECURITY INCOME (SSI) — Social Security federal and state program that provides income for needy elderly or disabled persons; requires a means test.

TELEPHONE TRIAGE — Sorting data given over the telephone by patient or family; determines the urgency and type of medical attention required.

THANATOLOGY — the study of death viewed from the biological, psychological, and sociological perspectives; includes values and traditions of changing society.

THEORIES — Ideas or plans about how something might work. In aging, ideas how and why body cells age.

TRAINED MEDICATION ASSISTANTS (TMA) — Persons trained in state approved programs to specifically administer medications in long term care facilities; usually experienced nursing assistants.

VULNERABLE ADULT — An adult who is in danger of losing health, finances, belongings, or life because of actions of others, or inability to care for self. Laws protecting these adults vary from state to state.

WEAR-AND-TEAR THEORY — Physical aging theory suggesting cells functioning in specialized tissues are confronted with abuses from use, such as degenerative joint disease.

WORK ETHIC — equates productivity with personal value; sometimes called the Protestant work ethic.

YOUNG OLD — Older adults between the ages of 65 and 74.

Bibliography

Articles

Abraham, Ivo.; Buckwalter, Kathleen; and Neundorfer, Marcia. "Alzheimer's Disease." *The Nursing Clinics of North America* 23, no. 1 (March 1988).

Andresen, Gayle P. "A Fresh Look at Assessing the Elderly." *RN* (June 1989): 28–39.

Brickfield, Cyril F. "The Future of Long-term Care." *Vital Speeches* (May 1, 1988): 442–444.

Brown, Margaret D. "Functional Assessment of the Elderly." *Journal of Gerontological Nursing* 14, no. 5 (May 1988): 13–17.

Burggraf, Virginia, and Barbara Donlon. "Assessing The Elderly." *American Journal of Nursing* 85, no.9 (September 1985): 974–984

Butler, Frieda R. "Minority Wellness Promotion: A Behavioral Self-management Approach." *Journal of Gerontological Nursing* 13, no.8 (August 1987): 23–28

Damrosch, Shirley, and Judith Strasser. "The Homeless Elderly in America." *Journal of Gerontological Nursing* 14, no. 10 (October 1988): 26–29.

Dreyfus, Joan. "Depression Assessment and Interventions in the Medically Ill Frail Elderly." *Journal of Gerontological Nursing* 14, no. 9 (September 1988): 27–36.

Fuller, Linda. "Reminiscence: Using Memories to Improve the Quality of Care for Elderly Patients." *Journal of Practical Nursing* (September 1988): 30–35.

Garner, Brenda. "Guide To Changing Lab Values in Elders." *Geriatric Nursing* (May/June 1989): 144–145.

Gibbs, Nancy. "Love and Let Die." *TIME* (March 19, 1990): 62–71.

Gomez, Gerda, and Efrain Gomez. "Dementia? or Delirium?" *Geriatric Nursing* (May/June 1989): 141–142.

Gozdziak, Elzbieta. "New Branches...Distant Roots: Older Refugees in the United States," *Aging* no. 359 (1989): 2–7.

"Grays on The Go." *TIME* (February 22, 1988): 66–70.

Grognet, Allene Guss. "Elderly Refugees and Language Learning." *Aging* no. 359 (1989): 8–-11.

Henderson, Carter. "Old Glory, America Comes Of Age." *The Futurist* (March–April 1988): 36–40.

Hollowell, Edward E., and James E. Eldridge. "The Right to a Natural Death." *The Journal of Practical Nursing* (September 1988): 44–47.

Jacob, John E. "Ageism." *Vital Speeches* (March 15, 1988): 332–335.

Keane, Sarah McDermott, and Sharon Sells. "Recognizing Depression in the Elderly." *Journal of Gerontological Nursing* 16, no. 1 (January 1990): 21–25.

Kolcaba, Katharine, and Carol Miller. "Geropharmacology Treatment." *Journal of Gerontological Nursing* 15, no. 5 (May 1989): 29–35.

Lamm, Richard D. "The Ten Commandments of an Aging Society." *Vital Speeches* (December 15, 1987): 133–139.

Lundy, Betty Mussell. "Connecting Body and Spirit, Parish Nurses are Ministering to the Whole Person." *The Lutheran* (October 12, 1988): 9–12.

McCracken, Ann. "Emotional Impact of Possession Loss." *Journal of Gerontological Nursing* 13, no. 2. (February 1987): 14–19.

McCracken, Ann L. "Sexual Practice by Elders: The Forgotten Aspect of Functional Health." *Journal of Gerontological Nursing* 14, no. 10 (October 1988): 13–17.

McHutchion, Edna, and Janice Morse. "Releasing Restraints, a Nursing Dilemma." *Journal of Gerontological Nursing* 15, no. 2 (February 1989): 16–21.

Montgomery, Carol. "What You Can Do for the Confused Elderly." *Nursing 87* (April): 55–56.

Nath, Charlotte; Sharon Murray; and Charles Ponte. "Lessons in Living with Type II Diabetes Mellitus." *Nursing 88* (August 1988): 44–49.

Nesbitt, Bonnie. "Nursing Diagnosis In Age-related Changes." *Journal of Gerontological Nursing* 14, no. 7 (July 1988): 7–12.

Parette, Howard, and Jack Hourcade. "Nursing Attitudes Toward Geriatric Alcoholism." *Journal of Gerontological Nursing* 16, no. 1 (January 1990): 26–31.

Rosenkoetter, Marlene M. "Is Retirement Making Your Patient Sick?" *RN* (July 1988): 17–19.

Ryan, Maura, and Joanne Patterson. "Loneliness in the Elderly." *Journal of Gerontological Nursing* 13, no. 5 (May 1987): 6–12.

Santo-Novak, Debra. "Seven Keys to Assessing the Elderly." *Nursing 88* (August 1988): 60–63.

Struble, Laura, and Lynn Sivertsen. "Agitation. Behaviors in Confused Elderly Patients." *Journal of Gerontological Nursing* 13, no. 11 (November 1987): 40–44.

Strumpf, Neville E. "A New Age for Elderly Care." *Nursing and Health Care* 8, no. 10. (October 1987): 445–448.

"The Search for The Fountain of Youth." *Newsweek* (March 5, 1990): 44–53.

Thomas, Evan. Reported by Ann Blackman, Washington; Cathy Booth, New York; Jon D. Hull, Los Angeles. "Growing Pains at 40." *TIME* (May 19, 1986): 22–41.

Westfall, Larry, and Richard Pavlis. "Why the Elderly Are so Vulnerable to Drug Reactions." *RN* (November 1987): 39–43.

Wordell, David. "Should You Crush That Tablet?", *Nursing 88* (January 1988): 48–49.

Books

Adler, Ronald B., and Neil Towne. *Looking Out/Looking In.* New York: Holt, Rinehart and Winston, 1987.

Alfaro, Rosalinda. *Application of Nursing Process, A Step-By-Guide*, 2nd ed. Philadelphia: J.B. Lippincott, 1990.

Blanchard, Kenneth, and Spencer Johnson. *The One Minute Manager.* New York: William Morrow and Company, 1982.

Blanchard, Kenneth, and Robert Lorber. *Putting the One Minute Manager to Work.* New York: William Morrow and Company, 1984.

Breitung, Joan Carson. *Caring for Older Adults.* Philadelphia: W.B. Saunders, 1987.

Butler, Robert N. *Why Survive? Being Old in America.* New York: Harper and Row, 1985.

Butler, Robert N., and Myrna I. Lewis. *Aging and Mental Health*, 3rd ed. St. Louis: C.V. Mosby, 1982.

Carpenio, Lynda Juall. *Nursing Diagnosis.* Philadelphia: J. B. Lippincott, 1987.

Carroll, David L. *When Your Loved One Has Alzheimer's.* New York: Harper & Row, 1989.

Curtain, Leah, and M.J. Flaherty *Nursing Ethics: Theories and Pragmatics.* Bowie, Maryland: R.J. Brady, 1982.

Davis, A. Jann. *Listening and Responding.* St. Louis: C.V. Mosby, 1984.

De Young, Lillian. *Dynamics of Nursing.* St. Louis: C.V. Mosby, 1985.

Douglass, Laura Mae. *The Effective Nurse, Leader, Manager.* St. Louis: C.V. Mosby, 1988.

Dychtwald, Ken. *Age Wave.* Los Angeles: Jeremy P. Tarcher, 1989.

Eliopoulos, Charlotte. *Gerontological Nursing* Philadelphia: J.B. Lippincott, 1987.

Kübler-Ross, Elisabeth. *On Death and Dying.* New York: McMillan Publishing, 1969.

Lakein, Alan. *How To Get Control Of Your Time And Your Life.* New York: The New American Library, 1973.

Mace, Nancy, and Peter Rabins. *The 36-Hour Day.* New York: Warner Books, 1981.

McNeely, R.L., and John L. Colen. *Aging in Minority Groups.* Beverly Hills, California: Sage Publications, 1983.

Metzger, Norman. *The Health Supervisor's Handbook.* Rockville, Maryland: Aspen Publishers, 1988.

Milliken, Mary Elizabeth. *Understanding Human Behavior: A Guide for Health Care Providers*, 4th Ed. Albany, New York: Delmar Publishers Inc., 1987.

Moore, Pat. *Disguised.* Waco, Texas: Word Books, 1985.

Northouse, Peter G., and Laurel L. Northouse. *Health Communication A Handbook for Health Professionals.* Englewood Cliffs, New Jersey: Prentice-Hall, 1985.

Peters, Tom. *Thriving on Chaos, Handbook for a Management Revolution.* New York: Alfred A. Knopf, 1987.

Potter, Diane Odell, Editorial Director. *Practices.* Nurse's Reference Library, Nursing 84 Books. Springhouse, PA: Springhouse Corporation, 1984.

Ringsven, Mary K., and Barbara M. Jorenby. *Basic Community and Home Care Nursing.* Albany, N.Y.: Delmar Publishers Inc., 1988.

Sullivan, Eleanor J., and Phillip J. Decker. *Effective Management in Nursing.* New York: Addison-Wesley, 1988.

U.S. Bureau of the Census. *Statistical Abstract of the United States: 1988*, 108th ed. Washington, D.C., 1987.

Zins, Sandra. *Aging in America: An Introduction to Gerontology.* Albany, New York: Delmar Publishers Inc., 1987.

Index